Neurology and Neurobiology

EDITORS

Victoria Chan-Palay
University Hospital, Zurich

Sanford L. Palay
The Harvard Medical School

ADVISORY BOARD

Albert J. Aguayo
McGill University

Günter Baumgartner
University Hospital, Zurich

Masao Ito
Tokyo University

Tong H. Joh
Cornell University Medical College, New York

Bruce McEwen
Rockefeller University

William D. Willis, Jr.
The University of Texas, Galveston

---

1 • **Cytochemical Methods in Neuroanatomy,** Victoria Chan-Palay and Sanford L. Palay, *Editors*

2 • **Basic Mechanisms of Neuronal Hyperexcitability,** Herbert H. Jasper and Nico M. van Gelder, *Editors*

3 • **Anorexia Nervosa: Recent Developments in Research,** Padraig L. Darby, Paul E. Garfinkel, David M. Garner, and Donald V. Coscina, *Editors*

4 • **Clinical and Biological Aspects of Peripheral Nerve Diseases,** Leontino Battistin, George A. Hashim, and Abel Lajtha, *Editors*

5 • **The Physiology of Excitable Cells,** Alan D. Grinnell and William J. Moody, Jr., *Editors*

6 • **Developing and Regenerating Vertebrate Nervous Systems,** Penelope W. Coates, Roger R. Markwald, and Alexander D. Kenny, *Editors*

7 • **Glutamine, Glutamate, and GABA in the Central Nervous System,** Leif Hertz, Elling Kvamme, Edith G. McGeer, and Arne Schousboe, *Editors*

8 • **Catecholamines,** Earl Usdin, Arvid Carlsson, Annica Dahlström, and Jörgen Engel, *Editors*. Published in three volumes: *Part A: Basic and Peripheral Mechanisms; Part B: Neuropharmacology and Central Nervous System—Theoretical Aspects; Part C: Neuropharmacology and Central Nervous System—Therapeutic Aspects*

9 • **Development of Visual Pathways in Mammals,** Jonathan Stone, Bogdan Dreher, and David H. Rapaport, *Editors*

10 • **Monoamine Innervation of Cerebral Cortex,** Laurent Descarries, Tomás R. Reader, and Herbert H. Jasper, *Editors*

11 • **The Neurobiology of Zinc,** C.J. Frederickson, G.A. Howell, and E.J. Kasarskis, *Editors*. Published in two volumes: *Part A: Physiochemistry, Anatomy, and Techniques; Part B: Deficiency, Toxicity, and Pathology*

12 • **Modulation of Sensorimotor Activity During Alterations in Behavioral States,** Richard Bandler, *Editor*

13 • **Behavioral Pharmacology: The Current Status,** Lewis S. Seiden and Robert L. Balster, *Editors*

14 • **Development, Organization, and Processing in Somatosensory Pathways,** Mark Rowe and William D. Willis, Jr., *Editors*

15 • **Metal Ions in Neurology and Psychiatry,** Sabit Gabay, Joseph Harris, and Beng T. Ho, *Editors*

16 • **Neurohistochemistry: Modern Methods and Applications,** Pertti Panula, Heikki Päivärinta, and Seppo Soinila, *Editors*

17 • **Two Hemispheres—One Brain: Functions of the Corpus Callosum,** Franco Leporé, Maurice Ptito, and Herbert H. Jasper, *Editors*

18 • **Senile Dementia of the Alzheimer Type,** J. Thomas Hutton and Alexander D. Kenny, *Editors*

19 • **Quantitative Receptor Autoradiography,** Carl A. Boast, Elaine W. Snowhill, and C. Anthony Altar, *Editors*

20 • **Ion Channels in Neural Membranes,** J. Murdoch Ritchie, Richard D. Keynes, and Liana Bolis, *Editors*

21 • **PET and NMR: New Perspectives in Neuroimaging and in Clinical Neurochemistry,** Leontino Battistin and Franz Gerstenbrand, *Editors*

22 • **New Concepts in Cerebellar Neurobiology,** James S. King, *Editor*

23 • **The Vertebrate Neuromuscular Junction,** Miriam M. Salpeter, *Editor*

24 • **Excitatory Amino Acid Transmission,** T. Philip Hicks, David Lodge, and Hugh McLennan, *Editors*

25 • **Axonal Transport,** Richard S. Smith and Mark A. Bisby, *Editors*

26 • **Respiratory Muscles and Their Neuromotor Control,** Gary C. Sieck, Simon C. Gandevia, and William E. Cameron, *Editors*

27 • **Epilepsy and the Reticular Formation: The Role of the Reticular Core in Convulsive Seizures,** Gerhard H. Fromm, Carl L. Faingold, Ronald A. Browning, and W.M. Burnham, *Editors*

28 • **Inactivation of Hypersensitive Neurons,** N. Chalazonitis and Maurice Gola, *Editors*

29 • **Neuroplasticity, Learning, and Memory,** N.W. Milgram, Colin M. MacLeod, and Ted L. Petit, *Editors*

30 • **Effects of Injury on Trigeminal and Spinal Somatosensory Systems,** Lillian M. Pubols and Barry J. Sessle, *Editors*

31 • **Organization of the Autonomic Nervous System: Central and Peripheral Mechanisms,** John Ciriello, Franco R. Calaresu, Leo P. Renaud, and Canio Polosa, *Editors*

32 • **Neurotrophic Activity of GABA During Development,** Dianna A. Redburn and Arne Schousboe, *Editors*

33 • **Animal Models of Dementia: A Synaptic Neurochemical Perspective,** Joseph T. Coyle, *Editor*

34 • **Molecular Neuroscience: Expression of Neural Genes,** Fulton Wong, Douglas C. Eaton, David A. Konkel, and J. Regino Perez-Polo, *Editors*

35 • **Long-Term Potentiation: From Biophysics to Behavior,** Philip W. Landfield and Sam A. Deadwyler, *Editors*

36 • **Neural Plasticity: A Lifespan Approach,** Ted L. Petit and Gwen O. Ivy, *Editors*

37 • **Intrinsic Determinants of Neuronal Form and Function,** Raymond J. Lasek and Mark M. Black, *Editors*

38 • **The Current Status of Peripheral Nerve Regeneration,** Tessa Gordon, Richard B. Stein, and Peter A. Smith, *Editors*

39 • **The Biochemical Pathology of Astrocytes,** Michael D. Norenberg, Leif Hertz, and Arne Schousboe, *Editors*

40 • **Perspectives in Psychopharmacology: A Collection of Papers in Honor of Earl Usdin,** Jack D. Barchas and William E. Bunney, Jr., *Editors*

41 • **Non-Invasive Stimulation of Brain and Spinal Cord: Fundamentals and Clinical Applications,** Paolo M. Rossini and Charles D. Marsden, *Editors*

42A • **Progress in Catecholamine Research, Part A: Basic Aspects and Peripheral Mechanisms,** Annica Dahlström, Haim Belmaker, and Merton Sandler, *Editors*

42B • **Progress in Catecholamine Research, Part B: Central Aspects,** Merton Sandler, Annica Dahlström, and Haim Belmaker, *Editors*

42C • **Progress in Catecholamine Research, Part C: Clinical Aspects,** Haim Belmaker, Merton Sandler, and Annica Dahlström, *Editors*

43 • **Dopaminergic Mechanisms in Vision,** Ivan Bodis-Wollner and Marco Piccolino, *Editors*

44 • **Developmental Neurobiology of the Frog,** Emanuel D. Pollack and Harold D. Bibb, *Editors*

45 • **The Lennox-Gastaut Syndrome,** Ernst Niedermeyer and Rolf Degen, *Editors*

46 • **Frontiers in Excitatory Amino Acid Research,** Esper A. Cavalheiro, John Lehmann, and Lechoslaw Turski, *Editors*

47 • **Cholecystokinin Antagonists,** Rex Y. Wang and Ronald Schoenfeld, *Editors*

48 • **Current Issues in Neural Regeneration Research,** Paul J. Reier, Richard P. Bunge, and Fredrick J. Seil, *Editors*

49 • **Extracellular and Intracellular Messengers in the Vertebrate Retina,** Dianna A. Redburn and Herminia Pasantes-Morales, *Editors*

CURRENT ISSUES IN
NEURAL REGENERATION
RESEARCH

International Symposium on Neural Regeneration (1987: Asilomar Conference Center)

CURRENT ISSUES IN NEURAL REGENERATION RESEARCH

Proceedings of an International Symposium on Neural Regeneration Held at the Asilomar Conference Center, Pacific Grove, California, December 6–10, 1987

Editors

Paul J. Reier

Departments of Neurosurgery
and Neuroscience
University of Florida
College of Medicine
Gainesville, Florida

Richard P. Bunge

Departments of Anatomy
and Neurobiology
Washington University
School of Medicine
St. Louis, Missouri

Fredrick J. Seil

Office of Regeneration
Research Programs
VA Medical Center
and
Department of Neurology
Oregon Health Sciences University
School of Medicine
Portland, Oregon

ALAN R. LISS, INC., NEW YORK

Address all Inquiries to the Publisher
Alan R. Liss, Inc., 41 East 11th Street, New York, NY 10003

Copyright © 1988 Alan R. Liss, Inc.

Printed in the United States of America

Under the conditions stated below the owner of copyright for this book hereby grants permission to users to make photocopy reproductions of any part or all of its contents for personal or internal organizational use, or for personal or internal use of specific clients. This consent is given on the condition that the copier pay the stated per-copy fee through the Copyright Clearance Center, Incorporated, 27 Congress Street, Salem, MA 01970, as listed in the most current issue of "Permissions to Photocopy" (Publisher's Fee List, distributed by CCC, Inc.), for copying beyond that permitted by sections 107 or 108 of the US Copyright Law. This consent does not extend to other kinds of copying, such as copying for general distribution, for advertising or promotional purposes, for creating new collective works, or for resale.

Library of Congress Cataloging-in-Publication Data

International Symposium on Neural Regeneration (1987 : Asilomar Conference Center)
　　Current issues in neural regeneration research : proceedings of an International Symposium on Neural Regeneration held at the Asilomar Conference Center, Pacific Grove, California, December 6–10, 1987 / editors, Paul J. Reier, Richard P. Bunge, Fredrick J. Seil.
　　　p. cm.— (Neurology and neurobiology ; v. 48)
　　Includes bibliographies and index.
　　ISBN 0-8451-2752-7
　　1. Nervous system—Regeneration—Congresses. I. Reier, Paul J.
II. Bunge, Richard P., 1932-　　. III. Seil, Fredrick J. IV. Title.
v. Series.
　　[DNLM: 1. Nerve Regeneration—Congresses. Wl NE337B v. 48 / WL 102 I664c 1987]
QP363.5.I58 1987
591.1'88—dc19
DNLM/DLC
for Library of Congress　　　　　　　　　　　　　　　　　　　　　　88-23161
　　　　　　　　　　　　　　　　　　　　　　　　　　　　　　　　　　　　CIP

Contents

Contributors	xi
Preface Paul J. Reier, Richard P. Bunge, and Fredrick J. Seil	xvii
Acknowledgments	xix

NEURONAL RESPONSE TO INJURY

Neuronal Response to Injury Stephen G. Waxman	3
Synthesis of Cytoskeletal Proteins by Axotomized and Regenerating Motoneurons W. Tetzlaff, F.D. Miller, and M.A. Bisby	13
Cytoskeleton of the Regenerating Axon Irvine G. McQuarrie	23
Effect of GM1 Ganglioside Administration on the Axotomy Response of Rat Rubral Neurons Kevin D. Barron	33
Some Responses of Sensory Neurons to Peripheral Nerve Injury P.M. Richardson, V.M.K. Verge, and R.J. Riopelle	47
Target-Dependence of Spinal Motoneurons John B. Munson, Robert C. Foehring, and George W. Sypert	55

NEURONAL RESCUE

Neuronal Rescue in CNS Lesions Silvio Varon, Theo Hagg, and Marston Manthorpe	67
Target-Specific Requirements of Immature Axotomized CNS Neurons for Survival and Axonal Elongation After Injury Barbara Sypniewski Bregman	75
Testing the Trophic Factor Hypothesis in the Visual System Timothy J. Cunningham, Caroline Fisher, and Forrest A. Haun	89

Nerve Growth Factor Rescues Septal Cholinergic Neurons and Promotes Reinnervation of the Hippocampus in Rats With Partial Fimbrial Transections
Franz Hefti, Claudia N. Montero, and Deborah C. Mash 105

EXTRACELLULAR MATRIX AND CELL SURFACE INTERACTIONS

Extracellular Matrix and Cell Surface Interactions
Louis F. Reichardt 119

Establishment of a Two-Dimensional Neural Network in an Insect Wing
James B. Nardi 127

Cellular Biology of Neuronal Interactions With Fibronectin and Laminin
Paul Letourneau, Sherry Rogers, Irene Pech, Sally Palm, James McCarthy, and Leo Furcht 137

Laminin, Fibronectin, Collagen, and Their Receptors in Nerve Fiber Growth
S. Carbonetto, P. Douville, W. Harvey, and D.C. Turner 147

Glia-Derived Nexins and Neurite Outgrowth
Denis Monard 159

Maintenance of Axon Terminals at Synaptic Sites in the Absence of Muscle Fibers
Yung-mae M. Yao 167

Expression of Nerve Growth Factor Receptors on Schwann Cells After Axonal Injury
Eugene M. Johnson, Jr., H. Brent Clark, John B. Schweitzer, and Megumi Taniuchi 179

NEURONAL SURFACE MOLECULES

Structural Properties of Neuronal Surface Macromolecules
Richard U. Margolis 189

Regulatory Mechanisms in Nerve Growth Cones
Karl H. Pfenninger 199

Families of Neural Adhesion Molecules
Melitta Schachner 209

NCAM as a General Regulator of Cell Contact
Urs Rutishauser, Ann Acheson, Alison K. Hall, Dennis M. Mann, and Jeffrey Sunshine 229

Developmental Regulation of Expression of the Neural Cell Adhesion Molecules NCAM and L1
E. Bock, O. Nybroe, and D. Linnemann 237

ASTROCYTIC RESPONSE TO INJURY

Astrocytic Response to Injury
Lawrence F. Eng 247

Astrocyte Response to Growth Factors and Hormones: Early Molecular Events
Alaric T. Arenander, Robert Lim, Brian Varnum, Ruth Cole, Harvey R. Herschman, and Jean de Vellis 257

Astroglia and Plasminogen Activator Activity: Differential Activity Level in the Immature, Mature, and "Reactive" Astrocytes
Nurit Kalderon, Kenneth Ahonen, Anna Juhasz, Joseph P. Kirk, and Sergey Fedoroff 271

Immunosuppression as a Treatment for Acute Injury of the Central Nervous System
Dana Giulian 281

The Development of the Gliotic Plaque in Experimental Allergic Encephalomyelitis
Marion E. Smith and Lawrence F. Eng 291

The Control of Astrocyte Populations in Rat Brain
M. Nieto-Sampedro 301

Induced Regeneration of Dorsal Root Fibers Into the Adult Mammalian Spinal Cord
M. Kliot, G.M. Smith, J. Siegal, S. Tyrrell, and J. Silver 311

NEURAL STRUCTURAL REPAIR AND FUNCTIONAL RESTORATION

Successful Spinal Cord Regeneration: Known Biological Strategies
Jerald J. Bernstein 331

Plasticity and Recovery of Function After Injury to the Developing Spinal Cord of the Rat
Dennis J. Stelzner and James M. Cullen 343

Shortening of the Rat Spinal Column: A Method For Studying Coaptation of Cord Stumps
Luis de Medinaceli 361

Pathfinding by Regenerating Axons in the Lamprey Spinal Cord
Diana Lurie and Michael E. Selzer 369

Functional and Non-Functional Regeneration in the Spinal Cord of Adult Lampreys
Avis H. Cohen and Margaret T. Baker 387

Index 397

Contributors

Ann Acheson, Neuroscience Program, Department of Developmental Genetics and Anatomy, Case Western Reserve University School of Medicine, Cleveland, OH 44106 **[229]**

Kenneth Ahonen, The Rockefeller University, New York, NY 10021 **[271]**

Alaric T. Arenander, Departments of Biological Chemistry, Anatomy, and Psychiatry, Laboratory of Biomedical and Environmental Sciences, Mental Retardation Research Center and Brain Research Institute, UCLA School of Medicine, Los Angeles, CA 90024 **[257]**

Margaret T. Baker, Section of Neurobiology and Behavior, Cornell University, Ithaca, NY 14853 **[387]**

Kevin D. Barron, Medical Research Service, Veterans Administration Medical Center and Department of Neurology, Albany Medical College, Albany, NY 12208 **[33]**

Jerald J. Bernstein, Laboratory of Central Nervous System Injury and Regeneration, Veterans Administration Medical Center, and Departments of Neurosurgery and Physiology, The George Washington University School of Medicine, Washington, DC 20037 **[331]**

M.A. Bisby, Department of Medical Physiology, University of Calgary, Calgary, Alberta, Canada T2N 4N1 **[13]**

E. Bock, The Protein Laboratory, University of Copenhagen, DK-2200 Copenhagen, Denmark **[237]**

Barbara Sypniewski Bregman, Department of Anatomy, University of Maryland School of Medicine, Baltimore, MD 21201 **[75]**

Richard P. Bunge, Departments of Neurology and Anatomy, Washington University School of Medicine, St. Louis, MO 63110 **[xvii]**

S. Carbonetto, Neuroscience Unit, Montreal General Hospital Research Institute, McGill University, Montreal, Canada H3G 1A4 **[147]**

H. Brent Clark, Department of Laboratory Medicine, Memorial Medical Center, Springfield, IL 62781 **[179]**

Avis H. Cohen, Section of Neurobiology and Behavior, Cornell University, Ithaca, NY 14853 **[387]**

Ruth Cole, Laboratory of Biomedical and Environmental Sciences, Mental Retardation Research Center, UCLA School of Medicine, University of California, Los Angeles, CA 90024 **[257]**

The numbers in brackets are the opening page numbers of the contributors' articles.

xii / Contributors

James M. Cullen, Department of Anatomy and Cell Biology, SUNY Health Science Center, Syracuse, NY 13210 **[343]**

Timothy J. Cunningham, Department of Anatomy, The Medical College of Pennsylvania, Philadelphia, PA 19129 **[89]**

Luis de Medinaceli, Microsurgical Research Center, Medical College of Hampton Roads, Norfolk, VA 23507 **[361]**

Jean de Vellis, Departments of Anatomy and Psychiatry, Laboratory of Biomedical and Environmental Sciences, Mental Retardation Research Center, and Brain Research Institute, UCLA School of Medicine, University of California, Los Angeles, CA 90024 **[257]**

P. Douville, Neuroscience Unit, Montreal General Hospital Research Institute, McGill University, Montreal, Canada H3G 1A4 **[147]**

Lawrence F. Eng, Department of Pathology, Stanford University School of Medicine, Stanford, CA 94305; and Department of Pathology, Veterans Administration Medical Center, Palo Alto, CA 94304 **[247, 291]**

Sergey Fedoroff, University of Saskatchewan, Saskatoon, Saskatchewan, Canada S7N 0W0 **[271]**

Caroline Fisher, Department of Anatomy, The Medical College of Pennsylvania, Philadelphia, PA 19129 **[89]**

Robert C. Foehring, Department of Neuroscience, College of Medicine, University of Florida, Gainesville, FL 32610 **[55]**

Leo Furcht, Departments of Laboratory Medicine and Pathology, University of Minnesota, Minneapolis, MN 55455 **[137]**

Dana Giulian, Department of Neurology and Program of Neuroscience, Baylor College of Medicine, Houston, TX 77030 **[281]**

Theo Hagg, Department of Biology, School of Medicine, University of California San Diego, La Jolla, CA 92093 **[67]**

Alison K. Hall, Neuroscience Program, Department of Developmental Genetics and Anatomy, Case Western Reserve University School of Medicine, Cleveland, OH 44106 **[229]**

W. Harvey, Neuroscience Unit, Montreal General Hospital Research Institute, McGill University, Montreal, Canada H3G 1A4 **[147]**

Forrest A. Haun, Department of Anatomy, The Medical College of Pennsylvania, Philadelphia, PA 19129 **[89]**

Franz Hefti, Department of Neurology, University of Miami School of Medicine, Miami, FL 33101 **[105]**

Harvey R. Herschman, Department of Biological Chemistry and Brain Research Institute, UCLA School of Medicine, University of California, Los Angeles, CA 90024 **[257]**

Eugene M. Johnson, Jr., Department of Pharmacology, Washington University School of Medicine, St. Louis, MO 63110 **[179]**

Anna Juhasz, The Rockefeller University, New York, NY 10021 **[271]**

Nurit Kalderon, The Rockefeller University, New York, NY 10021 **[271]**

Contributors / xiii

Joseph P. Kirk, The Rockefeller University, New York, NY 10021 **[271]**

M. Kliot, Department of Neurosurgery, Columbia Presbyterian Medical Center, New York, NY 10033 **[311]**

Paul Letourneau, Departments of Cell Biology and Neuroanatomy, University of Minnesota, Minneapolis, MN 55455 **[137]**

Robert Lim, Department of Biological Chemistry, UCLA School of Medicine, University of California, Los Angeles, CA 90024 **[257]**

D. Linnemann, The Protein Laboratory, University of Copenhagen, DK-2200 Copenhagen, Denmark **[237]**

Diana Lurie, The Department of Neurology, and The David Mahoney Institute of Neurological Sciences, University of Pennsylvania School of Medicine, Philadelphia, PA 19104-4283 **[369]**

Dennis M. Mann, Neuroscience Program, Department of Developmental Genetics and Anatomy, Case Western Reserve University School of Medicine, Cleveland, OH 44106 **[229]**

Marston Manthorpe, Department of Biology, School of Medicine, University of California San Diego, La Jolla, CA 92093 **[67]**

Richard U. Margolis, Department of Pharmacology, New York University Medical Center, New York, NY 10016 **[189]**

Deborah C. Mash, Department of Neurology, University of Miami School of Medicine, Miami, FL 33101 **[105]**

James McCarthy, Departments of Laboratory Medicine and Pathology, University of Minnesota, Minneapolis, MN 55455 **[137]**

Irvine G. McQuarrie, Division of Neurosurgery and Department of Developmental Genetics, Case Western Reserve University, and Neural Regeneration Center, Veterans Administration Medical Center, Cleveland, OH 44106 **[23]**

F.D. Miller, Department of Preclinical Neurosciences, Research Institute of Scripps Clinic, La Jolla, CA 92037 **[13]**

Denis Monard, Friedrich Miescher Institut, CH-4002 Basel, Switzerland **[159]**

Claudia N. Montero, Department of Neurology, University of Miami School of Medicine, Miami, FL 33101 **[105]**

John B. Munson, Department of Neuroscience, College of Medicine, University of Florida, Gainesville, FL 32610 **[55]**

James B. Nardi, Department of Entomology, University of Illinois, Urbana, IL 61801 **[127]**

M. Nieto-Sampedro, Department of Psychobiology, University of California, Irvine, CA 92717 **[301]**

O. Nybroe, The Protein Laboratory, University of Copenhagen, DK-2200 Copenhagen, Denmark **[237]**

Sally Palm, Departments of Laboratory Medicine and Pathology, University of Minnesota, Minneapolis, MN 55455 **[137]**

Irene Pech, Departments of Cell Biology and Neuroanatomy, University of Minnesota, Minneapolis, MN 55455 **[137]**

Karl H. Pfenninger, Department of Cellular and Structural Biology, University of Colorado School of Medicine, Denver, CO 80262 **[199]**

Louis F. Reichardt, Department of Physiology and Howard Hughes Medical Institute, University of California, San Francisco, CA 94143-0724 **[119]**

Paul J. Reier, Departments of Neurosurgery and Neuroscience, College of Medicine, University of Florida, JHM Health Center, Gainesville, FL 32610 **[xvii]**

P.M. Richardson, Division of Neurosurgery, Montreal General Hospital and McGill University, Montreal, Quebec, Canada H3G 1A4 **[47]**

R.J. Riopelle, Division of Neurology, Queen's University, Kingston, Ontario, Canada K7L 3N6 **[47]**

Sherry Rogers, Department of Anatomy, University of New Mexico, Albuquerque, NM 87131 **[137]**

Urs Rutishauser, Neuroscience Program, Department of Developmental Genetics and Anatomy, Case Western Reserve University School of Medicine, Cleveland, OH 44106 **[229]**

Melitta Schachner, Department of Neurobiology, University of Heidelburg, Heidelburg, Federal Republic of Germany **[209]**

John B. Schweitzer, Division of Neuropathology, Department of Pathology, University of Tennessee, Memphis, TN 38163 **[179]**

Fredrick J. Seil, Office of Regeneration Research Programs, VA Medical Center; and Department of Neurology, Oregon Health Sciences University School of Medicine, Portland, OR 97201 **[xvii]**

Michael E. Selzer, The Department of Neurology, and The David Mahoney Institute of Neurological Sciences, University of Pennsylvania School of Medicine, Philadelphia, PA 19104-4283 **[369]**

J. Siegal, Department of Developmental Genetics, Case Western Reserve University, Cleveland, OH 44106 **[311]**

J. Silver, Department of Developmental Genetics, Case Western Reserve University, Cleveland, OH 44106 **[311]**

G.M. Smith, Department of Developmental Genetics, Case Western Reserve University, Cleveland, OH 44106 **[311]**

Marion E. Smith, Department of Neurology, Veterans Administration Medical Center, Palo Alto, CA 94304 **[291]**

Dennis J. Stelzner, Department of Anatomy and Cell Biology, SUNY Health Center, Syracuse, NY 13210 **[343]**

Jeffrey Sunshine, Neuroscience Program, Department of Developmental Genetics and Anatomy, Case Western Reserve University School of Medicine, Cleveland, OH 44106 **[229]**

George W. Sypert, Department of Neuroscience, College of Medicine, University of Florida, Gainesville, FL 32610 **[55]**

Megumi Taniuchi, Department of Pharmacology, Washington University School of Medicine, St. Louis, MO 63110 **[179]**

W. Tetzlaff, Department of Medical Physiology, University of Calgary, Calgary, Alberta, Canada T2N 4N1 **[13]**

D.C. Turner, Department of Biochemestry and Molecular Biology, SUNY Medical Center at Syracuse, Syracuse, NY 13210 **[147]**

S. Tyrrell, Department of Developmental Genetics, Case Western Reserve University, Cleveland, OH 44106 **[311]**

Brian Varnum, Department of Biological Chemistry, UCLA School of Medicine, University of California, Los Angeles, CA 90024 **[257]**

Silvio Varon, Department of Biology, School of Medicine, University of California San Diego, La Jolla, CA 92093 **[67]**

V.M.K. Verge, Division of Neurosurgery, Montreal General Hospital and McGill University, Montreal, Quebec, Canada H3G 1A4 **[47]**

Stephen G. Waxman, Department of Neurology, Yale University School of Medicine, New Haven, CT 06510; and Neuroscience and Regeneration Research Center, Veterans Administration Medical Center, West Haven, CT 06516 **[3]**

Yung-mae M. Yao, Department of Neurobiology, Stanford University School of Medicine, Stanford, CA 94305 **[167]**

Preface

Recent technological advances in neurobiology and other biomedical disciplines have led to a wealth of new information concerning the cellular, molecular, and physiological properties and responses of neurons and their supporting glia to injury or disease in both the central and peripheral nervous systems. Such progress has also fostered a greater appreciation for the prospect of someday reversing the devastating functional deficits associated with various neuropathological conditions. Thus, important strides have been made in our understanding of several fundamental issues, including: the intrinsic growth properties of neurons in the mature brain and spinal cord; conditions that influence the extent and quality of axonal regeneration or functional plasticity; the potential for replacing degenerated neuronal populations through transplantation; and, the role of neuronotrophic factors, especially nerve growth factor, in promoting axonal regeneration and neuronal survival.

This volume highlights some of the recent advances that have been made in these and related areas of neural regeneration research. The chapters represent invited presentations pertaining to six major topics discussed at an international symposium held at the Asilomar Conference Center, Pacific Grove, California, December 6–10, 1987. It is hoped that each chapter, along with the introductory overview to each topic section, will provide to both the basic scientist and clinician some useful interdisciplinary perspectives regarding axonal growth, neuronal survival, neuron-glial interactions, and functional and anatomical plasticity as demonstrated by a variety of experimental approaches and models. In addition, we hope that this volume will serve to inspire further creativity and investigation in a field that has experienced dramatic practical and conceptual gains in recent years.

Paul J. Reier
Richard P. Bunge
Fredrick J. Seil

Acknowledgments

The Asilomar Conference, a successor to a similar symposium held in December, 1985, was sponsored by the Medical Research service of the U.S. Veterans Administration (Dr. Ralph E. Peterson, Director), the Paralyzed Veterans of America (Mr. R. Jack Powell, Executive Director), and the National Institutes of Health (Dr. Murray Goldstein, Director, NINCDS). The cosponsorship of these organizations and their dedicated support of neural regeneration research is gratefully acknowledged.

The Program Planning Committee consisted of members of the VA Office of Regeneration Research Programs Advisory Board and staff, including Drs. Kevin D. Barron, Bruce M. Carlson, Lawrence F. Eng, Irvine G. McQuarrie, Paul J. Reier, Fredrick J. Seil, David L. Stocum and Betty G. Uzman, and the Associate Director for Research of the Medical and Research Affairs Department of the Paralyzed Veterans of America, Ms. Anne W. Zimmer.

It is unfortunate that, because of space constraints, the abstracts of the posters presented at the symposium could not be included, though these scientific presentations were a critical and exciting part of the symposium and contributed significantly to its success. We wish to take this opportunity to recognize the poster presenters for their participation and their important contributions to the stimulating discussions at this conference.

NEURONAL RESPONSE TO INJURY

NEURONAL RESPONSE TO INJURY

Stephen G. Waxman, M.D., Ph.D.

Department of Neurology, Yale University
School of Medicine, New Haven, CT. 06510
and Neuroscience and Regeneration Research
Center, VA Medical Center, West Haven, CT 06516

In briefly discussing the neuronal response to injury, this introductory chapter will focus on certain aspects of adaptive neuronal mechanisms, i.e., those that subserve neuronal survival and regeneration. A number of steps are necessarily involved in the neuron's response to injury if functional recovery is to ensue. These include the perikaryal response, which in some cells includes chromatolysis (Lieberman, 1971; Baron, 1983; Grafstein, 1983). Notably, marked changes in excitability occur in the cell bodies of some neurons following axonal transection; for example, abnormal dendritic excitability, possibly related to "overproduction" of ion channels destined for the axon, is observed in the motor neuron cell body following severance of its axon (Kuno and Llinas, 1970; Eccles et al, 1958). It is interesting, in this context, that regeneration after axonal transection occurs more rapidly if the neuron has first been exposed to a "priming" lesion, possibly as a result of the initiation of reparative activities in the perikaryon in response to the initial lesion (Grafstein and McQuarrie, 1978; McQuarrie and Grafstein, 1981).

If functional recovery is to occur as a result of neuronal regeneration, it must include regrowth of a new axon, and there is thus a need for studies on the development and regeneration of the axonal cytoskeleton, as well as mechanisms such as axoplasmic transport which serve to maintain the newly formed neuronal process; this is discussed by several authors elsewhere in this volume. It is also essential that the regenerating axon travel beyond potential barriers (glial scar, glia limitans) and that the regenerating axon be guided to the correct target. Notably, regrowth to the correct target is not necessarily constrained to occur via a recapitulation of the previous pathway; in some cases regenerating CNS axons are guided to the correct target, where they apparently form functional synaptic connections so as to mediate some degree of functional recovery, although they travel to these targets via unconventional pathways (Kalil, 1988).

Since the function of axons is to carry action potentials from one site to another in the nervous system, it is also necessary for growing and regenerating axons to establish the capability for electrogenesis and action potential transmission. Moreover, since it is becoming clear that, in mammals, different types of axons exhibit different modes of electrogenesis which are reflected in axonal coding properties (e.g., accommodation) (Bowe et al, 1985), the regenerating axon must not only develop electrical excitability, but also the correct electrophysiological properties. Finally, in order for functional recovery to occur, regenerating neurons must form synaptic connections with appropriate targets, and there must be incorporation of the regenerated neurons into functional neuronal circuits.

Other chapters in this volume will focus on the perikaryal response, axonal cytoskeleton and axonal transport, mechanisms that guide growing and regenerating axons to appropriate targets, and formation of synaptic connections. The purpose of this chapter is to comment on the development of electrical excitability in regenerating neurons.

It is now well established that mammalian neurons exhibit a variety of conductances, corresponding to different types of voltage-sensitive and ligand-gated ion channels (Adams, 1982; Lipton and Tauck, 1986). The axon itself is no exception. Even in simple unbranched axons, such as in mammalian optic nerve or peripheral nerve, there are a multiplicity of channels, including voltage-sensitive sodium channels responsible for the depolarization phase of the action potential, and several distinct types of potassium channels (Kocsis et al, 1986). Notably, the potassium conductances appear to subserve different functional roles, a 4-AP-sensitive potassium conductance mediating repolarization of the action potential, and a TEA-sensitive conductance participating in the modulation of interspike intervals during repetitive firing (Kocsis et al, 1987). Thus, the regenerating neuron is faced with the problem of producing a variety of types of channels, as well as transporting these channels to the correct part of the neuron and inserting and anchoring them in the membrane. Moreover, it has been shown that neuronal firing properties depend not only on the _number_ of channels added to the membrane, but also on the precise _spatial distribution_, with movement of channels in the range of microns having significant effects, e.g., on the invasion of action potentials into regions of low safety factor (Waxman and Wood, 1984). Thus, in addition to the requirement for biosynthesis of appropriate numbers of channels of each type, there is a requirement for control of spatial aspects of excitable membrane assembly in regenerating neurons.

It is likely that any given neuron exhibits a variety of types of excitable membrane, with varying distributions and densities of ion channels. It is not yet known how the production of these various types of membrane is regulated. However, it does appear that membrane assembly is a _sequential_ and _spatially distributed_ process, in which a lipid bilayer framework is initially synthesized and added to the plasma membrane, with subsequent modification via the insertion of ion channels in appropriate numbers and types (Waxman and Black, 1985; Pfenninger, 1982; Griffin et al, 1981). Modulation of ion channel type and density appears to occur under local control and in this context, the axonal cytoskeleton (Ellisman, 1979; Waxman and Quick, 1978) and/or extracellular milieu (Waxman and Ritchie, 1985) may play a role.

In responding to the need for increased production of membrane constituents, the neuronal cell body plays an important role in axonal regeneration. An important, and still unanswered, question concerns the nature of the signals which initiate the perikaryal response to injury. Although the nature of this signal has not yet been delineated, it appears that injury to the axon _per se_ can result in alterations in the neuronal perikaryon. Thus, for example, Waxman and Anderson (1982) have studied the retrograde axon reaction in neuronal perikarya following axotomy in the electric organ of the gymnotid teleost _Sternarchus albifrons_. Axons in the electric organ have the distinction of being asynaptic, i.e., ending blindly without forming a synaptic ending (Bennett, 1971; Waxman et al, 1972). Interestingly, the cell bodies of origin of these asynaptic axons show several distinct characteristics of retrograde reaction of the perikaryon (including eccentricity of nuclei, large bundles of neurofilaments that are not observed in normal perikarya of these cells, a marked increase in number and size of dense bodies in the affected perikarya, and large arrays of parallel rough endoplasmic reticulum never observed in normal cells) in response to transection of the axon. Thus, at least some neuronal perikarya can undergo retrograde reaction following axotomy without the loss of synaptic terminals. These findings are consistent with those of Watson (1968) who showed that when axons are injured and prevented from regenerating by a ligation, a second injury evokes a retrograde response in the perikaryon. It remains possible that substances produced distally within, or in the neighborhood of, the asynaptic axons may be transported back to the cell body and that loss of such factor(s) may play a role in the retrograde reaction. However, loss of a trophic substance derived from postsynaptic elements or from the presynaptic terminal is not a prerequisite for perikaryal alteration.

Finally, it is important to briefly turn attention to the duration of the neuronal response to injury. It is well-established that, in successful axonal regeneration (e.g., in uncomplicated peripheral nerve injuries), the regrowing axon extends at a rate of several microns per day, finally establishing synaptic contact in the periphery. It might have been expected that, following the completion of this peripheral synapse formation, the neuronal response would abate since regrowth was finished. However this has not turned out to be the case. Recent electrophysiological studies indicate that, even in long term (> 1 year) regenerated axons in the rat sciatic nerve which have reestablished functional synaptic connections, there is a persistence of relatively immature electrophysiological properties. Thus, application of the potassium channel blocking agent 4-aminopyridine leads to stimulus-evoked burst activity in long-term regenerating fibers (Kocsis and Waxman, 1983). This is in marked contrast to normal developing fibers, where this unstable physiological behavior is attenuated as the developing axons and their myelin sheaths mature (Kocsis et al, 1983).

Morphological studies, at both the light and electron

microscope level, have recently delineated the structural basis for these unexpected abnormalities in physiological organization of regenerated fibers. These studies demonstrate persistent myelin remodelling in regenerated fibers, with displacement of some Schwann cell internodes and disruption of paranodal axo-Schwann cell junctions, providing an abnormal pathway from the extracellular space to the (formerly) internodal regions (Hildebrand et al, 1985, 1986). This "unmasks" 4-aminopyridine-sensitive potassium channels, which are normally covered by the myelin sheath and sequestered from the extracellular space by a compact axon-Schwann cell paranodal junction.

It is likely that, in these long-term regenerated fibers, there is reorganization in terms of ion channels within the axon membrane as myelin remodelling progresses. It is known that, despite the persistent remodelling of myelin along these fibers, conduction is maintained (Kocsis and Waxman, 1983). The normal internodal membrane contains a low density of voltage-sensitive sodium channels (Ritchie and Rogart, 1977; Waxman, 1977; Waxman and Ritchie, 1985). Following damage to the myelin or disruption of the paranodal axo-glial junction internode, reorganization of the exposed internode can occur so that conduction is maintained through the demyelinated fiber. This probably involves redistribution of sodium channels, or the production of new channels (Ritchie and Rogart, 1977; Waxman, 1977; Bostock and Sears, 1978). Thus, it is likely that, even following successful regeneration of the axon and reestablishment of synaptic connections with appropriate targets, there is still a need for compensatory activities in the perikaryon which serve to maintain ion channel distributions and densities that are sufficient to insure action potential conduction. We are led to inquire as to the effects of this sustained demand for synthesis of proteins involved in neuronal membrane organization. To the degree that the neuronal perikaryon responds to this demand, it must maintain a higher-than-normal level of protein synthesis.

In this context, it should be recalled that recent studies on the post-polio syndrome suggest that it occurs most commonly in individuals who have sustained significant functional recovery. This raises the question of whether, even in neurons which have "successfully" sprouted so as to reinnervate peripheral targets, there is a persistent metabolic and/or biosynthetic load on the neuronal cell body. Such a load might predispose the cell body to secondary damage and contribute to the late deterioration seen in some patients after apparently successful recovery from poliomyelitis. If this is the case, it would emphasize the mutual interdependence of perikaryon, axon, and associated glial cells in maintenance of the neuron and would suggest that studies on stabilization of axo-glial interactions following nerve regeneration might provide insight into mechanisms which would minimize late deterioration following apparently successful sprouting.

ACKNOWLEDGEMENTS

Work in the author's laboratory has been supported in part by the Medical Research Service, Veterans Administration, and by grants from the National Multiple Sclerosis Society (RG-1912) and the National Institutes of Health (NS-24931). We also thank the Allen Charitable Trust and the Paralyzed Veterans of America for support.

REFERENCES

Adams, P. (1982): Voltage-dependent conductances in vertebrate neurons. Trends Neurosci., 5:116-119.

Barron, K.D. (1983): Axon reaction and central nervous system regeneration. In: Nerve, Organ, and Tissue Regeneration: Research Perspectives. Seil, F.J. (ed.), pp. 3-36, Academic Press, New York.

Bennett, M.V.L. (1971): Electric organs. In: Fish Physiology, Vol.5. Hoar, W.J. and Randall, D.J. (eds.), pp. 347-491, Academic Press, New York.

Bostock, H., and Sears, T.A. (1978): The internodal axon membrane: electrical excitability and continuous conduction in segmental demyelination. J. Physiol. (Lond.), 280:273-301.

Bowe, C.M., Kocsis, J.D. and Waxman, S.G. (1985): Differences between mammalian ventral and dorsal spinal roots in response to blockade of potassium channels during maturation. Proc. Roy. Soc. Lond. B., 224:355-366.

Eccles, J.C., Libet, B., and Young, R.R. (1958): The behavior of chromatolyzed motoneurones studied by intracellular recording. J. Physiol. (Lond.), 143:11-40.

Ellisman, M. (1979): Molecular specializations of the axon membrane at nodes of Ranvier are not dependent upon myelination. J. Neurocytol., 8:719-735.

Grafstein, B. (1983): Chromatolysis reconsiderd: A new view of the reaction of the nerve cell body to axon injury. In: Nerve, Organ, and Tissue Regeneration: Research Perspectives. Seil, F.J. (ed.), pp. 37-50, Academic Press, New York, pp. 37-50.

Grafstein, B. and McQuarrie, I.G. (1978) The role of the nerve cell body in axonal regeneration. In: Neuronal Plasticity, Cotman, C.W. (ed.), pp. 155-195, Raven Press, New York.

Griffin, J.W., Price, D.L., Drachman, D.B. and Morris, J. (1981): Incorporation of axonally transported glycoproteins into axolemma during nerve regeneration. J. Cell Biol., 88:205-214.

Hildebrand, C., Kocsis, J.D., Berglund, S. and Waxman, S.G. (1985): Myelin sheath remodelling in regenerated rat sciatic nerve. Brain Research, 358-163-170.

Hildebrand, C., Mustafa, G.Y., and Waxman, S.G. (1986): Remodeling of internodes in regenerated rat sciatic nerve: Electron microscopic observations. J. Neurocytol., 15:681-692.

Kalil, K. (1988): Regeneration of pyramidal tract axons. In: Functional Recovery in Neurological Disease. Waxman, S.G., (ed.), Raven Press, New York (in press).

Kocsis, J.D. and Waxman, S.G. (1983): Long-term regenerated nerve fibres retain sensitivity to potassium channel blocking agents. Nature, 304:640-642.

Kocsis, J.D., Gordon, T.R., and Waxman, S.G.(1986): Mammalian optic nerve fibers display two pharmacologically distinct potassium channels. Brain Research, 393:357-361.

Kocsis, J.D., Eng, D.L., Gordon, T.R., and Waxman, S.G.

(1987): Functional differences between 4-aminopyridine and tetraethlyammonium-sensitive potassium channels in myelinated axons. Neuroscience Letters, 75:193-198.

Kocsis, J.D., Ruiz, J.A. and Waxman, S.G. (1983): Maturation of mammalian myelinated fibers: Changes in action potential characteristics following 4-aminopyridine application. J. Neurophysiol. 50:449-463.

Kuno, M. and Llinas, R (1970): Enhancement of synaptic transmission by dendritic potentials in chromatolyzed neurons. J. Physiol. (Lond.), 210:807-821.

Lieberman, A.R. (1971): The axon reaction: A review of the principal features of perikaryal responses to axon injury. Intl. Rev. Neurobiol., 14:49-124.

Lipton, S. and Tauck, D.L. (1986): Voltage-dependent conductances in solitary ganglion cells dissociated from the rat retina. J. Physiol. (Lond.), 385:361-391.

McQuarrie, I.G. and Grafstein, B. (1981): Effect of a conditioning lesion on optic nerve regeneration in goldfish. Brain Research, 216:253-264.

Pfenninger, K.H. (1982): Transport and insertion of membrane components into processes of growing neurons. Neurosci. Res. Prog. Bull., 20:73-79.

Ritchie, J.M. and Rogart, R.B. (1977): Density of sodium channels in mammalian myelinated fibers and nature of the axonal membrane under the myelin sheath. Proc. Natl. Acad. Sci. U.S.A., 74:211-215.

Watson, W. (1968): Observations on the nucleolar and total cell body nucleic acid of injured nerve cells. J. Physiol. (Lond.), 196:655-676.

Waxman, S.G. (1977): Conduction in myelinated, unmyelinated, and demyelinated fibers. Arch. Neurol., 34:585-590.

Waxman, S.G. and Anderson, M.J. (1982): Retrograde axon

reaction following section of asynaptic nerve fibers. *Cell and Tissue Research*, 223:487-492.

Waxman, S.G. and Black, J.A. (1985): Membrane structure of vesiculotubular complexes in developing axons in rat optic nerve: Freeze-fracture evidence for sequential membrane assembly. *Proc. Roy. Soc. Lond. B.*, 225:357-363.

Waxman, S.G. and Quick, D.C. (1978): Intra-axonal ferric ion-ferrocyanide staining of nodes of Ranvier and initial segments in central myelinated fibers. *Brain Research*, 144:1-10.

Waxman, S.G. and Ritchie, J.M. (1985): Organization of ion channels in the myelinated nerve fiber. *Science*, 228:1502-1507.

Waxman, S.G. and Wood, S.L. (1984): Impulse conduction in inhomogeneous axons: Effects of variation in voltage-sensitive ionic conductances on invasion of demyelinated axon segments and preterminal fibers. *Brain Research*, 294:111-122.

Waxman, S.G., Pappas, G.D. and Bennett, M.V.L. (1972): Morphological correlates of functional differentiation of nodes of Ranvier along single fibers in the neurogenic electric organ of the knife fish *Sternarchus*. *J. Cell Biol.*, 53:210-224.

SYNTHESIS OF CYTOSKELETAL PROTEINS BY AXOTOMIZED AND REGENERATING MOTONEURONS

W. Tetzlaff, F.D. Miller and M.A. Bisby

Departments of Medical Physiology, University of Calgary, Calgary, Alberta, Canada T2N 4N1 (W.T., M.A.B.) and Preclinical Neurosciences, Research Institute of Scripps Clinic, La Jolla, CA 92037, USA (F.D.M.)

INTRODUCTION

The cell body reaction (CBR) to axotomy may represent a reordering of synthetic priorities to sustain regeneration of the axon (Grafstein and McQuarrie, 1978). Changes in synthesis of cytoskeletal proteins would be expected, not only because outgrowth and maturation of new axon requires new cytoskeleton, but also because there are changes in the axonal transport of these proteins following axotomy (Hoffman and Lasek, 1980; Hoffman et al., 1985). Lasek and collaborators (Black and Lasek, 1979; Lasek et al., 1981; Wujek and Lasek, 1983) have shown a correlation between regeneration rate and velocity of slow component b of axonal transport, which in peripheral nerves contains both actin and tubulin (Oblinger et al., 1987). They suggest that the primary determinant of axonal elongation is the slow axonal transport of the cytoskeleton, which is both synthesized and assembled in the cell body. Since neurofilaments move with slow component a, significantly slower than slow component b, the neurofilaments and the microtubules or actin microfilaments must also slide past each other (Lasek, 1986). Thus interactions between cytoskeletal elements are also likely to be important.

Peripheral nerve regeneration involves the formation of growth cones at nodes of Ranvier, elongation of axons along guides provided by Schwann cells, formation of connections with target cells, myelination of regenerated axons, and growth in axonal calibre. Our objective was to study the time-course of changes in cytoskeletal protein synthesis following axotomy to determine how these changes relate to events in the regeneration sequence.

PROTEIN SYNTHESIS IN THE RAT FACIAL NUCLEUS FOLLOWING AXOTOMY

12 h - 21 d after facial axotomy (either a brief crush or a resection of the nerve just distal to the stylomastoid foramen), L[35S] methionine was applied to the facial nuclei, and the rats were killed after a further 2 h. Microdissected facial nuclei were prepared for two-dimensional electrophoresis and fluorography. Densitometric analysis of the fluorographs revealed a number of proteins whose synthesis increased or decreased following axotomy. One of the most obvious increases occurred in a protein which was identified as GFAP (Tetzlaff et al., 1988), in confirmation of earlier immunocytochemical studies (Graeber and Kreutzberg, 1986). While this result emphasized that axotomy also produces metabolic changes in the surrounding glial cells, it warned us not to interpret changes in synthesis of actin and tubulin as reflecting exclusively the behaviour of neurons.

The overall results of this study are summarized in Fig. 1: actin and tubulin (α and β combined) synthesis increased, while neurofilament synthesis decreased. The increase in actin synthesis occurred within 1 d of axotomy, and in crushed nerves began to return to normal by 7 d. In resected nerves, actin synthesis continued to increase at 7 days, but by 21 d had returned to control levels. There was no increase in tubulin synthesis 1 d post-axotomy, but by 3 d synthesis increased and in crushed nerves reached a plateau between 7 and 14 d, returning to normal by 21 d. In resected nerves, tubulin synthesis was still elevated at 21 d. Synthesis of the 68 and 150 kD neurofilament proteins declined significantly within 1 d, but in crushed nerves it recovered after 3 d, returning to normal by 21 d. No recovery occurred in resected nerves.

In facial nerve, axons regenerate past the crush site by 1 d, and grow at 4.2 mm/d, so that the recovery of whiskers movement begins at 11 d and is normal by 14 d (Tetzlaff and Kreutzberg, 1984). Many of the changes involved in the CBR reverse on successful regeneration (Grafstein and McQuarrie, 1978), and this is also the case

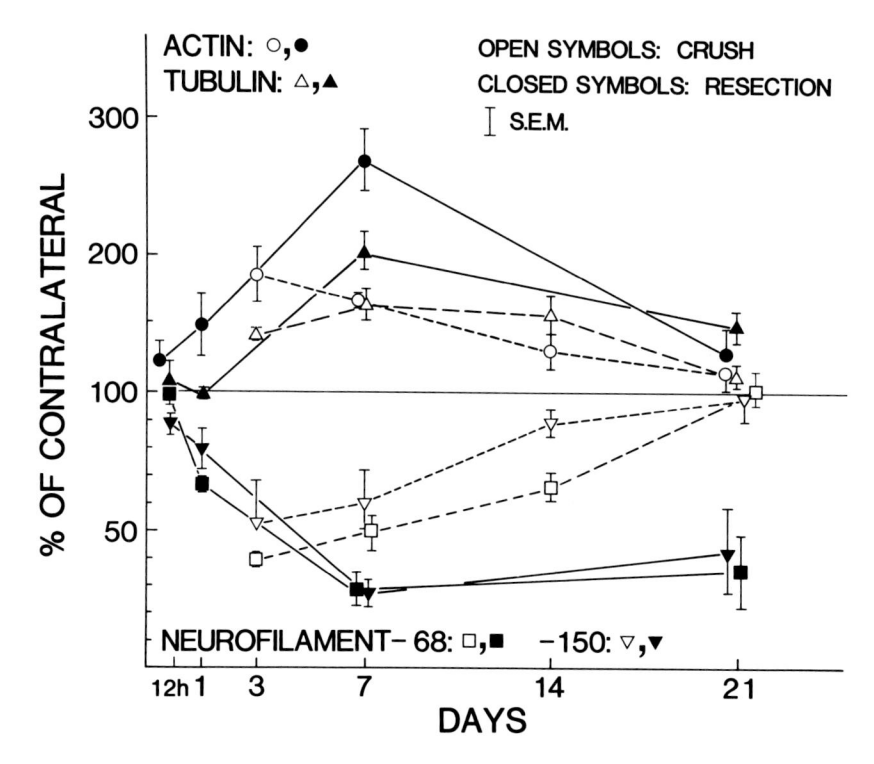

Figure 1. Changes in synthesis of cytoskeletal proteins in facial nucleus following axotomy.

for these cytoskeletal protein changes. Regeneration may permit the resumption of retrograde transport to the cell body of unidentified target-derived trophic factors. However, for actin and neurofilament synthesis, recovery begins between 3 and 7 d, before the regenerating axons have contacted their targets. In this case, the retrograde trophic factor may be derived from cells in the distal nerve rather than postsynaptic targets (Richardson and Ebendal, 1982; Heumann et al., 1987).

The obstruction to regeneration provided by resection results in an exaggerated CBR, most notably for actin. However, a recovery to normal levels of actin synthesis occurred by 21 d, even if regeneration was not successful, so there must be an additional control mechanism operating, apart from retrograde trophic control. The differential time course of the changes in synthesis of these cytoskeletal proteins, and the differential effect of success/failure of regeneration suggest that the CBR is not an "all-or-nothing" response regulated by a single mechanism, but instead is regulated by several different types of signals.

These changes correlate quite well with the events of regeneration: the early increase in actin may reflect an increased demand for actin in growth-cone formation and function (Bunge, 1986), which is necessary only during the initial phase of axon outgrowth. Impeding regeneration leads to a profusion of axonal sprouts (Shawe, 1955). The sustained increase in tubulin synthesis may be related to provision of the microtubule cytoskeleton for elongating and maturing axons. The decrease in neurofilament synthesis is associated with a reduction in proximal axon calibre (Hoffman et al., 1985). The subsequent recovery of neurofilament synthesis in regenerating neurons will result in a recovery of axon calibre, but in non-regenerating cells the maintained depression will be associated with maintained reduced axon calibre and decreased conduction velocity (Davis et al., 1978).

Though synthesis of neurofilaments is profoundly depressed, we found, using an antibody which binds independent of the state of phosphorylation, that neurofilament protein immunoreactivity in facial motoneurons did not decrease. Others have reported increased cell body neurofilament content (e.g. Sinicropi and McIlwain, 1983; Moss and Lewcowicz, 1983). Axotomy leads to abnormal phosphorylation of cell body neurofilaments (Rosenfeld et al., 1987; Goldstein et al., 1987) which might impair their participation in axonal transport so that they accumulate in the cell body in spite of reduced synthesis: indeed, their accumulation might even be the signal which suppresses synthesis.

IN-SITU HYBRIDIZATION WITH cDNA PROBES FOR CYTOSKELETAL mRNAs

In the foregoing discussion there has been the tacit assumption that the changes observed in actin and tubulin were neuronal. However, there could be a glial contribution, particularly since, as shown by GFAP, axotomy also provokes changes in protein synthesis in the surrounding glial cells. A second issue is the mechanism by which these changes in protein synthesis are effected. Both issues can be addressed by in situ hybridization experiments, in which the increased mRNA levels for actin and tubulin can be localized to neuronal or glial cells. Changes in mRNA levels could indicate that the control of synthesis is exerted at the transcriptional level, but alterations in mRNA stability must also be considered. In these studies we have used cDNA probes derived by hexa-nucleotide primer labelling ([35S] CTP) from the following clones: (i) mouse Mα1 α-tubulin cDNA (Lewis et al., 1985); (ii) mouse NF 68 cDNA (Lewis and Cowan, 1985); (iii) the mouse NF 150 cDNA (Julien et al., 1986); (iv) α-actin cDNA from mouse skeletal muscle (Minty et al., 1981). In situ hybridization was performed on cryostat sections of rat brainstem cut through the facial nucleus so that control and axotomized neurons could be compared on the same section.

As previously described for sensory neurons (Hoffman et al., 1987), the decrease in neurofilament protein synthesis in facial motoneurons was associated with decreased NF 68 and NF 150 mRNA expression (Fig. 2). Similarly, the increase in actin and tubulin synthesis was associated with increased mRNA expression within neuronal cell bodies. There were no detectable changes in the background labelling associated with glial cells. The changes in labelling with the various probes followed the time course of the changes in protein synthesis: thus, elevated levels of α-tubulin mRNA persisted longer than elevated levels of actin mRNA.

Our interest in the changes in cytoskeletal gene expression during regeneration led us to examine the differential expression of α-tubulin genes. Two α-tubulin mRNAs, Tα1 and T26, are expressed in the nervous system. Tα1 is enriched in embryonic brain, but expressed at only low levels in adult brain, while T26 expression does not change significantly during development (Miller et al., 1987). RNA probes were generated from an embryonic Tα1 α-tubulin cDNA after subcloning the non-coding 3' region into a PGEM4 vector using the SP6 RNA polymerase promoter. Subcloning the total cDNA clone (coding and non-coding) yielded a probe for total α-tubulin. To detect T26 mRNA, a 30 nucleotide oligonucleotide complementary to part of the 3' non-coding region of the T26 mRNA was used.

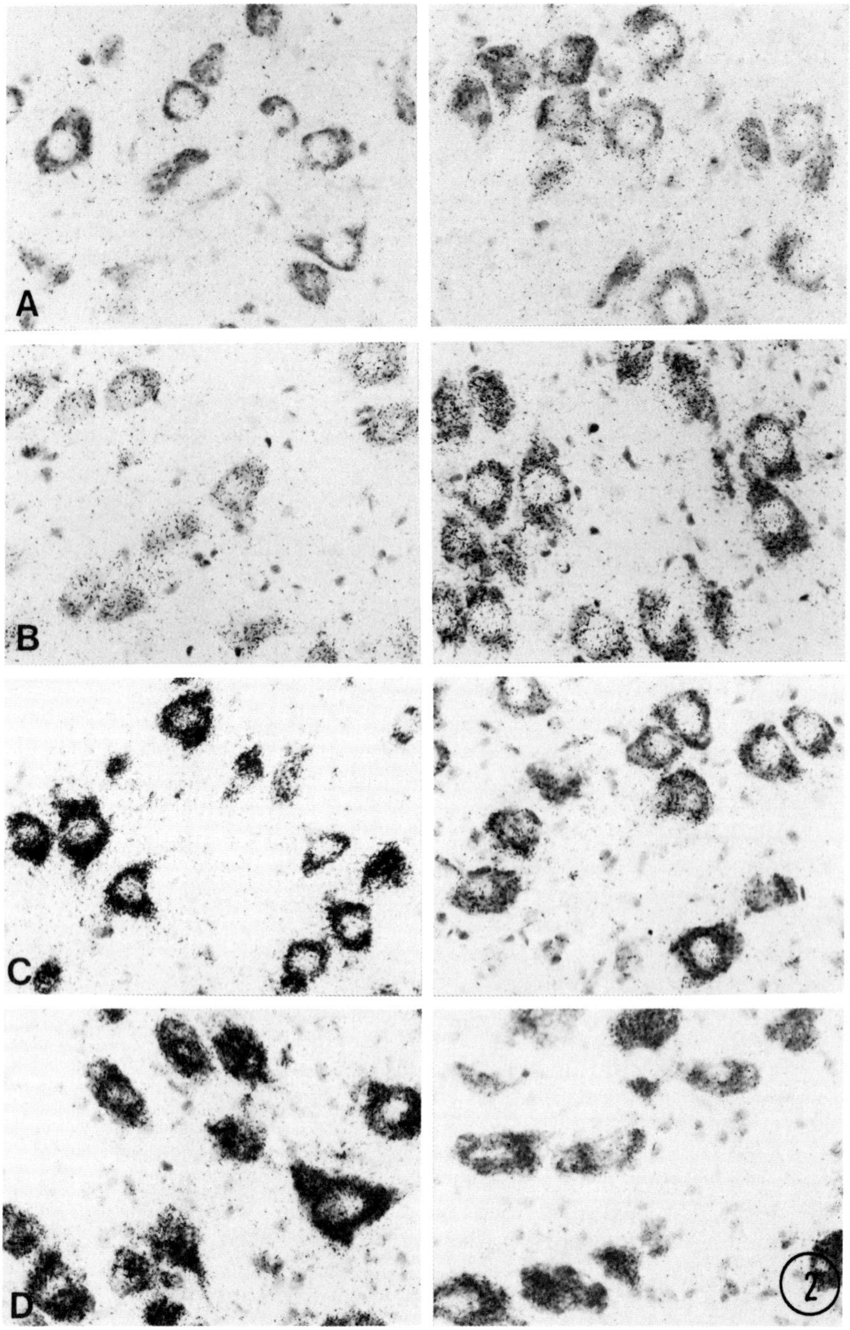
A
B
C
D
2

We found that within 4 h of axotomy performed 1.5 cm from the facial nucleus increased levels of Tα1 mRNA could be detected. Levels of Tα1 mRNA peaked 3 to 7 d following axotomy and thereafter declined. Surprisingly, levels of total α-tubulin mRNA were actually depressed up to 12 h postaxotomy and only slightly increased at 1 d. Levels of T26 mRNA remained constant. We believe that the increased tubulin synthesis observed during regeneration is due solely to increased production of the isotype coded by the Tα1 mRNA. This isotype probably differs only from that coded by T26 mRNA in the substitution of a single amino-acid, serine to glycine (Miller et al., 1987), but this could remove a site for phosphorylation.

Possibly the Tα1 isotype is less susceptible to linkage with neurofilaments, so that in growing axons a greater proportion of tubulin is free to travel in SCb or faster phases of axonal transport and support axonal outgrowth, rather than becoming trapped in the slower moving SCa. The rapid and specific re-expression of the embryonic Tα1 tubulin gene following axotomy provides direct support for the time-honoured concept that regeneration of neurons involves a reprise of the developmental programme (Van Biervliet, 1900). This is further underlined by the finding that axotomy of the facial nerve also induces re-expression of a developmentally regulated histone gene (Miller et al., 1988).

CYTOSKELETAL PROTEIN SYNTHESIS AND THE CONDITIONING LESION EFFECT

Axons regenerate sooner and more rapidly after a test lesion (TL) if they received a previous conditioning lesion (CL) (see McQuarrie, this volume). It is believed that this is because the CL induces the metabolic changes in the neuron cell body which support regeneration, so that the

Figure 2. In situ hybridization in the facial nucleus. In A,B, and C left panel is the control (unoperated) nucleus, right panel is the contralateral axotomized nucleus from the same animal. A: α-actin cDNA, 5 d post-crush. B: Mα1 α-tubulin cDNA, 5 d post-crush. C: NF 68 cDNA, 5 d post-resection. In D, probe is NF 68 cDNA. Left, 7 d post-test lesion; right, 14 d post-conditioning lesion and 7 d post-test lesion producing in a further decline in NF synthesis.

neuron is already in the regenerating mode when the TL is made.

In the facial nerve a TL crush applied at the same site as a CL made 7 days earlier leads to a 40% increase in regeneration rate. We found that the second lesion (TL) did not provoke any further change in tubulin or actin synthesis as measured either by L[35S] methionine incorporation or tubulin and actin mRNA expression. However, the TL did induce a further decrease in neurofilament synthesis and mRNA expression (Fig. 2D): the in-situ hybridizations showed that this decrease was not due to cell death. Both neurofilament immunocytochemistry and ultrastructural examination of the proximal axons revealed that they contained fewer neurofilaments than axons receiving a TL only.

We speculate that a critical event in the regulation of axon outgrowth is the interaction between neurofilament proteins and tubulins (and/or actin) at the site of cytoskeleton assembly in the cell body. Tubulin trapped by neurofilaments is conveyed at the SCa velocity (< 1.5 mm/d) and unable to participate in axon outgrowth (~4 mm/d). In conditioned axons this interaction is already reduced at the time of the TL, due to the reduced neurofilament synthesis and increased tubulin Tα1 synthesis, so that tubulin can be more rapidly transported (Hoffman et al., 1985). After the TL the further reduced neurofilament synthesis may permit accelerated tubulin transport and faster regeneration.

Since we believe that the changes in cytoskeletal protein synthesis following axotomy are critical to nerve regeneration, it is obviously important to investigate these responses in non-regenerating CNS neurons.

ACKNOWLEDGMENTS

WT was supported by a Fellowship from the Alberta Heritage Foundation for Medical Research and FDM by a Fellowship from the Medical Research Council of Canada, which also provided operating funds to MAB. Drs. R. Milner and F. Bloom are thanked for helpful advice and stimulating discussions.

REFERENCES

Black MM, Lasek RJ (1979). Slowing of the rate of axonal regeneration during growth and maturation. Exp Neurol 63: 108-119.

Bunge MB (1986). The axonal cytoskeleton: its role in generating and maintaining cell form. Trends Neurosci 9: 477-482.

Davis LA, Gordon T, Hoffer JA, Jhamandas J, Stein RB (1978). Compound action potentials recorded from mammalian peripheral nerves following ligation or resuturing. J Physiol 285: 553-559.

Graeber MB, Kreutzberg GW (1986). Astrocytes increase in glial fibrillary acidic protein during retrograde changes of facial motor neurons. J Neurocytol 15: 363-373.

Grafstein B, McQuarrie IG (1978). The role of the nerve cell body in axonal regeneration. In Cotman CW (Ed), "Neuronal Plasticity", Raven Press, New York, pp. 155-195.

Goldstein ME, Cooper HS, Bruce J, Carden MJ, Lee VM-Y, Schlaepfer WW (1987). Phosphorylation of neurofilament proteins and chromatolysis following transection of rat sciatic nerve. J Neurosci 7: 1586-1594.

Heumann R, Korsching S, Bandtlow C, Thoenen H (1987). Changes of nerve growth factor synthesis in nonneuronal cells in response to sciatic nerve transection. J Cell Biol 104: 1623-1631.

Hoffman PN, Cleveland DW, Griffin JW, Landes PW, Cowan NJ, Price DL (1987). Neurofilament gene expression: a major determinant of axonal caliber. Proc Natl Acad Sci USA 84: 3472-3476.

Hoffman PN, Lasek RJ (1980). Axonal transport of the cytoskeleton in regenerating motor neurons: constancy and change. Brain Res 202: 317-333.

Hoffman PN, Thompson GW, Griffin JW, Price DL (1985). Changes in neurofilament transport coincide temporally with alterations in the caliber of axons in regenerating motor fibers. J Cell Biol 101: 1332-1340.

Julien J-P, Meyer D, Flavell D, Hurst J, Grosveld F (1986). Cloning and developmental expression of the murine neurofilament gene family. Molec Brain Res 1: 243-250.

Lasek RJ (1986). Polymer sliding in axons. J Cell Sci Suppl 5: 161-179.

Lasek RJ, McQuarrie IG, Wujek JR (1981). The central nervous system regeneration problem: neuron and environment. In Gorio A, Millesi H, Mingrino S (Eds.), "Posttraumatic Peripheral Nerve Regeneration", Raven Press, New York, pp. 59-70.

Lewis SA, Cowan NJ (1985). Genetics, evolution, and expression of the 68,000-mol-wt neurofilament protein: isolation of a cloned cDNA probe. J Cell Biol 100: 843-850.

Lewis SA, Lee MG-S, Cowan NJ (1985). Five mouse tubulin isotypes and their regulated expression during development. J Cell Biol 101: 852-861.

Miller FD, Naus CCG, Bloom FE, Milner RJ (1987). Isotopes of α-tubulin are differentially regulated during neuronal maturation. J Cell Biol (in press).

Miller FD, Tetzlaff W, Bisby M, Milner RJ (1988). Rapid induction of the major embryonic α-tubulin mRNA in adults following neuronal injury (submitted).

Minty AJ, Caravatti M, Robert B, Cohen A, Daubas P, Weydert A, Gros F, Buckingham ME (1981). Mouse actin messenger RNAs. J Biol Chem 256: 1008-1014.

Moss TH, Lewkowicz SJ (1983). The axon reaction in motor and sensory neurones of mice studied by a monoclonal antibody marker of neurofilament protein. J Neurol Sci 60: 267-280.

Oblinger MM, Brady ST, McQuarrie IG, Lasek RJ (1987). Cytotypic differences in the protein composition of the axonally transported cytoskeleton in mammalian neurons. J Neurosci 7: 453-462.

Richardson PM, Ebendal T (1982). Nerve growth activities in rat peripheral nerve. Brain Res 246: 57-64.

Rosenfeld J, Dorman ME, Griffin JW, Sternberger LA, Sternberger NH, Price DL (1987). Distribution of neurofilament antigens after axonal injury. J Neuropathol Exp Neurol 46: 269-282.

Shawe GDH (1955). On the number of branches formed by regenerating nerve-fibres. Br J Surg 42: 474-488.

Sinicropi DV, McIlwain DL (1983). Changes in the amounts of cytoskeletal proteins within the perikarya and axons of regenerating frog motoneurons. J Cell Biol 96: 240-247.

Tetzlaff W, Graeber MB, Bisby MA, Kreutzberg GW (1988). Increased glial fibrillary acidic protein synthesis in astrocytes during retrograde reaction of the axotomized rat facial nucleus. Glia (in press).

Tetzlaff W, Kreutzberg GW (1984). Enzyme changes in the rat facial nucleus following a conditioning lesion. Exp Neurol 85: 547-564.

Van Biervliet J (1900). La substance chromophile pendant le cours de developpement de la cellule neurveuse. Le Nevraxe 1: 33-35.

Wujek JR, Lasek RJ (1983). Correlation of axonal regeneration and slow component b in two branches of a single axon. J Neurosci 3: 243-251.

CYTOSKELETON OF THE REGENERATING AXON

Irvine G. McQuarrie

Division of Neurosurgery and Department of Developmental Genetics, Case Western Reserve Univ., and Neural Regeneration Center, Veterans Admin. Medical Center, Cleveland, OH 44106

INTRODUCTION

The axonal cytoskeleton, as revealed by scanning electron microscopy of rapidly frozen nerves, is organized in a complex manner (Hirokawa, 1982; Schnapp and Reese, 1982). The fibrillar macromolecules of the axon are the same as those found in other cell types: intermediate filaments, microtubules, and microfilaments. In neurons, however, these have a unique composition and complexity. The intermediate filament proteins that form neurofilaments differ substantially from those of other cell types, and approximately 50% of axonal microtubules cannot be disassembled by cold temperatures or micromolar calcium (Weber and Geisler, 1985; Sahenk and Brady, 1987). The close association between microtubules and neurofilaments, providing axial organization, is apparently responsible for the extreme asymmetry of the axon.

There is substantial evidence indicating that neurofilaments function primarily to maintain the radius of axons, particularly in large axons which conduct action potentials rapidly (Hoffman et al., 1988). Microtubules form sinuous "streets" through the axoplasm that carry membranous tubulo-vesicular elements from the Golgi apparatus in the perikaryon to the axon terminal at the fast transport rate of 200-400 mm/day (Lasek et al., 1984). Tubulo-vesicular elements are used to renew axonal membranes (axolemma and smooth endoplasmic reticulum) and to make synaptic vesicles at the axon terminal. Neurofilaments and microtubules advance much less rapidly, as part of slow transport, at a rate of 0.2-6 mm/day. Neurofilaments and most of the microtubules move as a slower subcomponent of slow transport, called slow component a (SCa), at 0.2-1.7 mm/day; the remaining microtubules and most of the dimeric tubulin move with a faster subcomponent, called slow component b (SCb), at 2-6 mm/day (McQuarrie et al., 1986; Brady and Black, 1986).

These cytoskeletal elements (subunits and polymers) advance in association with other proteins that can be assembled into fibrillar polymers: actin, spectrin, and non-muscle myosin (McQuarrie et al., 1986). In addition, slow transport conveys the proteins which regulate assembly; these include calmodulin and a class of microtubule-associated proteins (MAPs) called tau factors (McQuarrie, 1988a). Another important group of proteins that moves with slow transport are the glycolytic enzymes (Oblinger et al., 1987). These are characteristic of SCb and include neuron-specific enolase, aldolase, pyruvate kinase, and creatine kinase. In general, proteins that support "export" functions are carried by fast transport and those that support "housekeeping" functions (e.g. maintenance of the cytoskeleton) are carried by slow transport.

AXOTOMY AND TRANSPORT CHANGES

During axonal regeneration, the rate of outgrowth is limited by the rate at which a new cytoskeleton can be constructed behind the advancing growth cone (McQuarrie, 1983, 1988a). Several lines of evidence suggest that slow transport continues almost unimpeded following an axonal injury, so that a new "daughter" axon (sprout) is soon elaborated from the "parent" axon stump and advances at the upper end of the range for slow transport rates (McQuarrie, 1985; McQuarrie and Lasek, 1988). This means that the cytoskeleton of the regenerating axon must arise from materials already being conveyed by slow transport at the time of axonal injury (axotomy). The only exception is when the site of axotomy is located near the cell body: the increased amounts of housekeeping proteins, which are synthesized as part of the cell body reaction, would then be able to reach the daughter axon in time to augment the elongation phase of regeneration (McQuarrie, 1984, 1988b).

The change in transport of structural proteins in parent axons has been examined in several types of neurons (McQuarrie, 1988c). The common theme is that there are significant increases in the amounts of actin and tubulin moving with SCb, and decreases in the amounts of neurofilament proteins and tubulin moving with SCa (e.g. Hoffman and Lasek, 1980). Thus, the metabolic emphasis shifts from one of maintenance of the cytoskeleton in its mature state to one of growth and development of a new cytoskeleton. This response is common to all neurons that exhibit successful axonal regeneration. The cell body reaction presumably evolved at a time when organisms were small enough for axonal regeneration to benefit from it. Perhaps it simply represents a modification of the bacterial response to loss of a flagellum, since the changes in tubulin metabolism are remarkably similar to that seen following axotomy (McQuarrie, 1984).

SLOW TRANSPORT IN MATURE AXONS AND DAUGHTER AXONS

To study axonal transport, newly-synthesized proteins are radiolabeled at the level of the nerve cell body (Grafstein and Forman, 1980). This produces waves of radioactivity which move proximo-distally in the axon, each wave representing a rate-component of axonal transport. Fast transport is the most rapid, and conveys approximately 10% of the axonally transported radioactivity that is in protein. Labeled mitochondria form a wave of labeling that moves at the intermediate rate of 50-100 mm/day. Slow transport is represented by a large wave containing most of the total transported radioactivity. To study slow transport, the nerve must be long enough to separate the radioactivity in faster moving membranous organelles from that in slower moving cytoskeletal elements. Additionally, it is often necessary to separate SCb from SCa. Motor axons in the rat sciatic nerve have been found to meet these requirements (McQuarrie et al., 1986). These are also suitable for studying axonal regeneration: when a testing lesion is made far proximally, at the point where the L4 and L5 spinal nerves join, a 75 mm length of degenerated nerve is made available for studying slow transport in daughter axons (McQuarrie and Lasek, 1988).

In normal sciatic motor axons, SCa carries most of the labeled tubulin. This is postulated to represent moving microtubules since the peak of labeling is prominent, spreads minimally over time, and is cotransported with peaks of labeling for putative MAPs (Tytell et al., 1984). In motor axons of the rat sciatic nerve, the SCa peak advances at a rate of 1.3 mm/day. The SCb peak becomes evident as a shoulder of labeling that emerges from the front of the SCa wave by one week after isotope injection. The SCb peak consists mainly of cotransported peaks of labeling for actin, calmodulin, and tubulin; these advance at 3.1 mm/day (McQuarrie et al., 1986).

In the daughter axons of motor neurons that had been labeled 7 days prior to the testing lesion, the leading part of the SCb wave reaches the lesion site by the time that lesion is made (McQuarrie and Lasek, 1988). As the daughter axons elongate, labeled SCb proteins enter the sprouts unimpeded to label cytoskeletal elements. These separate into two groups that have the composition of SCa and SCb, with the slower peak advancing at 1.3 mm/day and the faster at 2.9 mm/day. This suggests that axonal regrowth is a continuation of normal processes, intrinsic to SCb, for maintaining the cytoskeleton of the axonal arbor. These processes may be particularly well developed in motor neurons, where the number of microtubules and the cross-sectional area of terminal axons is 10-fold greater than in the stem axon (Zenker and Hohberg, 1973).

SLOW TRANSPORT IN CONDITIONED DAUGHTER AXONS

The question, then, is how does SCb maintain the cytoskeleton? One approach is to examine the composition of SCb when axonal growth is accelerated. This can be done by using the conditioning lesion paradigm. After a conditioning interval of 7-14 days (which allows time to increase the synthesis of housekeeping proteins and augment the delivery of these to the axon via SCb), a testing lesion is made to examine the effect of SCb augmentation on axonal outgrowth (McQuarrie, 1986a, 1988b). Thus, the conditioning interval allows sufficient time for the cell body reaction to increase the synthesis of housekeeping proteins, and for SCb to carry these to the site of the testing lesion (Fig. 1):

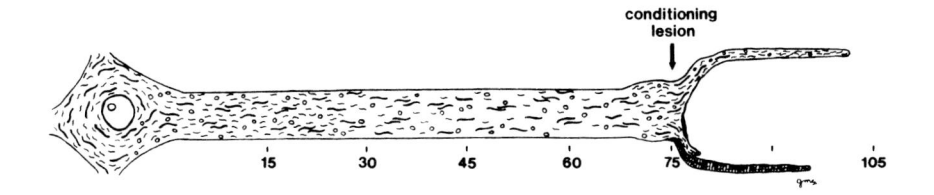

Fig. 1: Illustration of the conditioning lesion paradigm. In response to an axotomy (conditioning lesion) made one week earlier, the neuron has increased the synthesis of actin and tubulin moving with SCb (thin lines) and decreased the synthesis of tubulin and neurofilament proteins moving with SCa (thick lines). Fast-transported membranous materials are represented by small circles. To test the effect of this metabolic shift on axonal outgrowth, a testing lesion must be made such that it interacts with the increased amounts of SCb present in the axon (i.e., within 30 mm of the cell body). A testing lesion made at a greater distance (e.g. 60 mm) would produce daughter axons that would grow distally at about the same rate as SCb is carrying additional tubulin and actin toward them (approximately 4 mm/day). Thus, outgrowth would be complete before this additional support could arrive. (Distances are in mm.)

The effect of such an augmentation is to increase the fraction of daughter axons that survive, and to increase the rate at which these advance, compared to observations made after a testing lesion alone (McQuarrie, 1984, 1985, 1986a). For example, when nodes of Ranvier located 200-500 um proximal to a testing lesion of the rat sciatic nerve are examined by electron microscopy after a 9 hour interval, the incidence of cytoskeleton-containing daughter axons is 9% (McQuarrie, 1985). However, when the testing lesion is made 2 weeks after a conditioning lesion of the largest distal branch (carrying 35-39% of the myelinated axons), the incidence of daughter axons with cytoskeletal components is 33%. Thus, almost all of the conditioned axons are able to produce elongating daughter axons by 9 hours after a testing lesion. In this model and in other similar models, the daughter axons that emerge after a testing lesion appear to take advantage of an augmentation in SCb (McQuarrie and Grafstein, 1982; McQuarrie, 1984).

When the changes in composition of SCb in daughter axons are examined after a testing lesion in conditioned vs. sham-conditioned nerves, attention has been directed primarily to actin and tubulin (McQuarrie, 1986a; McQuarrie, 1988c). This is because a sizable literature documents an increase in the transport of these proteins via SCb in parent axons (reviewed in McQuarrie, 1988c). And, the data emerging from studies on rat motor neurons indicate that a sustained 2-fold increase in tubulin labeling occurs in conditioned daughter axons, associated with a less marked increase in actin labeling (McQuarrie, 1986a, 1988c). During the first week of outgrowth, there is also a marked increase in the amounts of calmodulin and a group of proteins enriched for putative MAPs entering daughter axons (McQuarrie, 1986b). Examples of this are shown (Figs. 2 and 3).

During the second week of outgrowth, the increases for calmodulin and putative MAPs are no longer apparent while increases for tubulin and actin have persisted. Taken together, the studies of SCb labeling in daughter axons suggest that calmodulin and putative MAPs become incorporated into (or closely associated with) cytoskeletal polymers as these are being formed, and that many of these subsequently move with SCa (McQuarrie, 1986b, McQuarrie and Lasek, 1988). Whether it is the availability of structural proteins that is rate-limiting for outgrowth, or the availability of regulatory proteins, remains to be investigated.

4 DAYS AFTER TESTING LESION

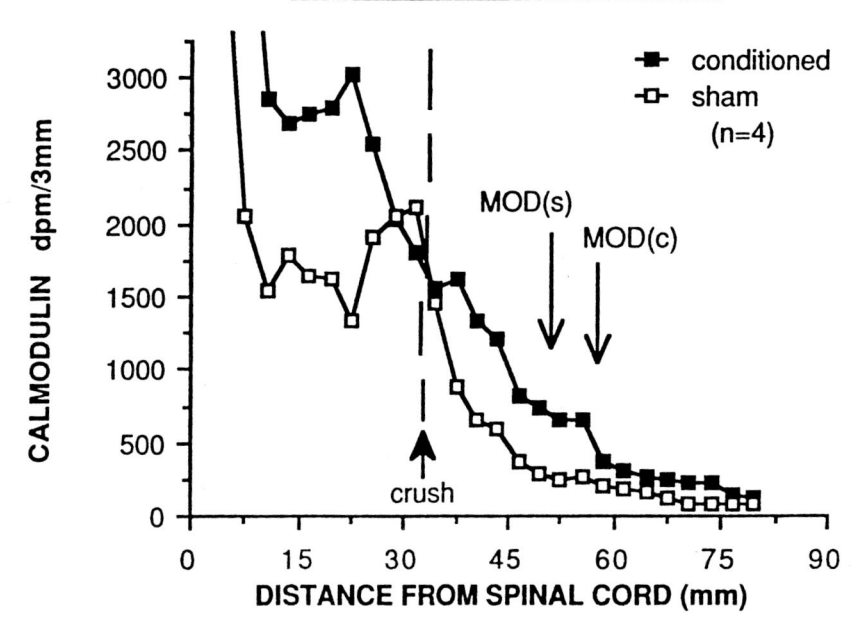

Fig. 2: The distribution of mean amounts of labeled calmodulin in motor axons of the rat sciatic nerve at 11 days after microinjection of the lumbar spinal cord with 35-S methionine. In 4 animals, a conditioning crush lesion was made at 90 mm from the spinal cord 7 days prior to isotope injection; 4 paired control animals received sham conditioning lesions. Rats weighed 170-200 g at the time of injection; the conditioning lesion group received 769 +/- 97 microCuries and the sham-conditioned group received 806 +/- 103 microCuries. A testing lesion was made at the junction of the L4 and L5 spinal nerves 7 days after isotope injection (14 days after the conditioning lesion). Animals were killed 4 days after the testing lesion (crush). Consecutive 3 mm nerve segments of the L4 and L5 ventral roots, L4 and L5 spinal nerves, and sciatic nerve were processed by SDS-PAGE, fluorography, and protein solubilization for liquid scintillation counting (McQuarrie et al., 1986). For plotted points, the SEM was less than 20% of the mean

in over 90% of nerve segments. The maximum outgrowth distances (MOD) for conditioned (c) and sham-conditioned (s) nerves are indicated by arrows; the MOD in each nerve was the most distal nerve segment carrying a peak of actin labeling co-located with a peak of labeling for putative MAPs at 58-67 kiloDaltons (kD). The MOD located by this method corresponds to the location of growth cones identified by labeling fast transport (McQuarrie and Lasek, 1988).

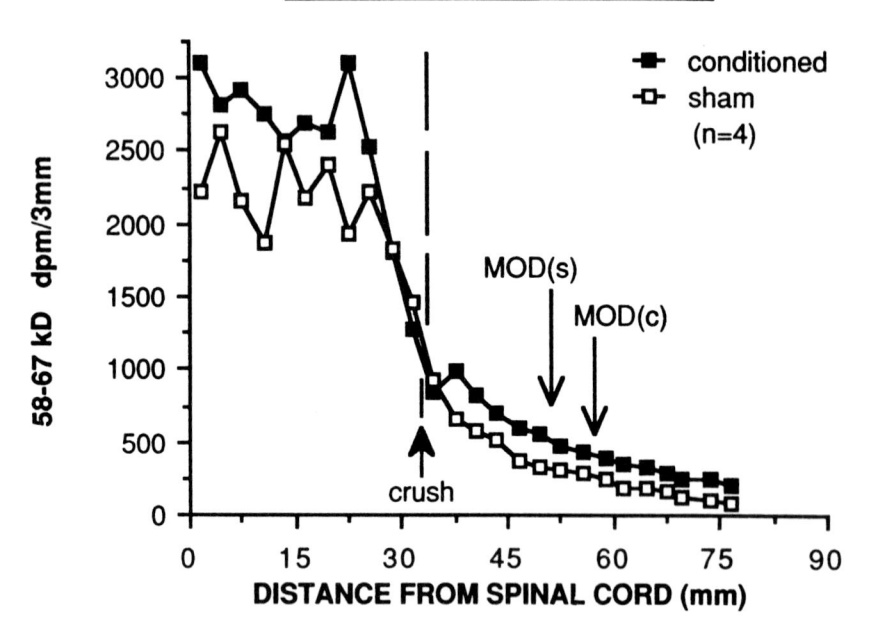

Fig. 3: The distribution of mean amounts of labeled polypeptides at 58-67 kD in motor axons of the rat sciatic nerve at 11 days after microinjection of the lumbar spinal cord with 35-S methionine (same nerves and legend as Fig. 2). The 58-67 kD group is enriched for putative MAPs of axonal microtubules, including tau factors and chartins (McQuarrie and Lasek, 1988).

REFERENCES

Brady ST, Black MM (1986). Axonal transport of microtubule proteins: Cytotypic variation of tubulin and MAPs in neurons. Ann New York Acad Sci 466:199-217.

Grafstein B, Forman DS (1980). Intracellular transport in neurons. Physiol Rev 60:1167-1283.

Hirokawa N (1982). Cross-linker system between neurofilaments, microtubules, and membranous organelles in frog axons revealed by the quick-freeze, deep-etching method. J Cell Biol 94:129-142.

Hoffman PN, Koo EH, Muma NA, Griffin JW, Price DL (1988). Role of neurofilaments in the control of axonal caliber in myelinated nerve fibers. In Lasek RJ, Black MM (eds): "Intrinsic Determinants of Neuronal Form and Function," New York: Alan R. Liss, pp 389-402.

Hoffman PN, Lasek RJ (1980). Axonal transport of the cytoskeleton in regenerating motor neurons: Constancy and change. Brain Res 202:317-333.

Lasek RJ, Garner JA, Brady ST (1984). Axonal transport of the cytoplasmic matrix. J Cell Biol 99:212s-221s.

McQuarrie IG (1983). Role of the axonal cytoskeleton in the regenerating nervous system. In Seil FJ (ed): "Nerve, Organ and Tissue Regeneration: Research Perspectives," New York: Academic Press, pp 51-88.

McQuarrie IG (1984). Effect of a conditioning lesion on axonal transport during regeneration: The role of slow transport. In Elam JS, Cancalon P (eds): "Axonal Transport in Neuronal Growth and Regeneration," New York: Plenum Press, pp 185-209.

McQuarrie IG (1985). Effect of a conditioning lesion on axonal sprout formation at nodes of Ranvier. J Comp Neurol 231:239-249.

McQuarrie IG (1986a). Structural protein transport in elongating motor axons after sciatic nerve crush: Effect of a conditioning lesion. Neurochem Pathol 5:153-164.

McQuarrie IG (1986b). Regulatory proteins enter axons ahead of microtubules. Soc Neurosci Abstr 12:513.

McQuarrie IG (1988a). Transport of cytoskeletal proteins into axonal sprouts during nerve regeneration. In Gordon T, Stein RB, Smith PA (eds): "The Current Status of Peripheral Nerve Regeneration," New York: Alan R. Liss, pp 25-34.

McQuarrie IG (1988b). Neuronal metabolic basis of the conditioning lesion effect. In Flohr H (ed):

"Post-Lesion Neural Plasticity," New York: Springer, in press.
McQuarrie IG (1988c). Axonal transport and the regenerating nerve. In Seil FJ (ed): "Neural Regeneration Research for the Clinician," New York: Alan R. Liss, in press.
McQuarrie IG, Grafstein B (1982). Protein synthesis and axonal transport in goldfish retinal ganglion cells during regeneration acceleration by a conditioning lesion. Brain Res 251:25-37.
McQuarrie IG, Lasek R J (1988). Transport of cytoskeletal elements from parent axons into regenerating daughter axons. J Neurosci, in press.
McQuarrie IG, Brady ST, Lasek RJ (1986). Diversity in the axonal transport of structural proteins: Major differences between optic and spinal axons in the rat. J Neurosci 6:1593-1605.
Oblinger MM, Brady ST, McQuarrie IG, Lasek RJ (1987). Cytotypic differences in the protein composition of the axonally transported cytoskeleton in mammalian neurons. J Neurosci 7:453-462.
Sahenk Z, Brady ST (1987). Axonal tubulin and microtubules: Morphologic evidence for stable regions on axonal microtubules. Cell Motil Cytoskel 8:155-164.
Schnapp BJ, Reese TS (1982). Cytoplasmic structure in rapid-frozen axons. J Cell Biol 94:667-679.
Tytell M, Brady ST, Lasek RJ (1984). Axonal transport of a subclass of tau proteins: Evidence for the regional differentiation of microtubules in neurons. Proc Natl Acad Sci (USA) 81:1570-1574.
Weber K, Geisler N (1985). Intermediate filaments: Structural conservation and divergence. Ann New York Acad Sci 455:126-143.
Zenker W, Hohberg E (1973). A-alpha nerve fibre: Number of neurotubules in the stem fibre and in the terminal branches. J Neurocytol 2:143-148.

EFFECT OF GM 1 GANGLIOSIDE ADMINISTRATION ON THE AXOTOMY RESPONSE OF RAT RUBRAL NEURONS

Kevin D. Barron

Medical Research Service, Veterans Administration Medical Center and Department of Neurology, Albany Medical College, Albany, New York 12208

INTRODUCTION

The axon reaction in mammalian intrinsic nerve cells (somas and processes confined to the CNS) frequently is manifest by cytoplasmic, nuclear and nucleolar shrinkage and a decline in RNA and protein synthesis (Barron, 1983; Barron et al, 1985). Frequently, cell death supervenes, sometimes within a few days (Barron, 1983; Barron et al, 1986), or the injured cell remains for long periods (Barron et al, 1986) in a shrunken, metabolically quiescent state. Axons originated by the axotomized intrinsic neurons are not at all or only abortively regenerated, unless special experimental manipulations are undertaken, such as are described in this Symposium. In contrast, axotomized extrinsic neurons, which have somas and processes in whole or in part external to the CNS and which include primary motor and sensory nerve cells, generally maintain stable cytoplasmic, nuclear and nucleolar dimensions or show hypertrophy of these cellular components (Barron, 1983). When atrophy occurs, as happens for the nuclei of feline cervical motoneurons after brachial plexotomy, it is transitory (Barron et al, 1982). Furthermore, extrinsic neurons often regenerate the distal stump of the severed axon spontaneously and reconnect with terminal end stations (Barron et al, 1982). Another difference between the axotomy responses of intrinsic and extrinsic mammalian neuronal populations is the conspicuously heightened uptake of ^{14}C-2-deoxyglucose in CNS tissue containing axotomized aggregations of the latter. However, in nuclei containing intrinsic nerve cells, the uptake of ^{14}C-2-deoxyglucose does not rise above control levels after axotomy (Rodichok et al, 1984).

Since the axon is dependent upon the parent soma both for maintenance and for growth, and since CNS regeneration is practically a matter of reconstitution of axons distal to a point of interruption (and ultimately their reconnection to appropriate end stations), the regressive nature of the response to axotomy by somas of intrinsic neurons is of concern to those interested in the CNS regeneration problem.

In recent years, a number of experimental interventions have been designed and applied to injured mammalian CNS that have prevented atrophy and necrosis of the axotomized intrinsic neuron. These include use of CNS transplants, implants of PNS attached to or inserted in CNS tissues, and administration of trophins and other agents that enhance biosynthesis (Bregman and Reier, 1986; Kromer, 1987; LaVie et al, 1987; Vidal-Sanz et al, 1987). The glycolipid, ganglioside GM1, promotes sprouting of axons in partially de-afferented CNS tissues (Gradkowska et al, 1986) and appears also to have a growth-promoting action on neurons of PNS and CNS in in vivo and in vitro systems (Gorio et al, 1984; Skaper et al, 1985). The systemic injection of GM1 is said also to prevent atrophy and necrosis of nerve cells in the substantia nigra after partial interruption of the nigro-striatal pathway (Toffano et al, 1984) and in the nucleus basalis after corticectomy (Cuello et al, 1986). Encouraged by these reports, we undertook an experimental study of a major descending motor system of rat spinal cord, the rubro-spinal tract (RST) and its nucleus of origin, the red nucleus (RN). The RST was interrupted unilaterally at C2-3 segment in animals injected with GM1 ganglioside (treated group) and in animals from which GM1 was withheld (untreated group). Over a postoperative survival period of 3-90 days, the spinal cord was studied histologically and the RN was examined by morphometric and quantitative cytochemical (RNA) techniques. The RST is completely crossed and can be reliably interrupted extracranially.

METHODS

Under methoxyflurane anesthesia (Metofane, Pitman Moore), thirty-five female Sprague-Dawley rats weighing 220-300 g underwent unilateral interruption of the RST by lateral funiculotomy at the C2-3 segmental level. The 21 individuals of the untreated, experimental group were sacrificed 3 (2), 7

(2), 10 (2), 14 (4), 28 (6), 60 (3) and 90 (2) days postoperatively. (Numbers in parenthesis refer to the number of rats killed at each listed postoperative survival period). A treated group, consisting of 14 operated animals divided into 4 sets, was injected with GM1, 30 mg/kg i.p. daily. The first and second sets, 4 rats in each set, began ganglioside injections 24 hours postoperatively and were killed 14 and 28 days after operation. In a third and fourth set, 3 rats/set, GM1 treatment began 1 hour after operation and continued for 14 or for 28 days with sacrifice on the 28th postoperative day in each instance. Six untreated, unoperated control rats completed the experimental series.

Rats were killed under sodium pentobarbital anesthesia by perfusion-fixation with 4% formaldehyde in 0.1 M phosphate buffer containing 0.9% NaCl, followed by Clarke's solution (ethanol-acetic acid, 3:1). The brain and spinal cord were then removed. A 3-4 mm slice of midbrain, containing the caudal pole of the RN, and blocks of the spinal cord through, above and below the operative lesion were immerse-fixed in Clarke's solution for 4 hours at room temperature and embedded in paraffin. Serial sections of the spinal cord blocks that contained the operative lesion were made at 10 µm either in a transverse or a longitudinal (sagittal) plane and stained by hematoxylin-eosin or Bodian techniques. Midbrain sections through the RN were cut serially at 6 µm beginning at the caudal pole of the nucleus and progressing rostrally for 300 µm. These were mounted in triplets on glass slides and stained for RNA by an azure B technique (Barron et al, 1982, 1985). In 12 animals, the serial sections of midbrain were carried forward to a level more than 500 µm rostral to the caudal extremity of the RN. Additionally, random sections of midbrain were stained in all animals to and beyond the oral pole of the nucleus of the oculomotor nerve. Morphometric measurements were made on the first 50 nucleolated rubral neurons encountered, beginning at the caudal pole on each side and moving rostrally. Neuronal profiles were projected onto paper with a Nikon Optiphot instrument and somal and nuclear outlines were drawn. The areas of somas and nuclei were measured by use of the Zeiss MOP III system. Cytoplasmic areas (soma-nucleus) were computed. Rubral nerve cell counts were done bilaterally on alternating triplets of 6 µm sections for the first caudorostral 300 µm of the RN. In 12 animals, neuronal counts utilized 3 additional triplets of azure B-stained sections at levels 360 µm, 432 µm and 504 µm rostrally. Neurons with split nucleoli ranged from 1-4% of the total and were corrected for. Nucleolar diameters were determined by filar micrometry.

Microspectrophotometric assay for RNA was by the Zeiss Cytoscan System (Barron et al, 1982, 1985), which is programmed for a Digital Equipment Corporation PDP-12 computer, until, toward the end of the experiment, the PDP-12 failed to function and this obsolescent instrument could not be repaired. Accordingly, the data for the 6 unoperated control animals was re-accumulated by the Zeiss Image Scan System which was applied also to measurements of RNA staining in rubral neurons of 2 untreated and 6 treated (3rd and 4th sets of GM1-injected series) 28-day survivals. The Cytoscan System expresses RNA content as total extinctions (TE) in arbitrary units per soma and per nucleolus. The cytoplasm (perikaryon) contains more than 95% of the somal RNA. The Image Scan yields densitometric values (OD) for each of cytoplasm and nucleolus. Nuclear RNA was not measurable by either method. Both techniques provided measures of cellular area. Neurons with somal areas of 200 μm^2 or less constitute 2-7% of rubral nerve cells in the caudal 300 µm of the RN and, on the assumption that these were interneurons, they were not assayed.

The data were analyzed statistically by a multiway analysis of variance program. In view of the multiple variables that were analyzed, including sidedness, treatment, length of survival etc., a level of $p < 0.01$ was selected as the indicator of statistical significance.

RESULTS

All lesions interrupted completely the right rubrospinal tract. The posterior funiculi and corticospinal tracts were spared. Of interest was the degree of axonal sprouting 14-28 days postoperatively. Newly generated axons ran predominantly a dorsoventral course through the lateral funiculus and appeared to derive mostly from posterior roots. By the 90th postoperative day such axons were rare. GM1 injection did not appear to influence this process.

In azure B stains (Fig. 1), the axotomy response was qualitatively manifest 3 days after funiculotomy and took the form of central chromatolysis. Chromatolytic change occurred exclusively in the RN contralateral to operation and appeared to affect virtually all nerve cells above the size of putative interneurons (somal areas < 200 μm^2). The latter had such a paucity of Nissl substance that chromatolysis could hardly have been recognized. Central chromatolysis was succeeded by cellular atrophy, partial restoration of lysed Nissl particles and, ultimately, by extreme shrinkage and loss of basophilia. Qualitatively, no neuroglial change was apparent.

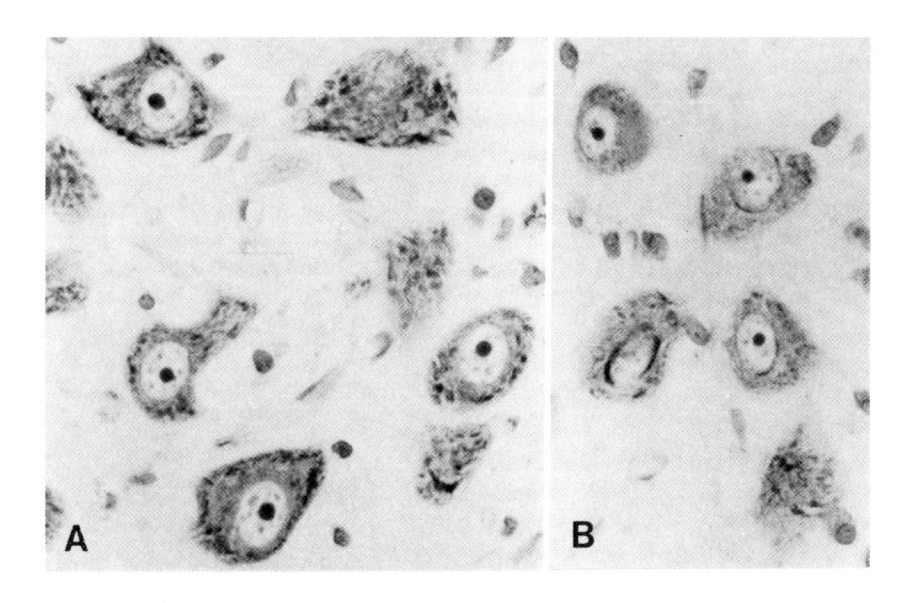

Figure 1. Note the Nissl pattern in nonaxotomized rubral neurons (A) of a 14-day postoperative survival and compare with axotomized side (B) where granules are few and fine and there are perinuclear basophilic rims.

Nerve cell counts did not disclose nerve cell loss to the 60th postoperative day. By 90 days postoperatively, although achromatic neurons of the axotomized RN could be recognized and areal measurements of individual nerve cells determined, the borders of the RN were difficult to separate from adjacent reticular formation and counts of rubral neurons were not carried out.

Morphometric assay of axotomized neurons of untreated animals showed significant cytoplasmic atrophy 7 days postoperatively (mean area in unoperated controls 418.9 μm^2 $\pm$ 10.1 vs 356 μm^2 $\pm$ 17.1) followed, at 10 days, by nuclear (108.4 μm^2s$\pm$ 1.5 vs 76.8 μm^2 $\pm$ 2.4) and nucleolar (mean diameters, 4.0 $\pm$ .05 μm vs 3.4 $\pm$ .06) shrinkage. Data for the soma (summed cytoplasmic and nuclear areas) is summarized in Figure 2. The atrophic process progressed relentlessly, but in a bimodal manner in the cytoplasm and the nucleolus, where regression analysis depicted a rapid phase of 2 weeks duration which was followed by a slow and steady decline. In contrast, the progression of nuclear atrophy was unimodal. On the axotomized side, 90 days after surgery, mean values for cytoplasm, nucleus and nucleolus were, respectively, 142.0 μm^2 $\pm$ 25, 56.1 $\pm$ 2.0 μm^2 and 2.7 $\pm$ .15 μm. GM1 treatment did not bring about significant changes in morphometric measures. Of some note was the significant decline in cytoplasmic area which occurred in non-axotomized neurons of untreated animals 3-28 days postoperatively. This was maximal on the 14th postoperative day (377.8 μm^2 $\pm$ 8.4).

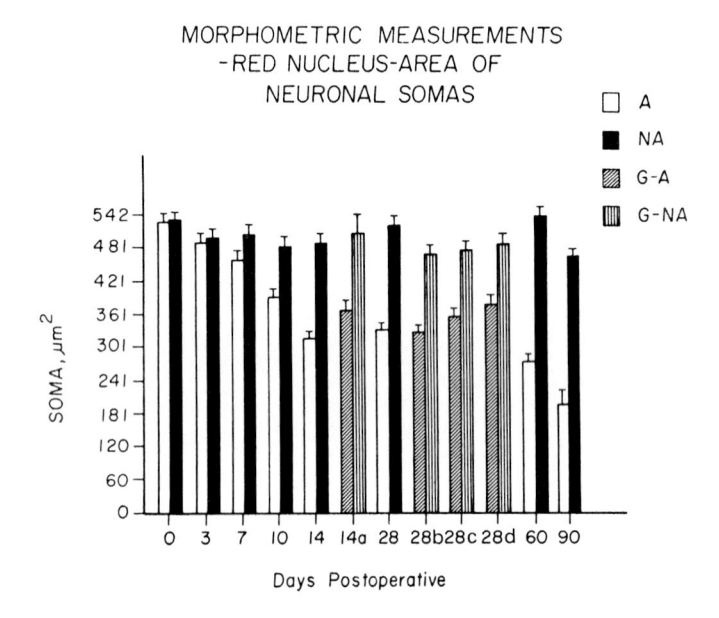

Figure 2. Data derive from the axotomized (A) and nonaxotomized (NA) sides of GM1-treated (G-A and G-NA) and untreated rats. GM1 had no statistically significant effect.

The somal (cytoplasmic) and nucleolar content of RNA decreased in axotomized neurons of untreated animals by both Cytoscan (TE) and Image Scan (OD) measurement. Twenty-eight days after section of the RST, the mean TE value for axotomized rubral nerve cells was 5159 ± 266 as compared to a value of 14834 ± 698 for the left side of the RN of unoperated control rats. Corresponding nucleolar values 28 days after tractotomy were 268 ± 12.2 vs 647 ± 25.1 (left RN of unoperated, control rat, all surgery being right-sided). Ganglioside treatment for 14 days had no statistically provable effect on cytoplasmic RNA whether animals were killed immediately on completion of a course of GM1 injections or two weeks after discontinuance of a 14-day treatment period. However, the loss of nucleolar RNA ordinarily apparent in axotomized neurons of untreated operates may have been partly prevented by 14-day courses of GM1 injections. GM1 treatment continued over 28 days and begun either the day following tractotomy or within 1 hour of operation clearly and significantly reduced the decline in RNA content ordinarily observed in the cytoplasm and the nucleolus of the rubral neuron after axotomy. Thus, 28 days postoperatively, the mean ODs for untreated rats were, for cytoplasm and nucleolus respectively, .080 ± .003 and .074 ± .002. These values may be compared with .108 ± .004 and .097 ± .004 for GM1 treated rats injected within 1 hour of lesioning and continued on GM1 until sacrifice 28 days after operation.

Cytoplasmic and nucleolar RNA declines were observed in non-axotomized rubral nerve cells of operated rats. These were reversed by GM1 injection.

DISCUSSION

The axotomy response in rat RN following unilateral interruption of the RST is not accompanied by neuronal death over the two postoperative months that we studied. Despite the pervasiveness of the axon reaction contralateral to tractotomy and the severity of the concomitant neuronal atrophy and RNA depletion, extensive qualitative survey failed to find any evidence of neuronal necrosis or neuronophagia, thereby confirming the results of actual counts of nerve cells. That consequential nerve cell death is absent in the axotomized RN during the 60 days that immediately succeed axotomy is based on experimental observations by us which are similar to those of Egan et al (1977a,b). Unlike these authors, however, we did not discover evidence of even a transient enlargement of axotomized rubral somas. Furthermore, in contrast to Goshgarian et al (1983), we did not find a reduction in neuronal numbers after tractotomy. However, their counts were done on frozen sections of 40 µm thickness and were very variable, the number of nerve cells retained in the axotomized RN 219 days after surgery being, as reported, greater than in 5 of the 7 tractotomized rats sacrificed during the first postoperative month. In the case of the pyramidal neurons of layer Vb of the primary sensorimotor cortex, axonal transection at a spinal cord level results in minimal effects (Barron et al, In Press). The axotomy response in mammalian central neurons is indeed quite unpredictable. In the thalamus and the retina (Barron et al, 1973, 1986), substantial nerve cell death is apparent within the first week after axotomy. It may be significant that the operative procedure for the thalamic and retinal studies was associated with insults unrelated to axotomy, including edema and ischemia (Barron, 1983; Barron et al., 1986). Some part of the relatively indolent nature of the injury reaction in cortical and rubral neurons axotomized at a spinal level may relate to the absence of factors extraneous to axonic interruption per se but induced by cranial operations, e.g. edema, ischemia etc. In any case, in contrast to the situation in the neonatal rat (Prendergast and Stelzner, 1976), the failure of regeneration of the rubrospinal tract in the adult animal cannot be attributed to neuronal necrosis.

The rapid depletion of cytoplasmic and nucleolar RNA in rubral neurons after axotomy is seen in other mammalian populations of central nerve cells (Barron, 1983; Barron, et al, 1985) and is believed to be an indication of an inherently degenerative, regressive response. Whether axotomized central neurons, under stimulus of special interventions e.g. those mentioned in the opening text of this article, would show RNA accumulation while regenerating axons into peripheral nerve implants (Vidal-Sanz et al, 1987) or fetal CNS transplants (Kromer, 1987) is quite unknown. However, it is well established that the successfully regenerating central neurons of the ganglion cell layer of retina of goldfish, a submammalian vertebrate, do accumulate RNA after axotomy. This accumulation precedes axonal outgrowth (Barron et al, 1985). In support of a generally regressive nature of axon reaction in mammalian central neruons, which may somehow be inherent in the response unless it is manipulated experimentally, is the observation that peripheral nerve cells, even when destined to die after axotomy, first accumulate RNA (Aldskogius et al, 1980) as though they were "programmed" to do so. In another population of mammalian peripheral neurons, the spinal motoneurons of cat, section of axons within the CNS is followed by regeneration of new neurites through an astrocytic scar within a CNS milieu (Risling et al, 1983), thus adding one more example of an apparently fundamental difference in the axon reaction of mammalian peripheral and central neurons. However, the axotomy response of central neurons may be modified powerfully by events at the lesion site (Barron, 1983; Vidal-Sanz et al, 1987) and by pharmacologic intervention (Hefti and Weiner, 1986).

The rationale for the use of GM1 in an attempt to promote CNS regeneration follows from literature reviewed in introductory paragraphs. Unfortunately, we could find no evidence that GM1 encouraged regeneration of the RST. Perhaps a longer course of GM1 administration might have led to axonal regrowth. Or perhaps fibers too fine, e.g. monoaminergic axons (Commissiong and Toffano, 1986), to be seen at the light microscopic level were regenerated. Bose et al (1986) have claimed promotion of axonal regeneration across a complete transverse section of the thoracic spinal cord performed 6 months before their experimental animals were sacrificed. They gave a 6 week course of GM1, 3.5 mg/kg daily, which was completed 4 months before the animals were killed. Their evidence for regeneration was based on retrograde transport to medullary neurons of HRP injected caudal to the transection site. No direct histological-histochemical proof of regeneration was provided, however.

The retardation of RNA depletion in axotomized rubral neurons of treated rats likely is a non-specific effect produced by GM1 on the axon reaction and is similar to other unspecified effects reported to occur with administration of this substance (Yates, 1986). No evidence for a direct metabolic role of GM1 in RNA metabolism can be inferred from this study.

The different regression slopes generated by plots over time of cytoplasmic and nucleolar dimensions, on the one hand, vs nuclear size on the other, may have fundamental significance for the nature of the axon reaction in rubral neurons. It is even conceivable that the different temporal patterns of atrophy evidenced by regression analysis may relate to a period, e.g. the first two weeks after injury, when measures undertaken to "rescue" axotomized neurons would need to be initiated. Whether similar plots could be generated during the axon reaction of other neuronal systems remains to be determined.

Alterations in morphometric and cytochemical parameters of the non-axotomized RN following unilateral operations have practical significance in that they point to hazards inherent in the use of ratios of axotomized/non-axotomized sides in this type of experimentation. However, the cause and the potential significance of the described changes in non-axotomized neurons are alike unknown.

The absence of substantial change in neuroglia of the axotomized RN has been alluded to in the description of experimental results and certainly differs from the neuroglial hypertrophy and hyperplasia so readily evident in the surround of rodent extrinsic neurons after axotomy (Aldskogius et al, 1980; Barron, 1983). This matter is under active investigation in our laboratory.

SUMMARY

1. Unilateral severance of the cervical rubrospinal tract (RST) induces cytoplasmic atrophy in neurons of the contralateral RN (red nucleus, magnocellular division) 7 days postoperatively with nuclear and nucleolar atrophy following on the 10th postoperative day. Atrophy of all 3 cellular elements is progressive through the 90th postoperative day, but exhibits a bimodal pattern in cytoplasm and nucleolus where a rapid phase through 14 days after tractotomy is followed by a slow relentless decline. Nuclear atrophy has a unimodal regression slope.

2. Nerve cell death was not identified through 60 days postoperatively.

3. RNA content of the neuronal cytoplasm and nucleolus declined progressively in the axotomized RN from the 7th (cytoplasm) and 14th (nucleolus) postoperative days. GM1 administration retarded this process, especially when continued a longer period (28 vs 14 days) and initiated earlier (within 1 hour of axotomy vs 24 hours).

4. Both the operative procedure and GM1 administration had demonstrable effects on morphometrical and cytochemical parameters of neurons of the non-axotomized RN ipsilateral to the severed RST.

5. No evidence of axonal regeneration across spinal cord lesions appeared either in treated or in untreated rats.

ACKNOWLEDGMENT

This research was supported by the Veterans Administration. Drs. M.P. Dentinger and R. Mankes rendered crucial assistance to the author.

REFERENCES

Aldskogius H, Barron KD, Regal R (1980). Axon reaction in dorsal motor vagal and hypoglossal neurons of the adult rat. Light microscopy and RNA-cytochemistry. J Comp Neurol 193:165-177.
Barron KD (1983). Axon reaction and central nervous system regeneration. In Seil FJ (ed): "Nerve, Organ and Tissue Regeneration. Research Perspectives," New York: Academic Press, pp 3-36.
Barron KD, Cova J, Scheibly ME, Kohberger R (1982). RNA content and morphometric measurements of axotomized feline cervical motoneurons. J Neurocytol 11:707-720.
Barron KD, Dentinger MP, Krohel G, Easton S, Mankes R (1986). Qualitative and quantitative ultrastructural observations on retinal ganglion cell layer of rat after intraorbital optic nerve crush. J Neurocytol 15:345-362.
Barron KD, Dentinger MP, Popp AJ, Mankes R (1988). Neurons of layer Vb of rat sensorimotor cortex atrophy but do not die after thoracic cord transection. J Neuropath Exp Neurol. In Press.
Barron KD, McGuinness CM, Misantone LJ, Zanakis MF, Grafstein B, Murray M (1985). RNA content of normal and axotomized retinal ganglion cells of rat and goldfish. J Comp Neurol 236:265-273.
Barron KD, Means ED, Larsen E (1973). Ultrastructure of retrograde degeneration in thalamus of rat. I. Neuronal somata and dendrites. J Neuropath Exp Neurol 32:218-244.
Bose B, Osterholm JL, Kalia M (1986). Ganglioside-induced

regeneration and re-establishment of axonal continuity in spinal cord-transected rats. Neurosci Lett 63:165-169.

Bregman BS, Reier PJ (1986). Neural tissue transplants rescue axotomized rubrospinal cells from retrograde death. J Comp Neurol 244:86-95.

Commissiong JW, Toffano G (1986). The effect of GM1 ganglioside on coerulospinal, noradrenergic, adult neurons and on fetal monoaminergic neurons transplanted into the transected spinal cord of the adult rat. Brain Res 380:205-215.

Cuello AC, Stephens PH, Tagari PC, Sofroniew MV, Pearson RCA (1986). Retrograde changes in the nucleus basalis of the rat, caused by cortical damage, are prevented by exogenous ganglioside GM1. Brain Res 376:373-377.

Egan DA, Flumerfelt BA, Gwyn DG (1977a). A light and electron microscopic study of axon reaction in the red nucleus of the rat following cervical and thoracic lesions. Neuropath Appl Neurogiol 3:423-439.

Egan DA, Flumerfelt BA, Gwyn DG (1977b). Axon reaction in the red nucleus of the rat. Perikaryal volume changes and the time course of chromatolysis following cervical and thoracic lesions. Acta Neuropath 37:13-19.

Gorio A, Ferrari G, Fusco M, Janigro D, Zanoni R, Jonsson G (1984). Gangliosides and their effects on rearranging peripheral and central neural pathways. CNS Trauma 1:29-37.

Goshgarian HG, Koistinen JM, Schmidt ER (1983). Cell death and changes in the retrograde transport of horseradish peroxidase in rubrospinal neurons following spinal cord hemisection in the adult rat. J Comp Neurol 214:251-257.

Gradkowska M, Skup M, Kiedrowski L, Calzolari S, Oderfeld-Nowak B (1986). The effect of GM1 ganglioside on cholinergic and serotinergic systems in the rat hippocampus following partial denervation is dependent on the degree of fiber degeneration. Brain Res 375:417-422.

Hefti F, Weiner WJ (1986). Nerve growth factor and Alzheimer's disease. Ann Neurol 20:275-281.

Kromer LF (1987). Nerve growth factor treatment after brain injury prevents neuronal death. Science 235:214-216.

Lavie V, Harel A, Doron A, Solomon A, Lobel D, Belkin M, Ben-Basat S, Sharma S, Schwartz M (1987). Morphological response of injured adult rabbit optic nerve to implants containing media conditioned by growing optic nerves. Brain Res 419:166-172.

Prendergast J, Stelzner DJ (1976). Changes in the magnocellular portion of the red nucleus following thoracic hemisection in the neonatal and adult rat. J Comp Neurol 166:163-172.

Risling M, Cullheim S, Hildebrand C (1983). Reinnervation of the ventral root L7 from ventral horn neurons following intramedullary axotomy in adult cats. Brain Res 280:15-23.

Rodichok LD, Barron KD, Popp AJ, Dentinger MP, Scheibly ME (1984). Glucose utilization is unchanged in red nucleus after axotomy. Brain Res 324:253-259.

Skaper SD, Katoh-Semba R, Varon S (1985). GM1 ganglioside accelerates neurite outgrowth from primary peripheral and central neurons under selected culture conditions. Dev Brain Res 23:19-26.

Toffano G, Savoini G, Moron F, Lombardi G, Calza L, Agnati LF (1984). Chronic GM1 ganglioside treatment reduces dopamine cell body degeneration in the substantia nigra after unilateral hemitransection in rat. Brain Res 296:233-239.

Vidal-Sanz M, Bray GM, Villegas-Perez MP, Thanos S, Aguayo AJ (1987). Axonal regeneration and synapse formation in the superior colliculus by retinal ganglion cells in the adult rat. J Neurosci 7:2894-2909.

Yates AJ (1986). Gangliosides in the nervous system during development and regeneration. Neurochem Path 5:309-329.

SOME RESPONSES OF SENSORY NEURONS TO PERIPHERAL NERVE INJURY

P.M. Richardson, V.M.K. Verge & R.J. Riopelle*

Division of Neurosurgery, Montreal General Hospital & McGill University, Canada H3G 1A4
*Division of Neurology, Queen's University, Can.

Successful regeneration of damaged axons depends not only on the glial environment in the field of growth but also on injury-induced changes within neurons. This latter contribution is demonstrated by two observations on the central axons of primary sensory neurons.

In one group of rats, the dorsal columns were divided at high cervical level and a segment of the right sciatic nerve was co-apted to the mid-dorsal surface of the spinal cord at the site of injury (Richardson & Issa, 1984; Fig 1).

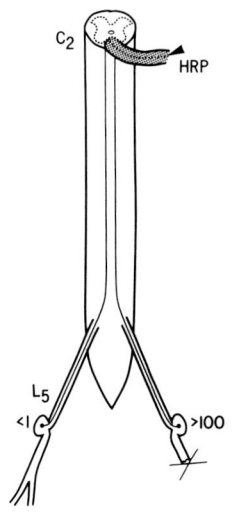

Figure 1. Neurons with cell bodies in the L5 DRG whose axons grew from the spinal cord to a peripheral nerve graft averaged less than one if the sciatic nerve was intact and greater than one hundred if the nerve was cut.

Two months later, the free end of the peripheral nerve graft was exposed in the subcutaneous tissue and injected with horseradish peroxidase (HRP) for retrograde labelling of neurons with axons growing into the graft. Dorsal column axons from most sensory neurons entered grafts no more frequently than other long spinal axons, for example rubrospinal or reticulospinal axons. However, the probability that long spinal axons from the fourth and fifth lumbar dorsal root ganglia (L4 & L5 DRG) would grow into a peripheral nerve graft was increased one hundredfold by sciatic nerve transection. Thus, peripheral nerve injury stimulates a regenerative propensity of sensory neurons which is manifest in dorsal column axons.

A second transganglionic effect of peripheral nerve injury (Richardson & Verge, 1987) is to accelerate the regeneration of crushed axons in the corresponding root. As measured by anterograde tracing with HRP, the rate of regeneration of crushed L5 dorsal root axons was tripled by sciatic nerve transection. In cross-sections of the L5 root 15mm from the crush site (Fig 2), the number of thinly myelinated new axonal processes was increased tenfold by a peripheral nerve injury. Axons in the L5 dorsal root regrow more quickly towards the spinal cord if the sciatic nerve is cut when or before the root is crushed.

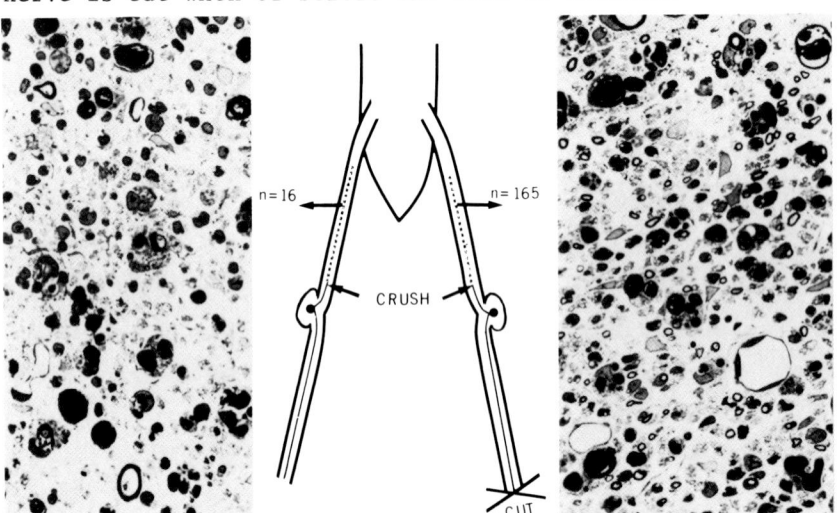

Figure 2. 18 days after crush injury of the L5 dorsal root, the mean number of new myelinated axons, 15mm from the crush site was 16 if the sciatic nerve was intact and 165 if the nerve was cut.

These two observations on primary sensory neurons corroborate other evidence that the regenerative state within neurons is activated by nerve injury. i) In conditioning experiments first described more than a decade ago (McQuarrie & Grafstein, 1973), peripheral nerve axons are seen to regenerate more rapidly following a previous distal injury to the same nerve. The magnitude of such conditioning effects is small presumably because the neuron is activated by the test lesion itself and the conditioning lesion gives only a headstart. Transganglionic enhancement of regeneration is more conspicuous because test injuries to the central axon of sensory neurons tend not to perturb the nerve cell body (Perry et al, 1983). ii) Following peripheral nerve injury, " supernumerary axons" sprout from the cell body of motoneurons for more than a mm through the spinal grey matter (Havton & Kellerth, 1987). iii) Injured axons from a crushed nerve expand further into denervated territory than do sprouting axons from uninjured nerves (Jackson & Diamond, 1984). iv) In bipolar S interneurons of leech segmental ganglia, an intact axon can be stimulated to sprout by elimination of its target cell and crushing of another branch of the sprouting neuron (Scott & Muller, 1980) but not by either injury in isolation. The observations on leech interneurons and rat sensory neurons are highly analogous.

The initial events in an injured nerve that trigger a regenerative propensity in sensory neurons have been examined in experiments involving peripheral nerve grafts to the spinal cord (Richardson & Verge, 1986; Table 1).

TABLE 1

Nature of test lesion	Left/Right	
	Test alone	Cut & test
Crush	.12	.67
Colchicine(1)	.17	.80
Colchicine(4)	.47	1.12
Distal cut	.28	
Resuture		.38

Left/right refers to the side-to-side ratio of neurons in L4 & L5 DRG with axons growing from spinal cord to peripheral nerve grafts. For each group of animals, the right side with sciatic nerve transection served as a control.

The fact that nerve crush is much less inductive than nerve transection directs attention to Schwann cells rather than target cells because the time for crushed axons to reestablish contact with target tissues exceeds the critical inductive period. The failure of proximal nerve crush or injection of colchicine to block the inductive signal from a cut nerve suggests that the initial signal is not a positive "injury factor" from reactive Schwann cells or hematogenous cells. By exclusion, loss of normal contact with non-neuronal cells along the distal nerve stump appears to be the critical factor in nerve injury that activates sensory neurons. Only the initial or triggering event has been investigated in these experiments: the final activation of neurons could follow directly or indirectly. The intraneuronal changes in gene expression and/or protein phosphorylation that lead to rapid or abundant axonal growth remain unknown (Benowitz & Routtenberg, 1987).

Several of the responses of sensory neurons to peripheral nerve injury have been attributed to a diminution in the normal retrograde supply of nerve growth factor (NGF) to the nerve cell body. More precisely, these retrograde reactions to axotomy are counteracted by exogenous NGF (Fitzgerald et al, 1985; Miyata et al, 1986; Rich et al, 1987). However, two results suggest that lack of NGF is not the major inductive signal for an enhanced regenerative propensity of injured sensory neurons. Administration of NGF to the cut end of the sciatic nerve did not mitigate the effects of nerve injury on the regeneration of central sensory axons (Richardson & Verge, 1986) and the NGF receptor density on sensory neurons is decreased not increased by peripheral nerve injury (Verge et al, 1986).

NGF receptors on sensory neurons have been examined by quantitative radioautography after incubation of tissue sections with ^{125}I-NGF (Richardson et al, 1986). With computer-assisted image analysis, the percentage of neuronal cross-sectional area covered by silver grains has been measured for hundreds of neurons. In normal rat L5 DRG incubated with 40pM ^{125}I-NGF, perikaryal labelling is markedly heterogenous ranging from 1-20 times background over non-neuronal regions of the ganglia. Scatchard analysis of the binding of several concentrations of ^{125}I-NGF to heavily labelled neurons yields a non-linear plot with some high-affinity sites half-maximally saturated at less than 50pM. When histograms of the labelling of all neurons

Responses of Sensory Neurons / 51

in selected sections are prepared, the data can be fitted to two normal curves, compatible with the existence of two subpopulations of sensory neurons with and without high-affinity receptors. Why some but not all sensory neurons (Dodd et al, 1983) express high-affinity NGF receptors is a question of developmental and functional interest which merits more rigorous exploration (Raivich et al, 1987).

Several weeks following transection of the sciatic nerve, labelling of neurons in the L5 DRG was consistently diminished as compared to the contralateral uninjured side (Verge et al, 1986; Fig 3).

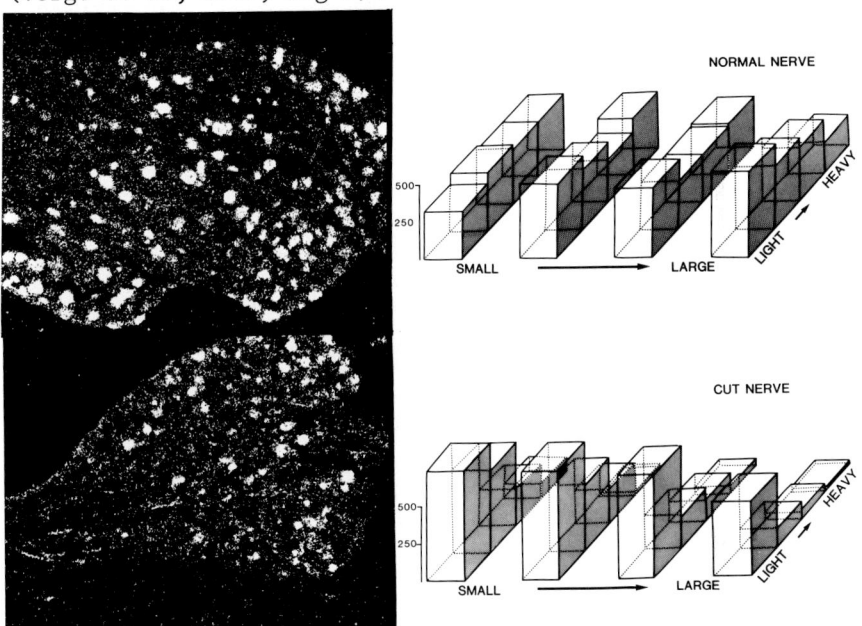

Figure 3. Darkfield photomicrographs (x30) show that the binding of ^{125}I-NGF to neurons in an L5 DRG is reduced after the sciatic nerve is cut. In histograms, both neuronal size and binding density are seen to decrease.

Radioautographs were quantitatively analyzed in two ways. Studies of the concentration dependence of binding to the most heavily labelled neurons indicated a 70% reduction in the density of high-affinity receptors with no change in affinity. Measurement of the diameter and labelling density for all neurons in selected radioautographs showed neuronal shrinkage and reduced binding of NGF plus death of 20% of the neurons (Arvidsson et al, 1986). Whether the loss of high-affinity NGF receptors represents selective death of an NGF-dependent neuronal subpopulation or decreased receptor synthesis in individual neurons remains to be ascertained. Nevertheless, the results exclude up-regulation of NGF receptors as a cause for the enhanced regeneration of sensory neurons after peripheral injury.

The activation of sensory neurons by peripheral nerve transection has been tacitly assumed to represent a direct response of individual neurons to axonal injury. However, most of the sciatic nerve injuries that stimulate the regrowth of central sensory axons also result in significant neuronal death in the L4 and L5 DRG. The possibility is now being considered that the cellular and molecular reactions to the death of some neurons in a spinal ganglion contribute to the regeneration of neurons that survive (Fig 4). A better understanding of how sensory neurons are stimulated to regenerate by peripheral nerve injury could lead to strategies for enhancing the regeneration of neurons in the central nervous system.

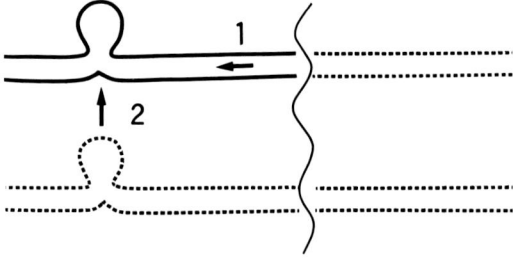

Figure 4. Following peripheral nerve injury, sensory neurons could be activated directly by axotomy(1) or indirectly through the death of other neurons in the same ganglion(2).

This work was funded by the NIH and MRC (Canada).

REFERENCES

Arvidsson J, Ygge J & Grant G (1986). Cell loss in lumbar dorsal root ganglia and transganglionic degeneration after sciatic nerve resection in the rat. Brain Res 373:15-21.
Benowitz LI & Routtenberg A (1987). A membrane phosphoprotein associated with neural development, axonal regeneration, phospholipid metabolism and synaptic plasticity. TINS 10:527-532.

Dodd J, Jahr CE, Hamilton PN, Heath MGS, Matthew WD & Jessell TM (1983). Cytochemical and physiological properties of sensory and dorsal horn neurons that transmit cutaneous sensation. Cold Spring Harbor Symp Quant Biol 48:685-695.
Fitzgerald M, Wall PD, Goedert M & Emson PC (1985). Nerve growth factor counteracts the neurophysiological and neurochemical effects of chronic sciatic nerve transection. Brain Res 332:331-341.
Havton L & Kellerth J-O (1987). Regeneration by supernumerary axons with synaptic terminals in spinal motoneurons of cats. Nature 325:711-714.
Jackson PC & Diamond J (1984). Temporal and spatial constraints on the collateral sprouting of low-threshold mechanosensory nerves in the skin of rats. J Comp Neurol 226:336-345.
McQuarrie I & Grafstein B (1973). Axon outgrowth enhanced by a previous nerve injury. Arch Neurol 29:53-55.
Miyata Y, Kashihara Y, Homma S & Kuno M (1986). Effects of nerve growth factor on the survival and synaptic function of Ia sensory neurons axotomized in neonatal rats. J Neurosci 6:2012-2018.
Perry GW, Krayanek J & Wilson DL (1983). Protein synthesis and rapid axonal transport during regrowth of dorsal root axons. J Neurochem 40:1590-1598.
Raivich G, Zimmermann A & Sutter A (1987). Nerve growth factor (NGF) receptor expression in chick cranial development. J Comp Neurol 256:229-245.
Rich KM, Luszcynski JR, Osborne PA & Johnson EM (1987). Nerve growth factor protects adult sensory neurons from cell death and atrophy caused by nerve injury. J Neurocytol 16:261-268.
Richardson PM & Issa VMK (1984). Peripheral injury enhances central regeneration of primary sensory neurons. Nature 309:791-793.
Richardson PM & Verge VMK (1986). The induction of a regenerative propensity in sensory neurons following peripheral axonal injury. J Neurocytol 15:585-594.
Richardson PM, Verge Issa VMK & Riopelle RJ (1986). Distribution of neuronal receptors for nerve growth factor in the rat. J Neurosci 6:2312-2321.
Richardson PM & Verge VMK (1987). Axonal regeneration in dorsal spinal roots is accelerated by peripheral axonal transection. Brain Res 411:406-408.

Scott SA & Muller KJ (1980). Synapse regeneration and signals for directed axonal growth in the central nervous system of the leech. Dev Biol 80:345-363.

Verge VMK, Richardson PM & Riopelle RJ (1986). Receptors for nerve growth factor on primary sensory neurons: quantitative radioautographic observations. Soc Neurosci Abstr 12:1095.

TARGET-DEPENDENCE OF SPINAL MOTONEURONS

John B. Munson, Robert C. Foehring and George W. Sypert

Department of Neuroscience, College of Medicine,
University of Florida, Gainesville, Florida 32610

INTRODUCTION

Axotomy results in many cytological and biochemical changes in both the cell body and the axon (e.g. Barron, 1983; see also this volume). Axotomy may also alter physiological properties of (e.g. Gustafsson & Pinter, 1984) and synaptic transmission to (e.g. Mendell 1984) the axotomized neuron. Over the past several years our laboratory has performed a number of investigations in which membrane electrical properties have been systematically characterized both in normal motoneurons (Mns) and in Mns disconnected from or reconnected to muscle following nerve section and resuture. A fundamental issue addressed by those studies was the extent to which normal Mn and muscle properties depend upon functional connection between them. In this chapter we summarize our recent experiments on the effects of axotomy and of reconnection on Mn electrical and synaptic properties, i.e. the target-dependence of normal Mn function (Foehring et al., 1986a,b, 1987a,b; Munson et al., 1985).

METHODS

In an initial procedure, muscle nerves of cats' medial gastrocnemius (MG) and lateral gastrocnemius-soleus (LGS) muscles were sectioned and then self- or cross-reunited. In terminal intracellular experiments 3 wk to 11 mo later, we studied electrical and synaptic properties of individual MG Mns functionally reconnected with the MG muscle, or with no functional reconnection. In one experiment the MG nerve was instead superfused with tetrodotoxin (TTX) by osmotic pump for 17 days (Munson et al., 1985). We measured axonal conduction velocity (CV: popliteal fossa to Mn), rheobase (I_{rh}: minimum 50 ms depolarizing current sufficient to generate action potentials), input resistance (R_N: voltage generated by 1 nA, 50 ms depolarizing current), afterhyperpolarization half-decay time (AHP; following action potential generated by 0.5 ms intracellular current pulse), and group I heteronymous excitatory postsynaptic potentials (EPSPs: generated by supramaximal electrical stimulation of the LGS nerve). Full details are published in Foehring et al. (1986a, 1987a).

RESULTS

MG Mns were studied in normal cats and at four stages following nerve resuture, as follows: <u>3-5 weeks</u>: at this stage, virtually no reinnervation of muscle had occurred, as evidenced by failure of tetanic intracellular stimulation of Mns to elicit electrical or mechanical response of the targeted muscle; <u>5-6 wks</u>: half of the Mns were now able to elicit weak muscle contraction; <u>9-10 wks</u>: ~75% of Mns elicited muscle contractions, which were largely normal; <u>9-11 mos</u>: ~90% of Mns elicited such muscle contractions. In the present report we compare the properties of normal MG Mns with the properties of those which reconnected with the MG muscle, and also with those which <u>failed</u> to reconnect with muscle, i.e. that remained axotomized, as evidenced by their inability to elicit muscle contraction.

Control values for the parameters measured are at the left of each of the plots of Fig. 1. Mean values changed for most of these parameters following axotomy, as follows:

<u>Motoneuron conduction velocity</u>: CV dropped quickly to 75% of control and thus remained for axotomized Mns. Mns reconnected with the MG muscle recovered their normal CV.

<u>Input resistance</u>: The R_N of axotomized Mns more than doubled, and remained increased over the survival time. Restoration of normal R_N followed reconnection with muscle.

<u>Rheobase</u>: The I_{rh} of Mns without functional connection with muscle averaged 1/5 to 1/2 of control values at various stages, but recovered fully if Mns reconnected with muscle.

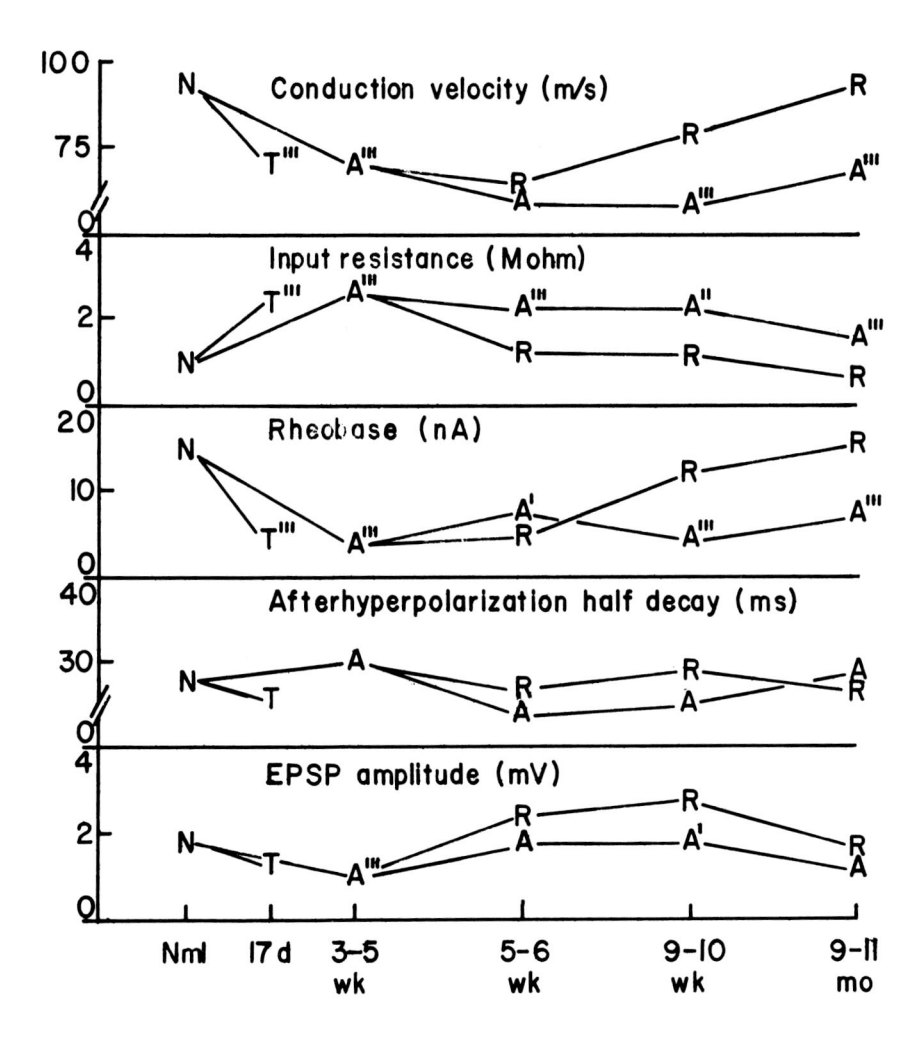

Fig. 1. Membrane electrical properties of normal (N), axotomized (A), and reconnected (R) MG Mns following nerve resuture, or following nerve block with TTX (T). Axotomized values differ from normal or from reconnected values, as appropriate: p<0.05 ('), p<0.001 (''),p<0.0001 (''').

Afterhyperpolarization: Mean values of AHP did not change following axotomy and reconnection; however the ranges of values were compressed by axotomy (cf Foehring et al., 1986a, b).

Excitatory postsynaptic potentials: Amplitudes of EPSPs were initially reduced following axotomy, but remained so in neither the reconnected or axotomized population.

Tetrodotoxin: The effects of 2 1/2 weeks' conduction block of the MG nerve with TTX precisely mimicked the effect of axotomy on each of the five measured parameters.

DISCUSSION

These results permit a number of conclusions, which will be discussed in the following paragraphs:

1) Axotomy alters most measured electrical properties of Mns. Normal Mns are characterized by specific combinations of electrical properties (Zengel et al., 1985). These differential clusters are no longer found following axotomy (Foehring et al., 1986a), an effect referred to as "dedifferentiation" by Kuno et al. (1974). This could signify the resumption of a growth state by the Mn (Watson, 1976), or reversion to undifferentiated neonatal- (Huizar et al., 1975) or slow-type Mns (Gustafsson & Pinter, 1984). The decline of CV of axotomized MG Mn axons has been attributed to reduced axonal diameter (Gillespie and Stein, 1984), perhaps resulting from reduced transport of neurofilament protein (Hoffman & Lasek, 1980). Axotomized MG Mns become more excitable to somatic current injection (decreased I_{rh}) and polarize more in response to current injection (increased R_N). Gustafsson & Pinter (1984) concluded that the post-axotomy increase in R_N is due to increased specific membrane resistivity, decreased surface area and altered dendritic geometry. While one would expect an inverse (i.e. Ohm's Law) relation between R_N and I_{rh}, the fact that axotomy reduced I_{rh} to about 1/4 of normal while R_N increased only 2.6 times (Fig. 1) indicates that the change in R_N cannot account fully for the change in I_{rh}. A major additional contribution is likely to be made by voltage-sensitive Na^+ channels newly inserted into the axotomized soma and dendritic membrane (Faber, 1984; Sernagor et al., 1986).

2) <u>Some Mns survive without functional connection with muscle.</u> While expression of normal mature Mn properties appears to depend upon functional connection with muscle, their mere survival, at least to 11 mo, does not (cf Gordon et al., 1980). The same is true of some muscle sensory fibers: Collins et al. (1986) found a population of muscle afferents lacking receptor innervation 9 mo after resuture of the MG nerve. CV was reduced for those non-reconnected muscle afferents (Fig 2), as for the present axotomized Mns.

3) <u>Electrical properties of Mns do not recover in the absence of functional reconnection with muscle.</u> At all postoperative times, Mns without reconnection displayed electrical properties similar to those of 3-5 wk axotomized Mns. In similar reinnervation experiments, Gordon & Stein (1982) found reduced action potential amplitudes of motor axons which did not elicit muscle contraction, but normal amplitudes in those that did. Kuno et al. (1974), however, reported that Mns <u>without</u> functional connection with muscle possessed normal AHP and CV. They concluded that merely the presence of the Mn axon in the muscle was sufficient for recovery. This apparent disagreement perhaps relates to post-operative times, kind of Mn, or detectability of muscle unit contraction (Foehring et al., 1986b). Alternatively, there may be two classes of non-reconnected Mns: those which fail to regenerate through the suture line, and those which regenerate into muscle but fail to reinnervate muscle fibers. Neither would be functionally connected, but the second could have access to trophic muscle substances.

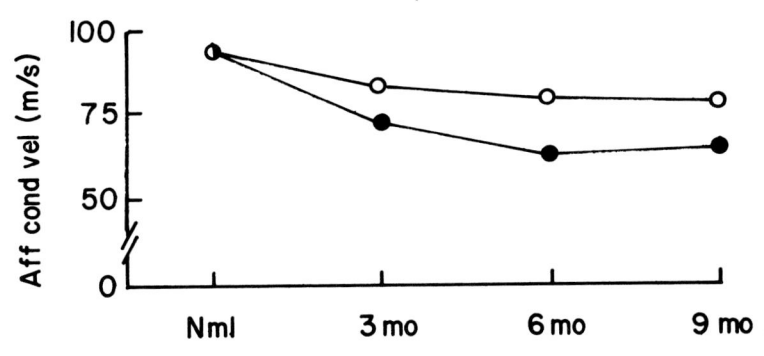

Fig. 2. Conduction velocity of MG muscle afferents reconnected (O) or not reconnected (●) to spindles or tendon organs in normal MG muscle and at 3 post-operative times in reinnervated MG muscle. (Data from Collins et al., 1986).

4) <u>MG Mns which re-establish functional connection with the MG muscle recover normal electrical properties.</u> Restoration of normal electrical properties has commenced at 9-10 wk, and is complete by 9-11 mo. The fact that most measures of electrical properties have recovered only partially in reconnected Mns 9-10 wk after resuture suggests that reconnection only initiates the recovery process, and that some weeks or months are required for full recovery. Is reconnection with muscle always <u>sufficient</u>, as well as necessary, for such restoration? In other experiments we have shown the importance of the <u>identity</u> of the muscle reinnervated: MG Mns which reinnervate the similarly 'fast' LG muscle also recover their normal properties, but those which reinnervate the 'slow' soleus may not (Foehring et al., 1987b). The fact that mean CV for reconnected muscle afferents did not recover fully (Fig. 2) may relate similarly to the fact that some regenerated afferent fibers reinnervated inappropriate targets (e.g. former muscle spindle afferents may innervate tendon organs: Collins et al., 1986), and may thus remain hypofunctional.

5) <u>Group I afferent --> Mn synaptic efficacy is reduced following Mn axotomy, and recovers whether or not functional reconnection with muscle occurs.</u> Single-fiber and composite group I EPSPs are reduced in amplitude in axotomized Mns (reviewed in Mendell, 1984). This apparently relates to the observation of Blinzinger & Kreutzberg (1968) and others (Barron, 1983) that microglia displace synaptic terminals from axotomized Mns. EPSP amplitude is normal following reconnection of the Mn with muscle (e.g. Mendell & Scott, 1975). Not previously reported, however, is our observation that composite group I EPSP amplitude recovers as well in Mns that <u>do not</u> reconnect with muscle. The fact that Mns axotomized for 200 days are activated during locomotion (Gordon et al., 1980) is further evidence for the continued efficacy of excitatory synaptic inputs to axotomized Mns. Altered Mn properties (see above) could contribute to the recovery of normal EPSP amplitude in axotomized Mns. Recovery of EPSP amplitude is even more remarkable when one considers that the LGS nerve, the source of the group I afferents in these experiments, was also sectioned and resutured (Methods). About 25-30% of such afferents fail to re-establish functional contact with receptors (Gallego et al., 1980; Collins et al., 1986), and afferents which do not reinnervate muscle may lose synaptic efficacy (Goldring et al., 1980). The apparently increased EPSP amplitude seen in

reconnected Mns at 9-10 wk (Fig. 1) could relate to the conclusion of Gallego et al. (1980) that sensory fibers which regenerate into muscle but do not reinnervate receptors generate enlarged EPSPs.

6) <u>Activity of the neuromuscular synapse or of the muscle appears essential to maintaining normal electrical properties of Mns.</u> Superfusion of the MG nerve with TTX altered MG Mn properties as did axotomy (Fig. 1). Such TTX interrupts neuromuscular transmission by blocking conduction of motor nerve impulses, and thereby blocks muscular activity. A role for muscle activity in the maintenance of Mn properties has been suggested by Czeh et al. (1978). They reported that block of the soleus nerve with TTX shortened the AHP of soleus Mns, but that electrical stimulation of the same nerve peripheral to, but not central of the block prevented that effect. Our results extend their findings by showing that such nerve block alters all of the parameters measured, and in a manner identical to the effect of surgical axotomy. While the specific mechanism of the effect can only be speculated upon, retrograde axonal transport of a substance acquired during neuromuscular transmission is an hypothesis consistent with the data. Mimicking of axotomy by interruption of axonal transport was previously reported by Pilar & Landmesser (1972) and by Purves (1976), who applied colchicine to post-ganglionic sympathetic nerves.

PERSPECTIVE

We have described many electrophysiological consequences of axotomy of cat Mns, and similar consequences of axotomy of other neuronal types. This does not mean, however, that the cat Mn can serve as the model of axotomy for all neurons. In fact, even the response of cat Mns may differ according to the lesion: the "partial spikes" seen in cat Mns after axotomy close to the soma (e.g. Sernagor, et al. 1986) are not seen after such axotomy performed in the periphery (e.g. Mendell et al., 1976). Furthermore, unlike for cat Mns, electrical properties (including input resistance and threshold) do not differ for normal vs. axotomized principal neurons of the guinea pig superior cervical ganglion (Purves, 1975). In addition, EPSPs disappear and cell death occurs when such neurons which are ligated and prevented from regenerating to a target. In another example, Gurtu & Smith (1988) found that CV of axotomized dorsal root ganglion cells of hamsters is not decreased, and may be increased from normal. Thus the same kind of neuron may respond differently in different species (cf Fig. 2 above; see also Aldskogius et al. 1985). Like cat Mns, these dorsal root ganglion cells responded to axotomy with reduced rheobase, and like superior cervical ganglion cells, they responded to axotomy with reduced invasion of the soma by action potentials. However, we found no greater failure of antidromic invasion in axotomized than in normal Mns (unpublished observations). These examples illustrate the point that attractive as the cat Mn is for such studies, the responses ascribed here to axotomy may not be assumed to be representative of the responses of other neurons in the same or other species, or even of the same neuron in other circumstances.

ACKNOWLEDGEMENTS

Helpful comments on an early version of this manuscript were made by Prof LM Mendell. Research support derived from NINCDS Grant NS-15913 and VA Grant MRS 821-103.

REFERENCES

Aldskogius, H, Arvidsson, J, Grant, G (1985). The reaction of primary sensory neurons to peripheral nerve injury with particular emphasis on transganglionic changes. Brain Res Rev 10: 27-46.
Barron, KD (1983). Comparative observations on the cytologic reactions of central and peripheral nerve cells to axotomy. In Kao, CC, Bunge, RP, Reier, PJ (eds): "Spinal cord reconstruction," New York: Raven, p 7-40.
Blinzinger, K, Kreutzberg, GW (1968). Displacement of synaptic terminals from regenerating motoneurons by microglial cells. Z Zellforsch 85: 145-157.
Collins, WF III, Mendell, LM, Munson, JB (1986). On the specificity of sensory reinnervation of cat skeletal muscle. J Physiol 375: 587-609.
Czeh, G, Gallego, R, Kudo, N, Kuno, M (1978). Evidence for the maintenance of motoneurone properties by muscle activity. J Physiol 281: 239-252.

Faber, DS (1984). Reorganization of neuronal membrane properties following axotomy. Exp Brain Res, Supp 9: 225-239.
Foehring, RC, Sypert, GW, Munson, JB (1986a). Properties of self-reinnervated motor units of medial gastrocnemius of cat. I. Long term reinnervation. J Neurophysiol. 55: 931-946.
Foehring, RC, Sypert, GW, Munson, JB (1986b). Properties of self-reinnervated motor units of medial gastrocnemius of cat. II. Axotomized motoneurons and time course of recovery. J Neurophysiol. 55: 947-965.
Foehring, RC, Sypert, GW, Munson, JB (1987a). Motor-unit properties following cross-reinnervation of cat lateral gastrocnemius and soleus muscles with medial gastrocnemius nerve. I. Influence of motoneurons on muscle. J Neurophysiol. 57: 1210-1226.
Foehring, RC, Sypert, GW, Munson, JB (1987b). Motor-unit properties following cross-reinnervation of cat lateral gastrocnemius and soleus muscles with medial gastrocnemius nerve. II. Influence of muscle on motoneurons. J Neurophysiol. 57: 1227-1245.
Gallego, R, Kuno, M, Nunez, R, Snider, WD (1980). Enhancement of synaptic function in cat neurones during peripheral sensory regeneration. J Physiol 306: 205-218.
Gillespie, MJ, Stein, RB (1983). The relationship between axon diameter, myelin thickness and conduction velocity during atrophy of mammalian peripheral nerves. Brain Res: 259: 41-56.
Gurtu, S, Smith, PA (1988). Electrophysiological characteristics of hamster dorsal root ganglion cells and their response to axotomy. J Neurophysiol (In the press).
Goldring, JM, Kuno, M, Nunez, R, Snider, WD. Reaction of synapses on motoneurones to restoration of peripheral sensory connexions in the cat. J Physiol 309: 185-198.
Gordon, T, Hoffer, JA, Jhamandas, J, Stein, RB (1980). Long-term effects of axotomy on neural activity during cat locomotion. J Physiol 303: 243-263.
Gordon, T, Stein, RB (1982). Reorganization of motor-unit properties in reinnervated muscles of the cat. J Neurophysiol 48: 1175-1190.
Gustafsson, B, Pinter MJ (1984). Effects of axotomy on the distribution of passive electrical properties of cat motoneurones. J Physiol 356: 433-442.
Hoffman, PL, Lasek, RJ (1980). Axonal transport of the cytoskeleton in regenerating motor neurons: constancy and change. Brain Res 202: 317-333.

Huizar, P, Kuno, M, Miyata, Y (1975). Differentiation of motoneurones and skeletal muscles in kittens. J Physiol 252: 465-479.

Kuno, M, Miyata, Y, Munoz-Martinez, EJ (1974). Differential reaction of fast and slow a-motoneurones to axotomy. J Physiol 240: 725-739.

Mendell, LM (1984). Modifiability of spinal synapses. Physiol Rev 64: 260-324.

Mendell, LM, Munson, JB, Scott, JG (1976). Alterations of synapses on axotomized motoneurones. J Physiol 255: 67-79.

Mendell, LM, Scott, JG (1975). The effect of peripheral nerve cross-union on connections of single Ia fibers to motoneurons. Exp Brain Res 22: 221-234.

Munson, JB, Foehring, RC, Sypert, GW (1985). Nerve block with tetrodotoxin mimics axotomy of cat MG motoneurons. Soc Neurosci Abstr 11: 1145.

Pilar, G, Landmesser, L (1972). Axotomy mimicked by localized colchicine application. Science 177: 1116-1118.

Purves, D (1975). Functional and structural changes in mammalian sympathetic neurones following interruption of their axons. J Physiol 252: 429-463.

Purves, D (1976). Functional and structural changes in mammalian sympathetic neurons following colchicine application to post-ganglionic nerves. J Physiol 259: 159-175.

Sernagor, E, Yarom, Y, Werman, R (1986). Sodium-dependent regenerative responses in dendrites of axotomized motoneurons in the cat. Proc Natl Acad Sci USA 83: 7966-7970.

Watson, WE (1976). "Cell Biology of Brain." London: Chapman & Hall.

Zengel, JE, Reid, SA, Sypert, GW, Munson, JB (1985). Membrane electrical properties and prediction of motor-unit type of medial gastrocnemius motoneurons in the cat. J Neurophysiol 53: 1323-1344.

NEURONAL RESCUE

NEURONAL RESCUE IN CNS LESIONS

Silvio Varon, Theo Hagg and Marston Manthorpe

Department of Biology, School of Medicine, M-001, University of California San Diego, La Jolla, California 92093

During development, neuronal populations undergo substantial cell losses when their axons reach and interact with their target territories (Hamburger and Oppenheim, 1982). Survival through this "developmental neuronal death" is thought to depend on the availability of specific neuronotrophic factors (NTFs), which are produced in the target territory and retrogradely transported by the axons to the cell somata to promote neuronal maintenance, general growth capabilities and/or functional performances. The discovery of Nerve Growth Factor, NGF, (Levi-Montalcini, 1987) has prompted, largely by use of in vitro neuronal test cultures, the search for other neuronotrophic proteins and the recognition of glial cells as additional NTF sources (Varon and Adler, 1981; Varon et al., 1984, 1988), as well as the investigation of a separate class of anchorage-dependent neurite promoting factors (NPFs) obtainable from glial and other cell cultures and from extracellular marix materials (Davis et al., 1985, 1987a).

A more general "neuronotrophic hypothesis" postulates that NTFs are equally important for adult neurons in the cenral nervous systems (CNS) (Varon et al., 1984, 1987). Deficits in the endogenous supply of NTFs, therefore, could result in adult CNS neuronal damages, be responsible for certain degenerative CNS pathologies (Varon, 1975; Appel, 1981; Varon et al., 1982; Hefti, 1983) and, possibly, also underlie the inability of mammalian CNS neurons to regenerate after traumatic lesions (Varon, 1977).

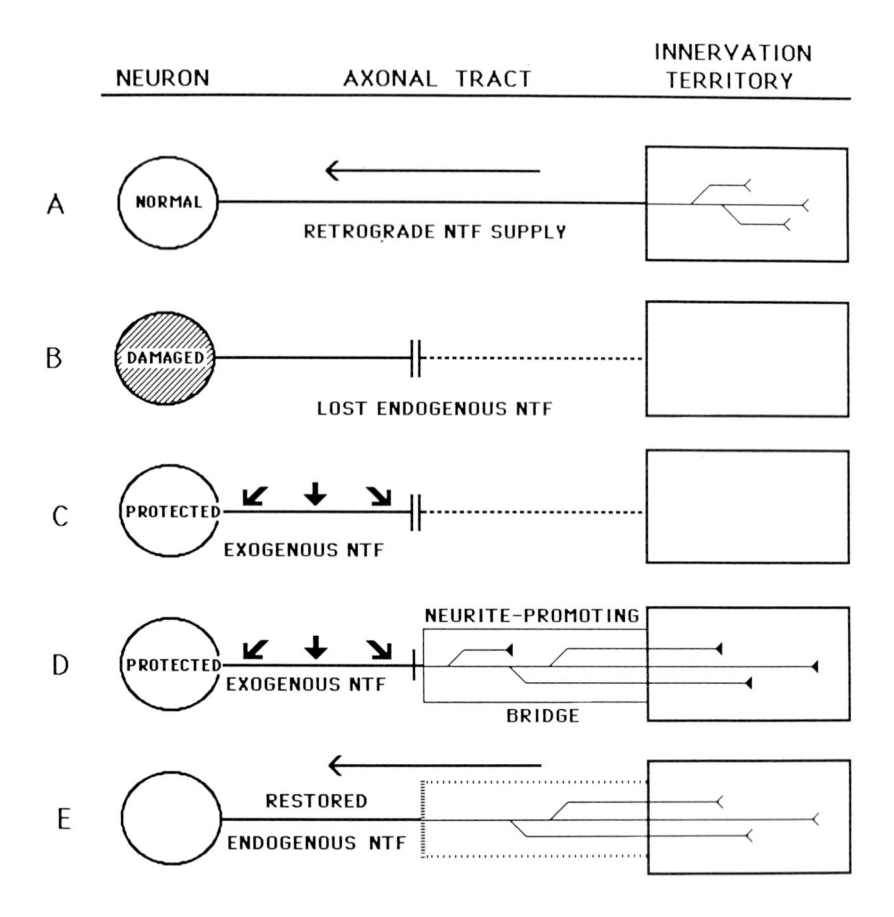

Figure 1. Endogenous and exogenous requirements for survival and axonal regeneration of axotomized neurons.

Figure 1 illustrates the concepts that will be explored in various CNS experimental systems in the following presentations of this section. If normal performances of a CNS neuron depend on an adequate retrograde delivery of NTFs from its innervation, or target, territory (A), then an experimental interruption of endogenous NTF delivery by axotomy (or by target territory damage) will result in discernible damage or even death of the nerve cell body (B). Concurrent administration of exogenous NTF, compensating for the loss of endogenous one, should protect the neuron from its axotomy-induced damages (C). Insertion into the lesion gap of a neurite-promoting bridge, together with exogenous NTF administration, could promote the regrowth of axons across the gap and into the target territory (D). The final outcome may be the recapture, by the new axons, of endogenous NTF supplies in the target territory and the consequent loss of the neuronal dependence on exogenous NTF administration. Ideally, reinnervation of the target territory could lead to the formation of new synapses and the restoration of functional networks.

Direct validation of some of these concepts has already been obtained with regard to cholinergic neurons in the basal forebrain of adult rats, the endogenous NTF for which is thought to be NGF itself. Cholinergic neurons in the medial septum and vertical diagonal band nuclei project to the hippocampal formation through the fimbria-fornix tract, while those in the Nucleus Basalis provide the main cholinergic innervation to the cerebral cortex. Transection of the fimbria-fornix leads to the disappearance of many of the cholinergic septal neurons, as visualized by their acetylcholinesterase or choline acetyltransferase (ChAT) contents, as well as a massive loss of cholinergic innervation in the hippocampal territory. The disappearance of septal cholinergic neurons is largely prevented by intraventricular administration of exogenous NGF (cf. Fig. 1 B, C) (Hefti, 1986; Williams et al., 1986; Kromer, 1987). Insertion into the lesion cavity of either fetal hippocampal tissue (Kromer et al., 1981) or extracelular matrix material from human placenta (Davis et al., 1987b) allows for the reappearance of cholinergic fibers in the hippocampus, and future experiments in which a bridge insertion is combined with exogenous NGF administration may lead to a greater cholinergic reinnervation of their target territory (cf. Fig. 1D). Chronic administration of exogenous NGF to aged rats corrects their impaired ability to peform cognitive tasks and brings about a size increase in nucleus basalis (and striatal) cholinergic neurons (Fischer et al., 1987).

Additional data in support of the neuronotrophic hypothesis for CNS neurons will be presented in the following papers. Bregman describes the loss of rubro-spinal neurons upon their axotomy by spinal cord transection in rat pups, their temporary protection by several tissue transplants into the spinal lesion and the specificity of target tissue for longer term protection. Cunningham addresses visual system components by combining in vitro and in vivo techniques to evaluate neuronotrophic and neurite promoting activities (and their underlying macromolecular factors) for dorsal lateral geniculate neurons from target-derived (cortical) cells. Hefti explores further the promotion by NGF of cholinergic septal neurons and cholinergic hippocampal innervation after unilateral and partial fimbrial transection in adult rats, and reports not only on the specificity of cholinergic neurons for an NGF response in the CNS but also on their enduring need for exogenous NGF administration -- possibly due to failure of regaining access to endogenous NGF supplies (cf. Fig. 1E).

These studies illustrate two important directions for current research in the field. One (Bregman, Cunningham) is to extend the applicability of the neuronotrophic hypothesis to additional CNS systems and additional NTFs. The other (Hefti) is to deepen our understanding of the septo-hippocampal model system, where both the trophic factor (NGF) and the selectively addressed neurons (septal cholinergic cells) are already identified. The latter system is under investigation by several other research groups, with largely concurrent results. Some discrepancies, however, are bound to surface among the several studies, which could either reflect minor differences in the experimental techniques or provide clues to yet unperceived aspects of the problem. Beside further methodologic improvements to secure a continuous and accurately defined delivery of the exogenous NGF, a major question needs additional attention, namely the question of axotomy-induced adult neuron death which remains a debated issue in several other experimental systems as well as human pathological conditions (e.g., Barron, 1983; McBride et al., 1987; Terry et al., 1981, 1987).

Neuronal cell death in the adult CNS is often assumed from, and monitored by, numerical reduction of neurons that fit particular criteria: location, soma size, cytochemical features (e.g., Nissl substance), ability to acquire or retain retrograde tracers, or subset-specific neuronal markers (transmitter-related, peptides, receptors) -- among others. In the septo-hippocampal model, septal cholinergic neurons and hippocampal cholinergic fibers are necessarily recognized by their cholinergic cytochemical propeties (acetylcholinesterase activity, ChAT immunoreactivity). The axotomy-induced disappearance of ChAT

-positive neurons, therefore, could result from a decline in their ChAT content below the present level of detectability rather than an actual neuronal death. It is known, for example, that peripheral neurons that are traditionally receptive to NGF action appear to require the factor for their survival only during a restricted prenatal or early postnatal period, even though they will continue to respond to NGF as adult cells by transmitter-related, or other, features (cf. Levi-Montalcini, 1987).

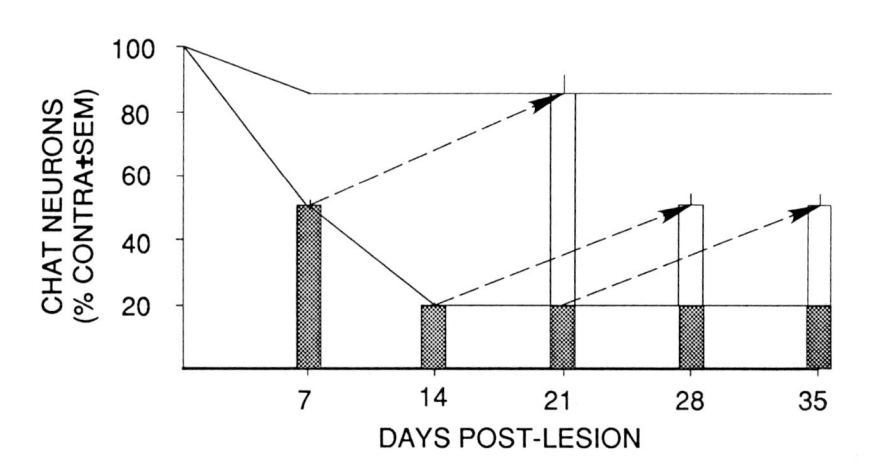

Figure 2. Effects on the number of ChAT-positive medial septum neurons of 14-day NGF treatments that are delayed by 7 to 21 days after fimbria-fornix transection. Solid lines = numerical losses without treatment (bottom) or with NGF started at lesion time (top). Broken lines = recoveries after delayed NGF. Bars = detectable ChAT-positive neurons at start (hatched) or end (open) of the delayed NGF treatments.

We have recently addressed this question by examining ChAT-positive neurons in the medial septum of adult rats subjected to complete unilateral fimbria-fornix transection and continuous intraventricular NGF infusions (Hagg et al., 1987). As shown in Figure 2, a 14-day NGF treatment which was only started 7 days after lesion, i.e., after a 50% disappearance of ChAT-positive neurons, not only prevents further numerical losses but reverses the previous loss back to the level protected by NGF supplied from lesion time on. Similarly, 14-day NGF treatments delayed by 14 or 21 days raise the numbers of ChAT-positive neurons from the residual level of 20% to at least 50% of the initial number. These data clearly show that the disappearance of medial septum cholinergic neurons following axotomy reflects -- at least for several days -- a reversible loss of their ChAT (or AChE) marker rather than irreversible degeneration and death.

An additional implication of these data is that NGF (and, thus, potentially other NTFs) includes among its trophic effects the promotion of _functional_ features such as transmitter enzyme competence. This fits well with the earlier observations in Hefti's group (1985) that NGF stimulates ChAT activity rather than survival in cultured septal neurons and our recent report of NGF-improved, cholinergically-mediated cognitive behaviors in aged rats (Fischer et al., 1987). A functional, rather than or in addition to a survival-supportive, benefit of NTF treatments encourages the expectation that the neuronotrophic hypothesis may well be extendable to pathological situations of the adult human brain and spinal cord.

ACKNOWLEDGEMENT: Supported by NINCDS grant NS-16349.

REFERENCES

Appel SH (1981). A unifying hypothesis for the cause of Amyotrophic Lateral Sclerosis, Parkinsonism, and Alzheimer disease. Ann Neurol 10:499-505.
Barron KD, (1983). Comparative observations on the cytologic reactions of central and peripheral nerve cells to axotomy. In Kao CC, Bunge RP, Reier PJ (eds): "Spinal Cord Reconstruction," New York: Raven Press, pp 7-40.
Davis GE, Varon S, Engvall E, Manthorpe M (1985). Substratum-binding neurite promoting factors: Relationships to laminin. Trends Neurosci 8:528-532.
Davis GE, Engvall E, Varon S, Manthorpe M (1987a). Human amnion membrane as a substratum for cultured peripheral and central nervous system neurons. Dev Brain Res 33:1-10.

Davis GE, Blaker SN, Engvall E, Varon S, Manthorpe M, Gage FH (1987b). Human amnion membrane serves as a substratum for growing axons in vitro and in vivo. Science 236:1106-1109.

Fischer W, Wictorin K, Bjorklund A, Williams LR, Varon S, Gage FH (1987). Amelioration of cholinergic neuron atrophy and spatial memory impairment in aged rats by nerve growth factor. Nature 329:65-68.

Hagg T, Vahlsing HL, Manthorpe M, Varon S (1987). Delayed intraventricular NGF infusion reverses axotomy-induced loss of medial septum ChAT-positive neurons. Soc Neurosci Abstr 13:922.

Hamburger V, Oppenheim RN (1982). Naturally occurring neuronal death in vertebrates. Neurosci Comment 1:39-55.

Hefti F (1983). Alzheimer's disease caused by a lack of nerve growth factor? Ann Neurol 13:109-110.

Hefti F (1986). Nerve Growth Factor promotes survival of septal cholinergic neurons after fimbrial transections. J Neurosci 6:2155-2162.

Hefti F, Hartikka JJ, Eckenstein F, Gnahn H, Heumann R, Schwab M (1985). Nerve Growth Factor increases choline acetyltransferase but not survival or fiber outgrowth of cultured fetal septal cholinergic neurons. Neurocience 14:55-68.

Kromer LF (1987). Nerve Growth Factor treatment after brain injury prevents neuronal death. Science 235:214-216.

Kromer LF, Bjorklund A, Stenevi U (1981). Regeneration of the septo-hippocampal pathways in adult rats is promoted by utilizing embryonic hippocampal implants as bridges. Brain Res 210:173-200.

Levi-Montalcini R (1987). The Nerve Growth Factor thirty-five years later. Science 237:1154-1162.

McBride RL, Feringa ER, Pruitt II JN (1987). Prelabeled red nucleus and sensory-motor cortex neurons 10 weeks after spinal cord transection. Soc Neurosci Abstr 13:920.

Terry RD, Peck A, DeTeresa R, Schechter R, Horoupian DS (1981). Some morphometric aspects of the brain in senile dementia of the Alzheimer's type. Ann Neurol 10:184-192.

Terry RD, DeTeresa R, Hansen LA (1987). Neocortical cell counts in normal human adult aging. Ann Neurol 21:530-539.

Varon S (1975). In vitro appoaches to the study of neural tissue aging. In Maletta G (ed): "Survey o the Aging Nervous System," DHEW Pub (NIH) 74-296, pp 59-76.

Varon S (1977). Neural growth and regeneration: A cellular perspective. Exp Neurol 54:1-6.

Varon S, Adler R (1981). Trophic and specifying factors directed to neuronal cells. Adv Cell Neurobiol 2:115-163.

Varon S, Manthorpe M, Longo FM (1982). Growth factors and motor neurons. In Rowland LP (ed): "Human Motor Neuron Diseases," Adv In Neurology, Vol 36, New York: Raven Press, pp 453-472.

Varon S, Manthorpe M, Williams LR (1984). Neuronotrophic and neurite promoting factors and their clinical potentials. Dev Neuroscience 6(2):73-100.

Varon S, Williams LR, Gage FH (1987). Exogenous administration of neuronotrophic factors in vivo protects central nervous system neurons against axotomy induced degeneration. In Seil FJ, Herbert E, Carlson BM (eds): "Neural Regeneration," Progress in Brain Research, Vol 71 Amsterdam: Elsevier, pp 191-201.

Varon S, Manthorpe M, Davis GE, Williams LR, Skaper SD (1988). Growth Factors. In Waxman SG (ed): "Functional Recovery in Neurological Disease," Advances in Neurology, Vol. 47, New York: Raven Press, pp 493-521.

Williams LR, Varon S, Peterson G, Wictorin K, Fischer W, Bjorklund A, Gage FH (1986). Continuous infusion of Nerve Growth Factor prevents basal forebrain neuronal death after fimbria-fornix transection. Proc Natl Acad Sci USA 83:9231-9235.

Current Issues in Neural Regeneration
Research, pages 75-87
© 1988 Alan R. Liss, Inc.

TARGET-SPECIFIC REQUIREMENTS OF IMMATURE AXOTOMIZED CNS NEURONS FOR SURVIVAL AND AXONAL ELONGATION AFTER INJURY

Barbara Sypniewski Bregman

Department of Anatomy, University of Maryland School of Medicine, Baltimore, Maryland 21201

INTRODUCTION

The response of immature CNS neurons to injury is not uniform. Although some developing pathways are capable of robust axonal growth following injury (for example, axonal sprouting, maintenance of exuberant connections, rerouting of late-developing axons), other immature neurons respond to injury by massive retrograde cell death. For example, after partial spinal cord lesions in newborn cats, immature corticospinal axons are able to grow around the site of the injury, to reach normal targets at caudal spinal cord levels (Bregman and Goldberger, 1982, 1983). In contrast, immature axotomized red nucleus neurons responded to this same injury by massive retrograde cell death (Bregman and Goldberger, 1982, 1983). At present, it is not clear why some injured immature CNS neurons are capable of considerable anatomical plasticity and sparing of function, while others die following injury. We are using neural tissue transplantation techniques to identify the rules which determine the response of immature CNS neurons to injury and to identify the alterations which lead to the more limited anatomical and functional reorganization characteristic of the mature CNS.

The reason that some immature central neurons are so sensitive to axotomy is not clear (see Lieberman, 1974; Barron, 1983 for reviews). One possibility is that for survival, the immature neurons are dependent upon their target for trophic support. The need for trophic support may itself vary with the developmental stage of the neuron. Studies in vitro have demonstrated relatively specific trophic support of nerve growth factor (NGF) for peripheral neurons of neural crest origin (Levi-Montalcini and Angeletti, 1968; Green and Shooter, 1980). NGF also supports the survival and differentiation of these neurons in vivo (Gorin and Johnson, 1979; Johnson et al, 1980; Yip and Johnson, 1984; Yip et al, 1984). After axotomy, exogenous NGF is able to delay the degeneration of some superior cervical ganglion neurons (Hendry and Campbell, 1975; Banks and Walter, 1977) or dorsal root gangion (DRG) neurons (Yip and Johnson, 1984; Yip et al 1984). In fact, some of the NGF essential for the survival of immature DRG neurons is of spinal cord origin, as indicated by the significant cell loss of immature DRG neurons after axotomy of their central process (Yip et al, 1984). Recent work indicates that some central neurons also respond to NGF (Shelton and Reichert, 1986; Kromer, 1987). More recently, in vitro studies have identified the presence of centrally derived factors (distinct from NGF) that affect the survival, growth and differentiation, or axonal outgrowth of central and peripheral neurons (Banker, 1980; Barde et al, 1982, 1983; Lindsay and Peters, 1984; Davies and Lindsay, 1984; Muller et al, 1984; Manthorpe et al, 1982). Immature CNS neurons deprived of target derived trophic support may fail to survive following axotomy.

The sensitivity of immature CNS neurons to axotomy may relate to their relative maturity. Mature CNS neurons may either be less dependent upon target-derived trophic support for their survival or may possess alternate sources of such support (for example, collateral projections). The response of immature neurons to axotomy suggests that they are at a critical stage in their development where they are dependent upon environmental factors (e.g. trophic substances) for their survival. If this is true, an intervention such as adding fetal spinal cord tissue at the site of an injury might act as a surrogate for the normal target to sustain these cells during a critical period of dependency. An alternative explanation for the sensitivity of immature neurons to axotomy may be their inability to re-establish connections across a glial scar or across a gap caused by the neonatal lesion. The axons may be influenced by the local environment at the site of the lesion (Reier et al, 1983). The axotomized neuron may initially respond to the lesion by axonal growth (sprouting, regeneration), but the terrain at the site of the lesion may prevent further axonal elongation. If the immature neuron is unable to regenerate and re-establish connections it may fail to survive. There is remarkable reorganization of the immature CNS after lesions alone, as evidenced by the plasticity of the corticospinal tract (Bernstein and Stelzner, 1983; Bregman and Goldberger, 1982, 1983). Even in the young animal, however, regenerating or late-growing undamaged axons do not grow through a glial scar or across a gap. Perhaps the presence of a transplant can provide a substitute terrain for growing axons, or modify the glial response at the site of injury and in that way modify the sequellae of neonatal lesions.

We have shown that after spinal cord damage at birth, transplants of fetal spinal cord tissue placed into the site of injury modify the response of immature neurons to injury by preventing the massive retrograde cell death of axotomized rubrospinal neurons (Bregman and Reier, 1986) and by supporting the growth of identified axons across the lesion site (Bregman, 1987 a,b). We have suggested that the transplants may rescue immature axotomized neurons by providing trophic support for the injured neurons and/or by providing a terrain which supports axonal elongation. It seems clear that both appropriate terrain and trophic factors may be required for the long term survival of immature axotomized CNS neurons. The aim of the current study was to determine the degree to which the requirements of immature axotomized neurons for survival are target specific. Immature axotomized neurons may be dependent upon very specific trophic support from their targets. Alternatively, a variety of immature tissues may possess some properties in common that can sustain the injured neurons.

EXPERIMENTAL PARADIGM

The experimental paradigm is illustrated in figure 1. Spinal cord hemisection was made at T6 in rat pups <48 hours of age. Transplants of embryonic target or non-target tissue were placed into the lesion site. The number of neurons in the red nucleus (RN) was used as our assay for cell survival. We compared the effects of target-

RED NUCLEUS NEURONS WERE AXOTOMIZED

BY MID-THORACIC HEMISECTION AT BIRTH

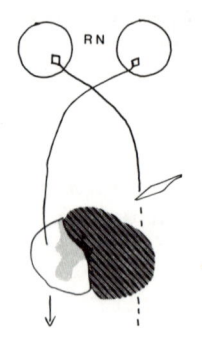

TRANSPLANTS WERE PLACED INTO THE LESION SITE

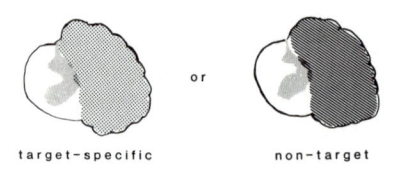

target-specific　　　or　　　non-target

RED NUCLEUS CELL COUNTS WERE MADE AFTER

ACUTE (7 DAYS) OR CHRONIC (30 DAYS) SURVIVAL

Figure 1. Schematic diagram illustrating the experimental paradigm to determine the effects of target and non-target tissue on the survival of immature axotomized red nucleus neurons. See text for details.

specific tissue on RN cell survival with that of a variety
of non-target tissues at acute (7 days post-operative,
dpo) and chronic (30 dpo) survival times. Embryonic
spinal cord tissue (from thoracic spinal cord of rats 14
days in gestation, E14) was the target-specific transplant
examined. Non-target transplants included the following:
cortex (E18), hippocampus (E18), cerebellum (E15), and
Schwann cells derived from littermate (newborn) sciatic
nerve segments. Control animals received one of the
following: 1) hemisection only, no transplant, 2)
hemisection plus gelfoam, collagen, or matrigel, or 3) no
lesion (normal littermates).

In a parallel series of experiments, we have examined
the time course of cell loss in the red nucleus after mid-
thoracic spinal cord hemisection. In this series, a
spinal cord lesion was made in rat pups (<24 hrs), and the
number of surviving RN neurons determined after 1-10, 14,
21, and 30 days (N=3 at each age). In each case the
number of neurons in the axotomized RN was compared with
that in unlesioned littermates.

TIME COURSE OF CELL LOSS AFTER AXOTOMY OF RED NUCLEUS NEURONS

In the control animals (normal littermates) there is
no change in the number of RN neurons during the time
period examined. Thus, during the postnatal time period
examined we do not see any naturally-occuring cell death
in the RN. After neonatal hemisection, the axotomized RN
undergoes massive retrograde cell loss (Prendergast and
Stelzner, 1976; Bregman and Reier, 1986). Midthoracic
hemisection resulted in a 50-60% cell loss in the
contralateral RN. In our experimental model, many of the
RN neurons remaining after mid-thoracic axotomy are in
fact not axotomized because they project to spinal cord
levels rostral to the mid-thoracic lesion. If one examines
only the RN neurons which project to caudal spinal levels,
the percentage of cell loss is much greater. Since it is
relatively easy to distinguish the boundaries of the RN as
a whole, but difficult to distinguish accurately by
position alone the forelimb/hindlimb boundaries within the
nucleus, we have chosen to examine cell loss and survival
within the entire nucleus. The cell loss was first
apparent by 24 hours after the axotomy and was complete by
5 days postoperative (Prendergast and Bates, 1981; Bregman

et al, in preparation). The number of neurons in the axotomized RN was similar at 7 days post-operative or 30 days post-operative with that seen after survival periods of up to 2 years.

TARGET AND NON-TARGET TRANSPLANTS SUPPORT THE TEMPORARY SURVIVAL OF IMMATURE AXOTOMIZED NEURONS

In all cases used for quantitative analysis of RN cell survival, the target and non-target transplants survived within the cord both at acute and chronic times. Both target and non-target transplants develop and mature within the lesioned spinal cord. The spinal cord transplants develop tissue specific cytological characteristics (Reier et al, 1986; Reier and Bregman, 1983). Similarly, the non-target transplants also develop many of the cytological characteristics that they exhibit during their development in situ. Both target and non-target transplants establish extensive areas of apposition with the host spinal cord. At acute survival periods, the presence of both target and a variety of non-target transplants prevented (or delayed) post-axotomy retrograde cell loss (Fig. 2). On the graph, each bar represents the mean ± SEM for 3-5 animals per group. Animals were included for quantitative analysis only if the transplant was in good apposition with the host spinal cord. In animals with hemisection only, or hemisection plus gelfoam, collagen, or matrigel, the retrograde cell loss in the RN was similar, i.e. approximately 1500 RN neurons remained. Of the CNS neuronal transplants examined, RN survival was greatest with spinal cord and hippocampal transplants, and somewhat less with cerebellar and cortical transplants. The sciatic nerves containing Schwann cells also supported the survival of axotomized RN neurons at acute survival times. Thus, at 7 days post-operative, both target specific transplants and non-target transplants were able to rescue immature axotomized red nucleus neurons.

PERMANENT SURVIVAL IS DEPENDENT UPON TARGET-SPECIFIC TRANSPLANTS

In contrast, at the chronic survial period examined (30 dpo), only target specific transplants (spinal cord)

RED NUCLEUS CELL SURVIVAL

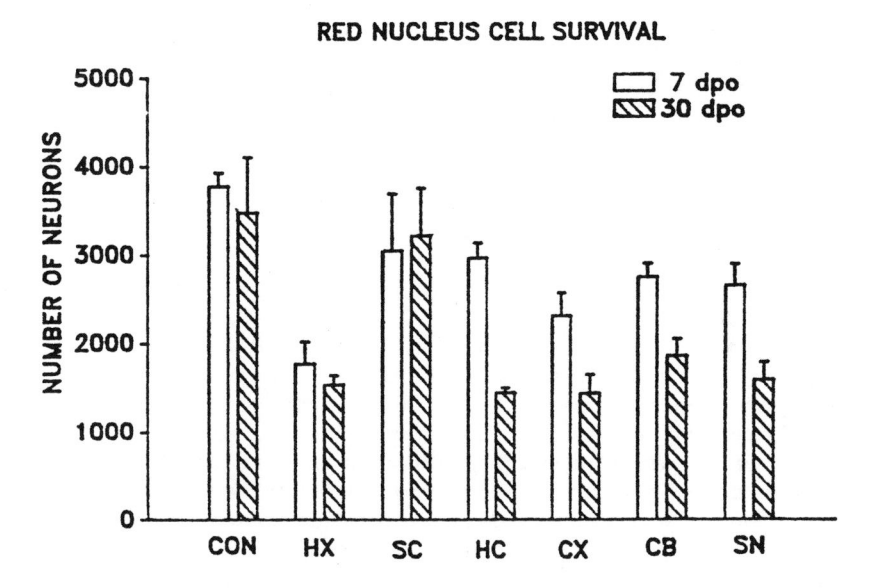

Figure 2. Comparison of the effects of target and non-target tissue on the survival of immature axotomized red nucleus neurons at acute (7 dpo) and chronic (30 dpo) survival times. Each bar represents the mean $\pm$ SEM for 3-5 animals in each group. Abbreviations: normal controls (CON); lesion only (HX); spinal cord (SC); hippocampus (HC); cortex (CX); cerebellum (CB); sciatic nerve (SN). At acute survival times both target and non-target transplants rescue the axotomized RN neurons, but the long term survival is target specific.

supported the survival of axotomized RN neurons (Fig. 2).
The number of RN neurons in animals with non-target
transplants was not significantly different from that seen
in animals with hemisection only. Consistently, cerebellar
transplants supported slightly more RN neurons than either
hippocampus, cortex, or sciatic nerve transplants. This
is intriguing, since a portion of RN neurons send
collaterals to both the spinal cord and to the cerebellum.
It remains to be determined whether this slight trend
toward survival with cerebellar transplants represents the
target specific rescuing of a sub-population of RN
neurons.

Many immature CNS neurons undergo massive cell loss
in response to target removal by axotomy. The role of
trophic support for injured immature neurons is also seen
after lesions in the developing visual system. Cunningham
and colleagues (Cunningham and Haun, 1984; Haun and
Cunningham, 1984; Repka and Cunningham, 1987) have
demonstrated that cortical transplants can provide
specific trophic support for lateral geniculate neurons
after removal of all of their normal cortical targets at
birth. Only target-specific transplants were able to
prevent cell loss, and the survival effect was observed
only temporary (i.e., 10 days). The difference observed
(i.e., only temporary rescue of LGN neurons even with the
target specific transplants, in contrast to the long term
rescue of RN neurons) may relate to the relative severity
of the injury to the immature neurons. The lateral
geniculate neurons are damaged much closer to the cell
body than are the RN neurons in the current study.
Alternatively, the trophic support provided by the
transplant may be necessary, but not sufficient, for the
long term survival of some cells after the lesions.

AXONAL ELONGATION

The immature red nucleus is not unique in its
response to axotomy. Other immature descending pathways
respond in a similar manner. For example, raphe-spinal,
vestibulospinal and coeruleospinal neurons undergo massive
retrograde cell loss after axotomy at birth, and these
neurons are rescued by the presence of target-specific
transplants at the site of injury. We have concentrated
on the red nucleus in the current studies simply because

it lends itself to quantitative analysis better than the other nuclei.

For the analysis of axonal elongation, we have chosen to use the raphe-spinal projection. We have used peroxidase-anti-peroxidase immunocytochemical techniques to examine the serotonergic projection to target and non-target transplants. One possibility suggested by the target specific rescuing of immature axotomized neurons is that the initial survival is mediated by diffusible trophic support, while the long term survival requires the subsequent axonal elongation and synaptogenesis, which may be target specific events. We have shown previously that transplants of fetal spinal cord tissue enhance the developmental plasticity of the serotonergic projection to the spinal cord both at the site of injury and within the host spinal cord caudal to the injury (Bregman, 1987 a,b). At survival periods of one month to one year after injury, serotonergic axons project throughout the spinal cord transplant (Bregman, 1987 a,b; Reier et al 1986). In the current study, the experimental paradigm was similar to that shown in figure 1. We made spinal cord lesions and transplants at birth and compared the serotonergic (5-HT) projection within the target (spinal cord) and non-target (cortex, hippocampus, cerebellum) transplants at acute (7 dpo) and chronic (30 dpo) survival times.

At chronic survival periods, 5-HT axons are observed only in the target-specific transplants. For example, although the hippocampal tissue in situ receives a serotonergic projection, at 30 days postoperative, there was no 5-HT projection to hippocampal transplants in a heterotopic position within the spinal cord. Thus, transmitter specificity per se is not sufficient to maintain the axonal projection (and neuronal survival). At acute survival periods, however, 5-HT axons were observed throughout both the spinal cord transplants and the cortex, hippocampus and cerebellar transplants within the cord. The time course of and conditions leading to the subsequent axonal retraction remain to be determined. Thus, immature serotonergic axons are capable of growing into both target and non-target tissue, but only the spinal cord transplants were capable of maintaining the projection.

SUMMARY AND CONCLUSIONS

At acute survival times, both target and non-target transplants are able to support the temporary survival of axotomized RN neurons. The permanent survival of axotomized RN neurons, however, is supported only by target specific transplants. These results suggest that components contained within a variety of immature tissues can substitute for the loss of the normal target immediately after injury. The permanent survival of the neurons may require that they establish specific synaptic connections within or caudal to the transplant. The stages of axonal elongation and synaptogenesis may be target specific. In the axonal elongation studies, each of our "non-target" transplants do receive a serotonergic projection in situ. Perhaps there is a hierarchy in the specificity requirements. For example, the serotonergic projection to the hippocampus arises from a different subset of raphe nucleui than does the spinal projection. Perhaps the trasmitter specificity is sufficient for initial axonal elongation, but particular target-recognition factors are required for the maintenance of the projection.

ACKNOWLEDGEMENTS

This work was supported by NIH grant NS19259 and by March of Dimes Birth Defects Foundation grant #1-1051. Barbara S. Bregman is supported by a Research Career Development Award NS01249 from the NINCDS. I thank Marietta McAtee and Andrea O'Neill for their outstanding technical assistance throughout the course of these studies. I am extremely grateful to Dr. Hynda Kleinman for generously supplying the matrigel used in these studies and to Drs. M. Blair Clark and Ellen Kunkel-Bagden for helpful discussion during the course of these studies.

REFERENCES

Banker GA (1980) Trophic interactions between astroglial cells and hippocampal neurons in culture. Science 209: 809-810.
Banks BEC, Walter SJ (1977) The effects of postganglionic axotomy and nerve growth factor on superior cervical

ganglia of developing mice. J Neurocytol 6: 287-297.
Barde YA, Edgar D, Thoenen H (1982) Purification of a new neuronotrophic factor from mammalian brain. EMBO J 1: 549-554.
Barde YA, Edgar D, Thoenen H (1983) New neuronotrophic factors. Ann Rev Physiol 45: 601-612.
Barron, KD (1983) Comparative observations on the cytologic reactions of central and peripheral nerve cells to axotomy. In: Spinal cord Reconstruction, CC Kao, RP Bunge, PJ Reier eds, Raven Press, New York, pp 7-40.
Bernstein, D.R. and Stelzner, D.J. 1983 Developmental plasticity of the corticospinal tract (CST) following mid-thoracic "over-hemisection" in the neonatal rat. J Comp Neurol 221: 371-385.
Bregman BS (1987 a) Development of serotonin immunoreactivity in the rat spinal cord and its plasticity after neonatal spinal cord lesions. Devel Brain Res 34: 245-263.
Bregman BS (1987 b) Spinal cord transplants permit the growth of serotonergic axons across the site of neonatal spinal cord transection. Devel Brain Res 34: 265-279.
Bregman BS, Goldberger ME (1983) Infant lesion effect: III. Anatomical correlates of sparing and recovery of function after spinal cord damage in newborn and adult cats. Devel Brain Res 9: 137-154.
Bregman BS, Goldberger ME (1982) Anatomical plasticity and sparing of function after spinal cord damage in neonatal cats. Science 217: 533-555.
Bregman BS, Reier PJ (1986) Neural tissue transplants rescue axotomized rubrospinal cells from retrograde death. J Comp Neurol 244: 86-95.
Cunningham TJ, Haun F (1984) Trophic relationships during visual system development. In: Development of Visual Pathways in Mammals, Alan Liss, Inc., New York, pp. 315-327.
Davies AM and Lindsay RM (1984) Neural crest derived spinal and cranial sensory neurones are equally sensitive to NGF but differ in their response to tissue extracts. Dev Brain Res 14: 121-127.
Donatelle JM (1977) Growth of the corticospinal tract and the development of placing reactions in the postnatal rat. J Comp Neurol 175: 207-232.
Gorin PD, Johnson EM (1979) Experimental autoimmune model of nerve gorwth factor deprivation: effects on

developing peripheral sympathetic and sensory neurons. Proc Natl Acad Sci 76: 5382-5386.
Greene LA, Shooter, EM (1980) The nerve growth factor: biochemistry, synthesis and mechanism of action. Ann Rev Neurosci 3:353-402.
Haun F, Cunningham TJ (1984) Cortical transplants reveal CNS trophic interactions in situ. Devel Brain Res 15: 290-294.
Haun F, Cunningham TJ (1987) Specific neurotrophic interactions between cortical and subcortical visual structures in developing rat: in vivo studies. J Comp Neurol 256: 561-569.
Johnson EM, Gorin PD, Brandeis LD, Pearson J (1980) Dorsal root ganglion neurons are destroyed by exposure in utero to maternal antibody to nerve growth factor. Science 210: 916-918.
Kromer LF (1987) Nerve growth factor treatment after brain injury prevents neuronal death. Science 235:214-216.
Levi-Montalcini R, Angeletti PU (1968) Nerve growth factor. Physiol Rev 48:534-569.
Lieberman AR (1974) Some factors affecting retrograde neuronal responses to axonal lesions. In: Essays on the Nervous System, R Bellairs and EG Gray eds. Oxford, Clarendon Press, pp 71-105.
Lindsay RM, Peters C (1984) Spinal cord contains neurotrophic activity for spinal nerve sensory neurons. Late developmental appearance of a survival factor distinct from nerve growth factor. Neurosci 12:45-51.
Manthorpe M, Longo FM, Varon, S (1928) Comparative features of spinal neuronotrophic factors in fluids collected in vitro and in vivo. J Neurosci Res 8:241-250.
Muller HW, Beckh S, Seifert W (1984) Neurotrophic factor for central neurons. Proc Natl Acad Sci 81: 1248-1252.
Prendergast J, Stelzner DJ (1976) Changes in the magnocellular portion of the red nucleus following thoracic hemisection in the neonatal and adult rat. J Comp Neurol 166: 163-172.
Prendergast J, Bates R (1981) The time course of the loss of red nucleus neurons as a result of T5-6 hemisection in the neonatal rats. Soc Neurosci Abstr 7: 292.
Reier PJ, Bregman BS (1983) Immunocytochemical demonstration of substantia gelatinosa-like regions and serotonergic axons in embryonic spinal cord transplants in the rat. Soc Neurosci Abstr 9: 696.

Reier PJ, Bregman BS, Wujek JR (1986) Intraspinal transplantation of embryonic spinal cord tissue in neonatal and adult rats. J Comp Neurol 247:275-296.

Reier PJ, Stensaas LJ, Guth L (1983) The astrocytic scar as an impediment to regeneration in the central nervous system. In: Spinal Cord Reconstruction. Kao CC, Bunge RP, Reier PJ eds, Raven Press, New York, pp 163-195.

Repka A, Cunningham TJ (1987) Specific neurotrophic interactions between cortical and subcortical visual structures in developing rat: in vitro studies. J Comp Neurol 256: 552-560.

Shelton DL, Reichert LF (1986) Studies on the expression of the nerve growth factor (NGF) gene in the central nervous system: level and regional distribution of NGF mRNA suggest that NGF functions as a trophic factor for several distinct populations of neurons. Proc Natl Acad Sci USA 83: 2714-2718.

Yip HK, Johnson, EM (1984) Developing dorsal root gangion neurons require trophic support from their central processes: evidence for a role of retrogradely transported nerve gorwth factor from the central nervous system to the periphery. Proc Natl Acad Sci 81: 6245-6249.

Yip HK, Rich, KM, Lampe, PA, Johnson, EM (1984) The effects of nerve growth factor and its antiserum on the postnatal development and survival after injury of sensory neurons in rat dorsal root ganglia. J. Neurosci 4: 2986-2992.

TESTING THE TROPHIC FACTOR HYPOTHESIS IN THE VISUAL SYSTEM

Timothy J. Cunningham, Caroline Fisher and Forrest A. Haun
Department of Anatomy, The Medical College of Pennsylvania, Philadelphia, PA 19129

INTRODUCTION

The "trophic factor hypothesis" was formulated originally to provide an explanation for the developmental relationship between the size of innervation zones in the peripheral nervous system and the numbers of neurons that ultimately project to these peripheral fields. Over the past several decades of research on peripheral nervous system development, it has been shown repeatedly that experimental manipulation of the amount of available synaptic space in the periphery (e.g. by limb extirpation or limb transplantation) results in corresponding adjustments in the number of neurons which innervate these regions (see reviews by Cunningham, 1982, Oppenheim, 1981, Jacobson, 1970). Even in the earliest of these studies, it was postulated that the explanation for this developmental relationship between neuron number and the size of innervation territory involved the existence of survival promoting chemicals (neurotrophic factors), synthesized and secreted by peripheral target cells (e.g. Shorey, 1909). Subsequent work has further suggested that a failure to compete for finite quantities of these neurotrophic factors results in the death of a proportion of the neurons originally generated, and subsequently, the appropriate matching of the number of surviving neurons to their peripheral domain.

More recent work utilizing tissue culture systems has now suggested the existence of many neurotrophic factors, agents that support the survival and/or the morphological and biochemical differentiation of both central and peripheral nervous system neurons (see reviews by Berg, 1984; Barde, et al.,

1983; Perez-Polo, et al., 1983). However, only one of these factors -Nerve Growth Factor (NGF) - has a defined physiological role as demonstrated by experimentation in vivo (Levi-Montalcini, 1982). NGF is a target-derived neurotrophic factor that supports the survival and differentiation of sensory and sympathetic ganglion cells of the peripheral nervous system. It appears to operate in developing and adult animals - systemic or local introduction of the factor will rescue ganglion cells degenerating naturally during development or degenerating because of axotomy or target deprivation in both developing and adult animals (Rich, et al., 1986; Hamburger, et al., 1981; Yip and Johnson, 1984; Hendry and Campbell, 1976). In adults NGF's survival promoting properties may also extend to certain populations of CNS cholinergic neurons (Kromer, 1987; Fischer et al., 1987; Hefti, 1986). These in vivo observations have been essential for recognizing NGF as a true endogenous neurotrophic factor. However, isolation and purification of NGF (which allowed such experiments to be conducted) depended on the availability of particularly rich sources of the factor: mouse sarcoma cells, with which the neurotrophic properties of NGF were first demonstrated in the grafting experiments of Beuker (1948); and the salivary glands (Cohen, 1960), a natural target for axons of sympathetic ganglion cells and the most common source of purified factor at present.

It is against this background that we can view the lack of similar progress in the search for specific neurotrophic molecules that are endogenous to the central nervous system. For the most part, in vivo models of neurotrophism in the CNS have not been widely used. One difficulty in the development of such models is the fact that CNS neurons generally do not have direct access to the contents of blood, which may make systemic delivery of putative trophic factors particularly difficult or ineffective. However, the major problem has been the identification of adequate sources of specific trophic agents that operate on specific subsets of CNS neurons. According to the classical view of the trophic factor hypothesis, the best source of a specific neurotrophic factor, that is, one which promotes the survival and growth of a particular population of neurons, should be the cells which form connections with those neurons. In vitro experiments on CNS neurons, in which neuron survival and neurite outgrowth are promoted by the presence of afferent sources or target structures, tend to support this view (e.g. Repka and Cunningham, 1987; Eagleson and Bennett, 1983; McCaffery, et al., 1982; Pollack and Muhlach, 1982; Nurcombe and Bennett, 1981; Bennett, et al., 1980; Bennett and Nurcombe, 1979). However, there are also several examples of trophic support provided to CNS neurons in vitro by the synthetic products of nonconnecting structures, nonneuronal cells, or cells of unknown origin (see reviews by Berg, 1984; Barde, et al., 1983, Perez-Polo, et al., 1983).

With these observations in mind, we have approached the question of CNS neurotrophism emphasizing both an in vivo assay, and the use of a system where lesion studies have shown strong dependencies between connecting neuron populations, both during development and in adulthood.

THE EFFECTS OF VISUAL CORTEX LESIONS ON THE DORSAL LATERAL GENICULATE NUCLEUS

The effects of visual cortex lesions on the dorsal lateral geniculate nucleus (dLGN) of rats are well documented (Cunningham, et al., 1987a; Haun and Cunningham, 1984;1987; Perry and Cowey, 1979; Cunningham, et al., 1979; Lashley, 1941). If the lesion is made in newborn rats, and includes all cortical projection zones for the dLGN, nearly all dLGN neurons degenerate and are removed in about 5 days. In adult rats, subtotal lesions of visual cortex have been studied most extensively. Because the projection is strictly topographic, a well defined zone of cells showing obvious degenerative changes appears in the dLGN following the lesion. The exact time course of neuron degeneration has not been worked out systematically after visual cortex lesions in adults but a proportion of the dLGN neurons which project to the lesion site actually disappear (as after infant lesions) by two weeks following the surgery. Nearly all the remaining neurons in the affected zone of the dLGN show some evidence of degenerative changes.

The reason for the death of dLGN neurons (or for that matter any neuron) after axotomy is not clear. We have argued previously that the trauma of axonal amputation and subsequent loss of cytoplasm is not by itself sufficient to explain axotomy-induced cell death (Cunningham, et al., 1987a). Since axotomy results in separating the neuron from its target, the lesion can also be viewed as a form of target deprivation. In developing systems, neuron death due to target deprivation is traditionally considered in terms of the trophic factor hypothesis; the lesion removes the source of a survival-promoting chemical which is synthesized by the target and transported to the cell body. It is reasonable to assume that adult neurons also require a supply of these factors to maintain their viability. However, because of the differences between immature and adult neurons in their response to axotomy, it appears that immature neurons depend more critically on such factors for survival, possibly because they have a higher rate of utilization of neurotrophic agents than do adult neurons (Jacobson, 1970).

IDENTIFYING A SOURCE OF NEUROTROPHIC FACTORS FOR DLGN NEURONS

Introduction of Survival Biases in Explant Co-Cultures

If immature neurons have a higher rate of utilization of neurotrophic factors, then it is reasonable to assume that they also have a higher rate of production of these factors. A plausible source of a neurotrophic factors for neurons of the dLGN would then be their immature cortical target cells. By allowing cortical explants to develop in vitro under a specific co-culturing regimen, we have obtained tissue that appears to be enriched with those particular developing cortical neurons that normally would be the targets for dLGN neurons when the pathway matures (Repka and Cunningham, 1987). For these experiments an explant of embryonic day 14 (E-14) posterior cortex tissue was placed in culture for 5 days with an explant of diencephalon (containing the presumptive dLGN neurons). Other cultures were established (from embryos of the same age) in which the cortical explants were grown with an explant of optic tectum or another cortical explant. The explants were placed on a substrate that allows them to adhere but is not conducive to neurite outgrowth so there was no contact between the tissue pieces. Any effects of one explant on the other therefore had to be due to the operation of diffusible factors.

Analysis of the composition of the cortical explants, in terms of cellular morphology, relative maturity of the cells, and their time of origin in vitro, suggested that diffusible trophic factors arise from the explants of the subcortical structures, and that these factors selectively support the survival of specific neuron populations in the developing neocortex explant. In the case of cortical explants co-cultured with diencephalon, it appears that the diencephalon exerts an afferent trophic influence on the developing cortex since the cortical explant contained mostly immature nonpyramidal neurons that normally occupy more superficial laminae in the cerebral cortex in vivo; many of these cells form the natural targets for thalamic projection neurons, including those of the dLGN. More importantly in the present context, such tissue should be the richest source of a specific neurotrophic factor for dLGN neurons in vivo since it is biased to contain a large proportion of their cortical target neurons.

Testing Trophic Activity of Cortical Cells In Vivo by Transplantation

As our initial test of the proposition that cortical cells could supply neurotrophic factors to dLGN neurons in vivo, we transplanted cell suspensions of cortical tissue (first cultured under the different conditions described above) into the cavity of a posterior cortex lesion in newborn rats. Five days later geniculate neuron survival was assayed and the effects of the "precultured" transplants were compared to tissue taken directly from the embryo and transplanted immediately (Haun and Cunningham, 1987). The most effective transplants, in terms of both surviving neuron-occupied volume of the dLGN and numbers of dLGN neurons labeled with [^{3}H]thymidine on E15 and E16 (late in neurogenesis), was cortical tissue that developed in explant culture with diencephalon. Similarly, cortical tissue first precultured with diencephalon also rescues the same population of dLGN neurons when transplanted into the cavity of an incomplete visual cortex lesion in an adult rat (Cunningham, et al., 1987a).

TESTING FOR THE EXISTENCE OF AN EMBRYONIC CELL-DERIVED NEUROTROPHIC FACTOR(S)

Delivery of Conditioned Culture Medium to the Lesion Site

If a neurotrophic factor (or factors) is synthesized by the transplant cells, then it is possible that the factor is present in the medium of the posterior cortex-diencephalon co-cultures. We have tested this possibility by supplying the medium of these cultures to newborn rats with visual cortex lesions (Cunningham, et al., 1987b). We find evidence for the existence of a macromolecule(s) in the culture medium that is able to mimic the effects of the cells when supplied to the site of the cortical lesion in infant rats with their entire visual cortex ablated (and preliminarily, also in adult rats with incomplete visual cortex lesions, see footnote 1). Furthermore, the molecule is a protein and appears to have an optimal concentration for its operation.

The details of the procedures used to prepare the conditioned medium fraction appear in Cunningham, et al. 1987b (a schematic illustration is presented in Figure 1). Briefly, the culture medium is filtered first through a 0.22μm Millex-GV filter (Millipore) and then by pressure ultrafiltration (Filtron Corp.) through membranes which retain macromolecules (8kD or 10kD molecular weight cut-offs). The macromolecular fraction is concentrated to some known value with this ultrafiltration procedure. The concentrate is then diluted to various levels in order to test the relationship between neurotrophic activity and concentration (see below).

The medium fraction is loaded into a carrier gel which will trap the medium and release it within the 5 day period of our assay. The gel is formed as a small chip or bead which is suitable for implantation into the cavity of a lesion to the posterior cortex of a newborn rat. We have tested gelfoam, polyacrylamide, and calcium-alginate as possible carriers for the conditioned medium fraction. The alginate gels release all proteins of the conditioned medium fraction rather quickly (over a 24hr period when placed in a dilute saline bath) but give the best and most consistent results in terms of neuron survival when implanted into the lesion (Cunningham, et al., 1987a; 1987b).

Assaying Geniculate Neuron Survival

As in the experiments on infant rats with tissue transplants, the neuron-occupied volume of the dLGN is measured 5 days after the lesion; rats with implants of alginate beads loaded with the conditioned medium fraction are compared to animals with a similarily prepared fraction of unconditioned culture medium. These simple volume measurements provide a rapid and reliable assay of the extent of dLGN neuron survival, and, if anything, underestimate the actual percentages of identified dLGN neurons (based on time of origin) that survive the lesion (see Cunningham and Haun, 1984).

While the lesions produce severe degeneration of the dLGN in all cases, there are marked differences between animals receiving conditioned medium implants and those receiving unconditioned medium implants. This difference is most pronounced in the more caudal parts of the nucleus as determined by serial reconstructions of the surviving dLGN in relation to adjacent thalamic nuclei (Fig. 2). When the conditioned medium fraction is loaded into the Ca-alginate gels

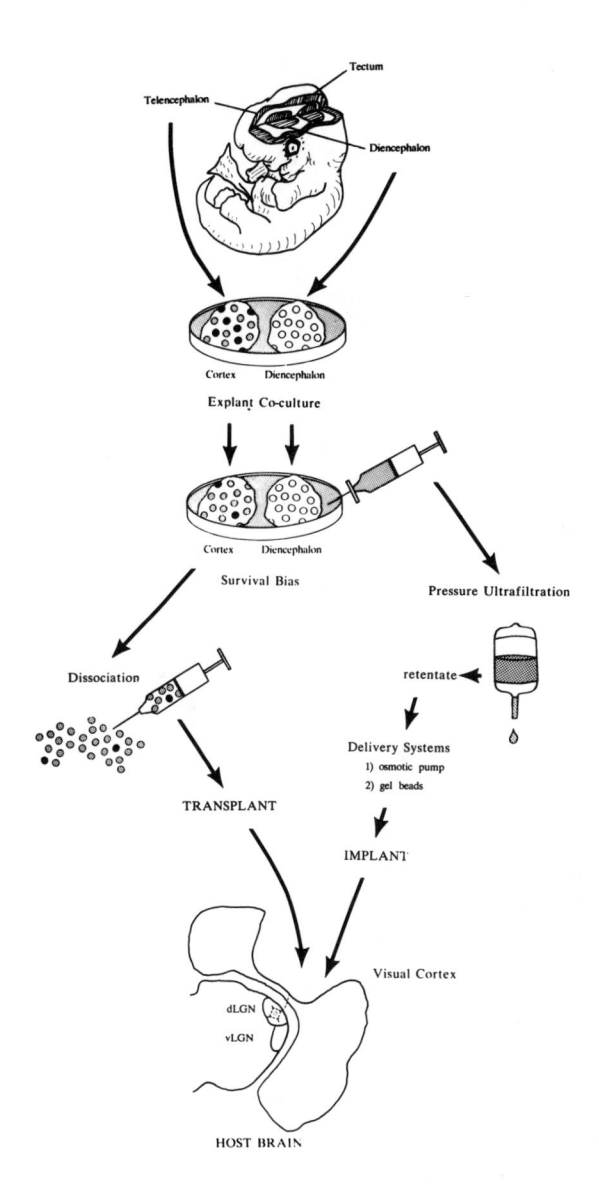

Fig. 1. Schematic showing our procedures for the production and testing of neurotrophic factors which promote the survival of dLGN neurons after lesions of the visual cortex. See text for details.

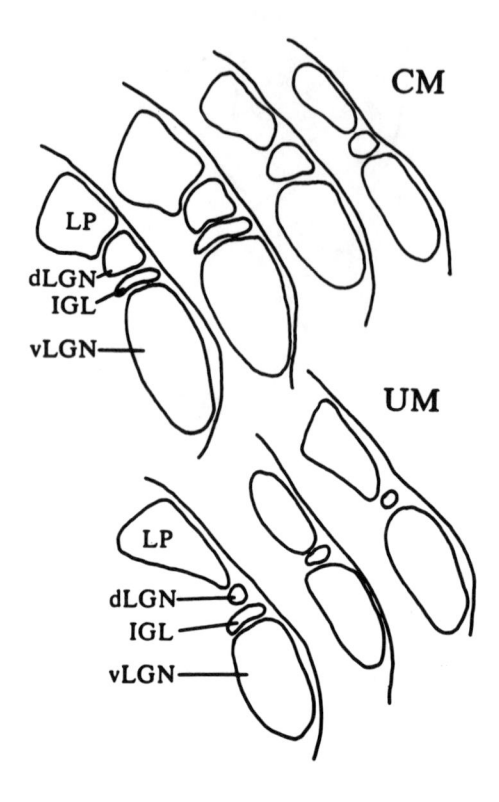

Fig. 2. Drawings of coronal sections through the lateral part of the posterior thalamus in postnatal day 6 rats receiving visual cortex lesions and implants of Ca-alginate beads at birth. CM: animal that received an implant of beads loaded with a macromolecular fraction of medium conditioned by co-cultures of cortex and diencephalon. UM: Animal that received an implant of beads loaded with the same fraction of unconditioned culture medium. In both cases the spacing of the sections is .12mm and the entire rostrocaudal extent of the dLGN is shown. LP - lateral posterior nucleus; IGL - intergeniculate leaflet; vLGN - ventral lateral geniculate nucleus.

at an optimal concentration (see below), up to 29% of the nucleus survives (mean 19.2 ± 6.1). Mean surviving dLGN volume for animals with implants of gels loaded with concentrated unconditioned medium is only 5.1 (± 1.3%). The extent of dLGN survival obtained with unconditioned medium is identical to that obtained after proteolysis of the conditioned medium fraction (10µg/ml pronase for 2 hrs. at 25⁰ with digestion of all proteins into amino acids and small peptides confirmed by gel electrophoresis, Cunningham, et al., 1987b). The fact that proteolysis destroys the trophic activity of the conditioned medium fraction indicates that the factor involved in supporting dLGN neuron survival after the lesion is a protein(s).[1]

The small degree of dLGN neuron survival found with concentrated unconditioned medium implants is similar to that found 5 days after a cortical lesion and no implant or transplant of any kind (Haun and Cunningham, 1984; 1987). The lack of any effect of unconditioned medium is interesting because our standard culture medium contains 5% fetal calf serum and a serum component is reported to support the survival of several CNS neuron types in vitro (Kaufman and Barrett, 1983). Our fraction of unconditioned medium should have contained this component (M_r = 55kD) so we can suggest that nonspecific serum factors may not support dLGN neuron survival in this in vivo system.

Importance of Conditioned Medium Concentration

We have recently determined that the survival-promoting activity of the factor or factors in the conditioned medium fraction decreases as the concentration of the medium increases (Fig. 3). The concentration of factor in the culture medium prior to ultrafiltration was arbitrarily set at X and then

---

[1] In preliminary experiments, we have also loaded the same macromolecular fraction of medium conditioned by cortex and diencephalon in an osmotic pump (No. 2001, Alzet) and delivered the medium to the cavity of a large but incomplete lesion of the visual cortex of adult rats. After a two week survival (when such a lesion results in a 60% loss of later-generated (E15 and E16 labeled) neurons in the affected area of the dLGN), we find that most of these cells are rescued (mean remaining = 95.4 ± 2.2%, N=3).

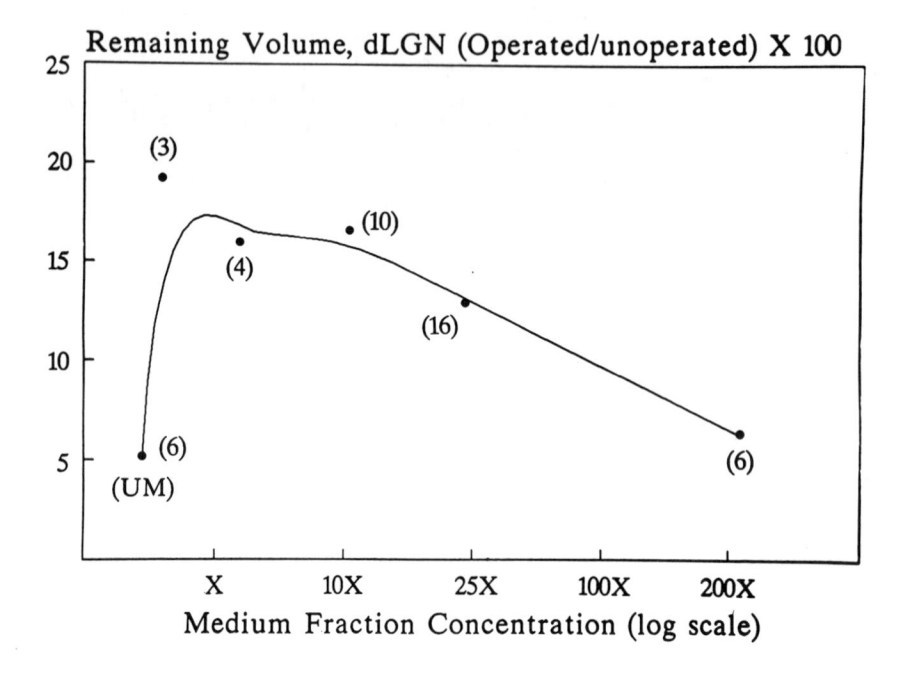

Fig. 3. Relationship of surviving neuron-occupied volume of dLGN and concentration of a macromolecular fraction of medium conditioned by co-cultures of cortex and diencephalon. Forty-five newborn rats received visual cortex lesions and implants of alginate beads loaded with the medium fraction at various concentrations. X - concentration of putative neuron survival factor in the conditioned medium prior to further concentration or dilution. (UM) - extent of dLGN survival in rats with implants of alginate beads loaded with unconditioned culture medium in which the concentration of the survival factor is assumed to be 0. Actual data ($\pm$ s.e.m.) for each point on the graph - UM (5.1 $\pm$ 1.3); 0.2X (19.2 $\pm$ 6.1); 2X (16.0 $\pm$ 4.7); 10X (16.6 $\pm$ 1.3); 25X (13.0 $\pm$ 1.0); 200X (6.3 $\pm$ 0.6).

following ultrafiltration the medium fraction was prepared so as to give concentrations of 0.2X, 2X, 10X, 25X, and 200X. Optimal neuron survival promoting activity is found at the 0.2X concentration while at 200X the amount of dLGN surviving the lesion is equivalent to unconditioned medium controls.

Other investigators have found a fall-off of neurotrophic activity in vitro as concentration of the putative factors increases. In some cases (e.g. Manthorpe, et al. 1982; Grau-Wagemans, et al., 1984) it has been suggested that the explanation for this fall-off in activity of conditioned medium is the existence of neurotoxic as well as neurotrophic factors in the medium; at higher concentrations the neurotoxic factors negate the effects of the neurotrophic factors. However, a similar concentration curve has been reported when neurite outgrowth is measured in the presence of various dilutions of purified NGF (Fenton, 1970). It seems unlikely that the lack of neurotrophic activity at high concentrations in these experiments is the result of neurotoxic factors. Therefore, until there is more definitive evidence for the co-existence of neurotrophic and neurotoxic factors in neurotrophically active media, we must assume that the action of neurotrophic factors is simply regulated strictly, and that this regulation includes an optimal concentration for biological activity. Regardless of the explanation for the relationship between concentration and activity for these neurotrophic agents, our results show that this relationship also exists when testing neurotrophic activity in vivo.

Specificity: The Effect of Medium Conditioned by Co-cultures of Hippocampus and Diencephalon

If the neurotrophic relationship that exists between the dLGN and the posterior neocortex is actually based on neuroanatomical connectivity and the factor(s) that exists is relatively specific to this pathway, then this agent should not be synthesized by an adjacent structure which does not connect directly to the dLGN nor should it be stimulated to do so in the presence of the diencephalon. This proposition was tested by allowing E14 hippocampus to develop in culture for 5 days with E14 diencephalon and then preparing the conditioned medium exactly as in the experiments on posterior cortex. The medium was loaded into the Ca-alginate gel and implanted into the cavity of a posterior cortex lesion. After 5 days, the amount of surviving dLGN is found not to be significantly different from animals receiving implants of unconditioned medium (Fig. 4).

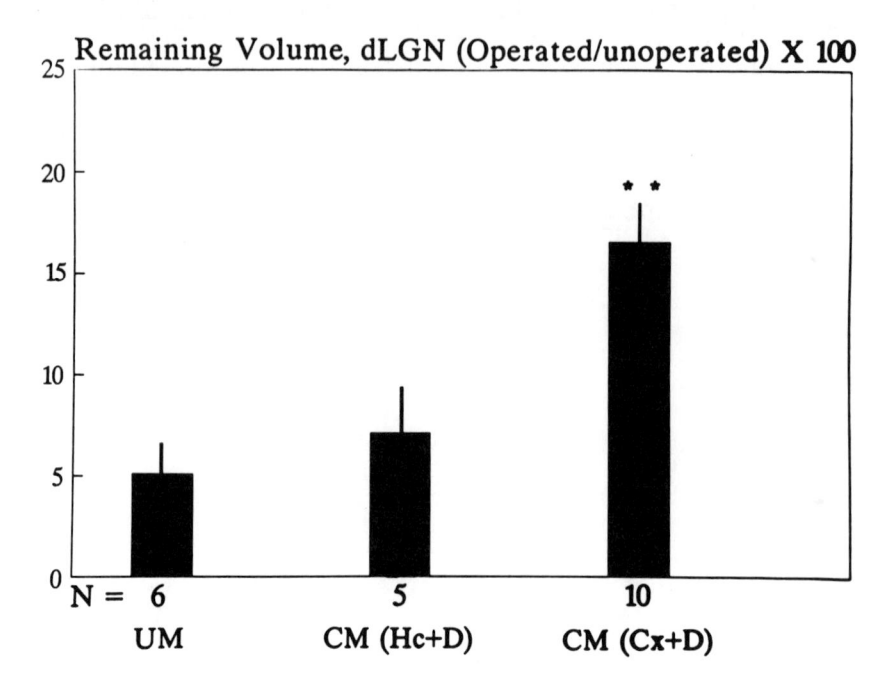

Fig. 4. Surviving neuron-occupied volume of the dLGN in rats with visual cortex lesions at birth and implants of alginate beads loaded with macromolecular fractions of: 1) unconditioned culture medium (UM - $5.1 \pm 1.3\%$ s.e.m.); 2) medium conditioned by co-cultures of hippocampus and diencephalon (Hc + D - $7.1 \pm 1.7\%$ s.e.m.); 3) medium conditioned by co-cultures of posterior cortex and diencephalon (Cx + D - $16.6 \pm 1.3\%$ s.e.m.). All fractions were loaded at the 10X concentration (see text).

This result suggests not only that there is some degree of specificity in the origin of the neurotrophic agent but also that it is not the diencephalic tissue alone that is responsible for production of the factor (rather, the cortical tissue alone or the combination of cortex and diencephalon).

CONCLUSIONS

These experiments suggest that a specific neurotrophic agent for a specific population of neurons in the CNS can be derived from explant cultures of a CNS structure with which the neurons normally connect. Based on our in vitro observations and the results of the implantation studies, it is suggested that a particularly good source of such an agent is explant co-cultures of the two connecting structures. In other words, the medium of co-cultures of diencephalon (which contains presumptive dLGN projection neurons) and posterior cortex should be particularly enriched with an agent that is neurotrophically active on dLGN neurons because the diencephalic explant biases the cortical explant to contain dLGN target cells. It remains to be determined however, whether this specific population of cortical neurons is actually the source of the trophic agent that promotes the survival of dLGN neurons in vivo. Furthermore, the suggestion that this approach to the production of specific neurotrophic agents is applicable generally, i.e., whether co-cultures of two embryonic structures that normally connect at some later stage in development are always a good source of a specific neurotrophic agent for at least one of the two, awaits testing in other nervous system pathways. Nevertheless, given the history of the trophic factor hypothesis, it seems a modest suggestion that physiologically relevant neurotrophic molecules are most likely to be present in medium conditioned by co-cultures of structures having direct connections in vivo.

ACKNOWLEDGEMENTS

We thank Bob Hackett for preparing the illustrations and for his expert technical assistance. This work was supported by grants NS16487 from NINCDS (T.J.C.) and MH41597 from NIMH (F.H.).

REFERENCES:

Barde, Y - A, Edgar D, Thoenen H (1983). New neurotrophic factors. Ann Rev Physiol 45: 601-612.

Bennett MR, Lai K Nurcombe V (1980). Identification of embryonic motoneurons in vitro: Their survival is dependent on skeletal muscle. Brain Res 190: 537-542.

Bennett MR, Nurcombe V (1979). The survival and development of cholinergic neurons in skeletal muscle conditioned media. Brain Res 173: 543-548.

Berg DK (1984). New neuronal growth factors. Ann Rev Neurosci 7: 149-170.

Bueker ED (1948). Implantation of tumors in the hind limb of the embryonic chick and the developmental response of the lumbosacral nervous system. Anat Rec 102: 369-389.

Cohen S (1960). Purification of a nerve growth promoting protein from the mouse salivary gland and its neurotoxic antiserum. Proc Nat Acad Sci USA 46: 302-311.

Cunningham TJ (1982). Naturally occurring neuron death and its regulation by developing neural pathways. In Bourne GH, Danielli JF (eds): "International Review of Cytology", Vol. 72, New York: Academic Press, pp. 163-186.

Cunningham TJ, Sutilla CB, Haun, F (1987a). Trophic effects of transplants following damage to the cerebral cortex. In Azmitia E, Bjorklund A (eds): " Cell and Tissue Transplantation to the Adult Brain", Ann New York Acad Sci, Vol. 495, New York: New York Academy of Sciences Press, pp. 153-168.

Cunningham TJ, Haun F, Chantler PD (1987b). Diffusible proteins prolong survival of dorsal lateral geniculate neurons following occipital cortex lesions in newborn rats. Dev Brain Res, In Press.

Cunningham TJ, Haun FA (1984). Trophic relationships during visual system development. In Stone J, Dreher B, Rapaport D (eds): "Development of Visual Pathways in Mammals", New York: Alan R. Liss, pp. 315-327.

Cunningham TJ, Huddelson C, Murray M (1979). Modification of neuron numbers in the visual system of the rat. J Comp Neurol 184: 423-434.

Eagleson KL, Bennett RM (1983). Survival of purified motor neurones in vitro: Effects of skeletal conditioned medium. Neurosci Lett, 38: 187-192.

Fenton EL (1970). Tissue culture assay of nerve growth factor and of the specific antiserum. Exp Cell Res, 59: 383-392.

Fischer W, Wictorin K, Bjorklund A, Williams LR, Varon S, Gage FH (1987). Amelioration of cholinergic neuron atrophy and spatial memory impairment in aged rats by nerve growth factor. Nature, 329: 65-68.

Grau Wagemans M -P, Selak I, Lefebvre PP, Moonen, G (1984). Cerebellar macroneurons in serum-free cultures: Evidence for intrinsic neuronotrophic and neuronotoxic activities. Dev Brain Res, 15: 11-19.

Hamburger V, Brunso-Bechtold JK, Yip JW (1981). Neuronal death in the spinal ganglia of the chick embryo and its reduction by nerve growth factor. J Neurosci, 1: 60-71.

Haun FA, Cunningham TJ (1987). Specific neurotrophic interactions between cortical and subcortical visual structures in developing rat: In vivo assay. J Comp Neurol, 256: 561-569

Haun F, Cunningham TJ (1984). Cortical transplants reveal CNS trophic interactions in situ. Dev Brain Res, 15: 290-294.

Hefti F (1986). Nerve growth factor promotes survival of septal cholinergic neurons after fimbrial transections. J Neurosci, 6: 2155-2162.

Hendry IA, Campbell J (1976). Morphometric analysis of rat superior cervical ganglion after axotomy and NGF treatment. J Neurocytol 5: 351-360.

Jacobson M (1970). "Developmental Neurobiology". Holt, Rinehart & Winston, New York.

Kaufman LM, Barrett JN (1983). Serum factor supporting long-term survival of rat central neurons in culture. Science, 220: 1394-1396.

Kromer LF (1987). Nerve growth factor treatment after brain injury prevents neuronal death. Science 235: 214-216.

Lashley, KS (1941). Thalamo-cortical connections of the rat's brain. J Comp Neurol, 75: 67-121.

Levi-Montalcini R (1982). Developmental neurobiology and the natural history of nerve growth factor. Ann Rev Neurosci, 5: 341-362.

Manthorpe M, Longo M, Varon S (1982). Comparative features of spinal neuronotrophic factors in fluids collected in vitro and in vivo. J Neurosci Res, 8: 241-250.

McCaffery CA, Bennett MR, Dreher B (1982). The survival of neonatal rat retinal ganglion cells in vitro is enhanced in the presence of appropriate parts of the brain. J Comp Neurol, 177: 519-528.

Nurcombe V, Bennett MR, (!981). Embryonic chick retinal ganglion cells identified in vitro. Exp Brain Res, 44: 249-258.

Oppenheim RW (1981). Neuronal cell death and some related regressive phenomena during neurogenesis: A selective historical review and progress report. In Cowan WM (ed): "Studies In Developmental Neurobiology", New York: Oxford, pp. 74-133.

Perry VH, Cowey A (1979). Changes in the retinofugal pathways following cortical and tectal lesions in neonatal and adult rats. Exp Brain Res, 35: 97-108.

Perez-Polo JR, de Vellis J, Haber B (1983). Growth and trophic factors. In "Progress in Clinical and Biological Research", Vol. 118. New York: Alan R. Liss.

Pollack ED, Muhlach WL (1982). Target control of neuronal development during formation of the spinal reflex. J Neurosci Res, 8: 343-355.

Repka A, Cunningham TJ (1987). Specific neurotrophic interactions between cortical and subcortical visual structures in developing rat: In vitro studies. J Comp Neurol, 256: 552-560.

Rich KM, Luszczynski JR, Osborne PA, Johnson EM (1986). NGF protects adult neurons after sciatic nerve injury. Soc Neurosci Absts, 12: 983.

Shorey ML (1909). The effect of the destruction of peripheral areas on the differentiation of the neuroblasts. J Exp Zool, 7: 25-63.

Yip HK, Johnson EM (1984). Developing dorsal root ganglion neurons require trophic support from their central processes: Evidence for the role of retrogradely transported nerve growth factor from the central nervous system to the periphery. Proc Nat Acad Sci USA, 81: 6245-6249.

NERVE GROWTH FACTOR RESCUES SEPTAL CHOLINERGIC NEURONS AND PROMOTES REINNERVATION OF THE HIPPOCAMPUS IN RATS WITH PARTIAL FIMBRIAL TRANSECTIONS.

Franz Hefti, Claudia N. Montero and Deborah C. Mash

Department of Neurology, University of Miami School of Medicine, Miami, Florida 33101

INTRODUCTION

Cholinergic neurons in medial septum, the nucleus of the diagonal band of Broca and the nucleus basalis form a continuum of cells which provide a wide-spread and topographically organized innervation for cortical and limbic structures (Mesulam et al., 1983). This group of neurons is trophically affected by nerve growth factor (NGF). NGF affects development of cholinergic neurons in the forebrain in a similar way as the development of peripheral sympathetic and sensory neurons. NGF promotes survival, neurite extension and expression of transmitter-specific enzymes of cholinergic neurons growing in vivo or in vitro (Gahwiler et al., 1987; Gnahn et al., 1983;, Hefti et al., 1985; Honegger and Lenoir, 1982; Mobley et al., 1985). The expression of NGF and its mRNA correlate with the anatomical distribution of basal forebrain cholinergic neurons (Korsching et al., 1985; Shelton and Reichardt, 1986; Whittemore et al., 1986 and Large et al., 1986). During the entire life-span, forebrain cholinergic neurons express receptors for NGF (Hefti et al., 1986; Johnson et al., 1987; Richardson et al., 1986; Springer et al., 1987).

The findings that adult cholinergic neurons express receptors for NGF and that this population of cells degenerates in human Alzheimer's disease prompted us to study the effects of NGF in animals with experimental lesions of forebrain cholinergic neurons. NGF was given intraventricularly to adult rats with partial transections of the fimbria which result in a partial lesion of the septo-hippocampal cholinergic pathway. This pathway was chosen because it represents the best characterized part of the ascending cholinergic projections from the basal forebrain and because the axons are easily accessible for lesioning in the fimbria. Partial rather than complete lesions of this pathway were chosen to be able to study effects of NGF on neuronal cell bodies in the septum as well as effects on surviving axons in the hippocampus. Furthermore, partial lesions leave a natural bridge between septum and hippocampus through which severed axons might regenerate. Initial observations revealed that intraventricular injections of NGF to such animals elevate both, hippocampal and septal ChAT activity (Hefti et al., 1984; Will and Hefti, 1985). Based on these findings we investigated in detail the effects of NGF administration on cholinergic cell bodies in the septum and cholinergic axons in the hippocampus. This chapter provides a summary of these studies and emphasizes recent data showing that long-term NGF treatment permanently rescues cholinergic neurons from lesion-induced degeneration and promotes the regrowth of cholinergic fibers into the denervated hippocampus.

EXPERIMENTAL SYSTEM: RATS WITH PARTIAL FIMBRIAL TRANSECTIONS

The experimental system used was described in detail elsewhere (Hefti et al., 1985; Hefti, 1986). Briefly, the lateral two-thirds of the fimbria were transected in adult female rats using a specially designed knife. A cannula was then implanted in the lateral ventricle ipsilateral to the lesion and fixed permanently. The animals were injected through the cannula twice a week with 5 μg of 2.5S NGF (purified from mouse salivary glands) or an equal amount of cytochrome c (which has similar biochemical properties as NGF but no activity on NGF receptors and serves as a control protein) in a volume of 5 μl of phosphate buffered saline containing 15 mg/ml of gentamycin. The first injection of NGF or cytochrome c was normally given at the day of lesioning. At various times after the lesion, NGF treated and control animals were taken for immunohistochemical analysis. In the septum, cholinergic neurons were visualized using choline acetyltransferase (ChAT) immunohistochemistry or acetylcholinesterase (AChE) histochemistry after pretreatment with DFP. In the hippocampus, cholinergic fibers were visualized using AChE histochemistry or quantitative autoradiography of [3H] hemicholinium-3 binding sites.

The amount of NGF given to lesioned rats represents a maximal amount which was determined from the highest permissible viscosity of the solution used for injections through small cannulas. A maximal amount was chosen, because distribution characteristics of injected NGF and its final concentration in the septal or hippocampal area were not known and could not be easily determined. Dose-response relationships were established in culture systems, in which the concentration of NGF was easily controlled. NGF was found to affect forebrain cholinergic neurons in culture at concentrations similar to the reported affinity of NGF receptors (Hefti et al., 1985). This finding suggests that NGF affects forebrain cholinergic neurons in vivo at concentrations similar to those mediating the well-known actions on peripheral sympathetic and sensory neurons.

SURVIVAL OF CHOLINERGIC NEURONS IN SEPTUM

Partial transection of the fimbria results in the loss of approximately 50% of the cholinergic neurons in the medial septal nucleus and the vertical limb of the diagonal band of Broca. The number of ChAT- and AChE positive cells and of large Nissl stained cells declines gradually during the first two weeks after lesioning and remains at a constant level thereafter. This cell loss is prevented by chronic bi-weekly intraventricular injections of NGF (Hefti, 1986). In rats with unilateral fimbrial lesions, there was no significant difference in the number of cholinergic cell bodies between lesioned and control sides. Similar findings were obtained in animals with complete transection of the fimbria which resulted in a more pronounced loss of septal cholinergic neurons (Kromer, 1986; Williams et al., 1986).

Our findings strongly suggest that fimbrial transections result in degeneration of cholinergic neurons and that NGF is able to counteract this degenerative process. However, the studies did not rule out the possibility that the lesions only down-regulated the expression of cholinergic marker enzymes and resulted in shrinkage of these cells. In such a situation, NGF administration would be expected to stimulate the expression of cholinergic markers to levels above the threshold of visibility. To test for this possibility, we delayed the NGF treatment in lesioned animals by two weeks, i.e., until a time point at which the disappearance of cholinergic cells had reached its maximum. The delayed administration did not result in re-appearance of cholinergic cells. This finding indicates that fimbrial transections indeed result in degeneration of cholinergic neurons and that NGF is able to prevent this degeneration.

SURVIVAL OF CHOLINERGIC NEURONS

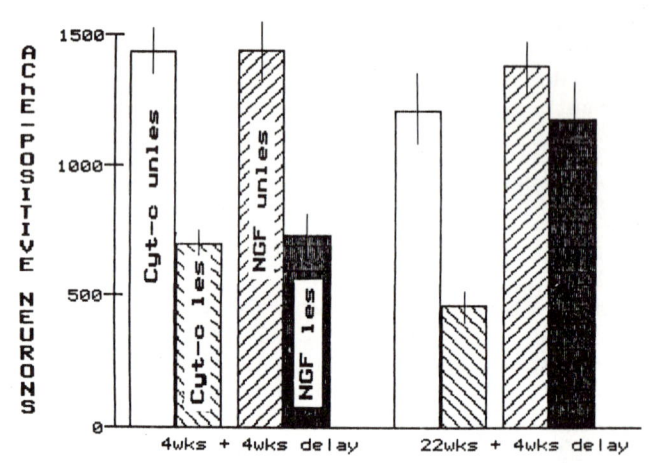

Figure 1. Permanent rescue of cholinergic cells in rats with partial fimbrial transections by long-term NGF treatment. The lateral two-thirds of the fimbria were transected unilaterally in adult rats. Animals then received chronic intraventricular injections of NGF (5µp twice weekly) or of a control protein. After 4 weeks or 22 weeks of treatment the rats were left without treatment for another period of 4 weeks and then taken for histochemical visualization of cholinergic neurons. Cholinergic cell bodies were counted in the medial septal nucleus and the vertical limb of the diagonal band of Broca. Bars indicate means ± S.E.M. of 6 rats. *Smaller than number measured on corresponding control sides ($p < 0.05$).

The protective effect of NGF most likely is due to a direct action of NGF on the cholinergic cells. Recently developed immunohistochemical methods, visualizing NGF receptors in rat and human brains, revealed that these receptors are exclusively located in cholinergic neurons (Hefti et al., 1986; Springer et al., 1987). After fimbrial transection in rats, NGF receptor positive cells disappear in parallel to the loss of ChAT positive neurons. This loss is prevented by injections of NGF. There is additional evidence in support of the view the effect of NGF is highly selective for cholinergic neurons. Septo-hippocampal GABAergic neurons degenerating after fimbrial transections are not rescued by NGF treatment. This is indicated by the fact that the number of glutamate decarboxylase (GAD) positive cells in the septum is reduced to an equal extent in NGF treated and lesioned control animals. Furthermore, intracerebral injections of NGF into rats with transections of the dopaminergic nigrostriatal pathway fail to promote the survival of dopaminergic neurons in the zona compacta of the substantia nigra.

During our initial studies, NGF was given bi-weekly during 4 weeks after lesioning. This chronic treatment was found to be necessary, since single injections of NGF at the day of lesioning or treatment during the first postoperational week were found to be ineffective. Furthermore, NGF treatment during 4 weeks was not able to permanently rescue the cholinergic neurons. When the injections were discontinued after 4 weeks and the animals were kept without treatment for another period of 4 weeks, there was a similar reduction in the number of cholinergic neurons in NGF treated and lesioned control animals (figure 1). In more recent studies, NGF treatment was continued for up to 22 weeks after lesioning. This long-term NGF treatment apparently was able to permanently rescue the cholinergic neurons in the medial septal nucleus and the diagonal band. No reduction in the number of cholinergic neurons was observed in lesioned rats receiving NGF during 22 weeks and left without NGF for another 4 weeks (figure 1).

GROWTH OF CHOLINERGIC FIBERS INTO DENERVATED HIPPOCAMPUS

Partial transections of the fimbria as performed in our studies result in a topographic and gradual reduction of the cholinergic innervation to the hippocampus. We earlier showed that the lesions decrease hippocampal ChAT activity and that this reduction progressively increases form the septal to the temporal pole of the hippocampus (Hefti et al., 1985). A similar progressive reduction was

HEMICHOLINIUM-3 BINDING SITES
[fmol/mg tissue]

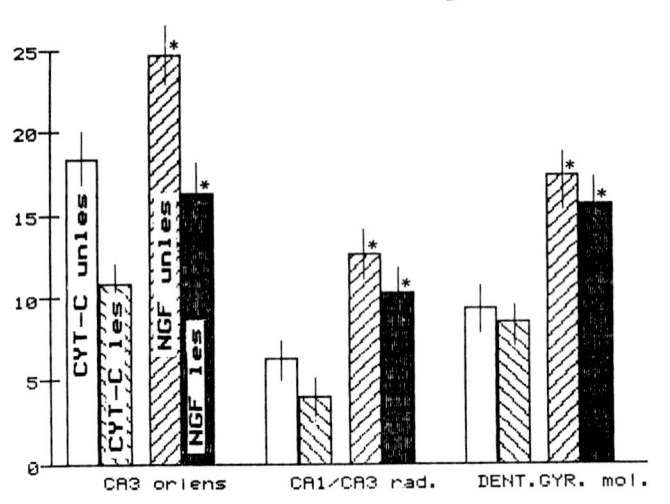

Figure 2: Effect of long-term NGF treatment on the density of cholinergic fibers in the hippocampus of rats with unilateral partial transections of the fimbria. Lesioned rats were treated during 22 weeks with NGF (5µg bi-weekly) or with a control protein. They were then taken for the visualization of [3H]hemicholinium-3 binding sites (a marker for cholinergic axons and terminals). Hippocampal sections were taken between antero-posterior levels A 3500 and A 4000 (Koenig and Klippel, 1963), i.e., at the level of the habenular nuclei. They were incubated with 7.5 nM of 3H-hemicholinium-3 and exposed to 3H-ultrafilm for quantitative autoradiography. Non specific binding was defined by the addition of 10 µM of unlabeled hemicholinium-3. Measurements were taken in the oriens layer of the CA3 region, the radiatum layer of the CA1/CA3 border region, and in the molecular layer of the dentate gyrus. Bars indicate means ± S.E.M. of 5 animals per group. *Significantly higher than corresponding value on lesioned sides of control animals (p<0.05).

found in the intensity of hippocampal AChE staining. NGF treatment of lesioned animals during 4 weeks elevated ChAT activity in the denervated hippocampus (Hefti et al., 1985). The magnitude of these increases depended on the extent of the lesion and was most pronounced near the temporal hippocampal pole, where the cholinergic denervation was maximal. Despite these elevations in biochemically measured ChAT activity, there was no difference in AChE staining intensity between NGF treated and lesioned control animals. These findings were taken to indicate that NGF treatment during 4 weeks stimulated ChAT expression in surviving cholinergic neurons but failed to promote regrowth of cholinergic neurites into the hippocampus.

In more recent studies, lesioned rats received chronic NGF treatment during 22 weeks. This long-term treatment resulted in a striking elevation of the density of cholinergic fibers in the denervated hippocampus. The difference between NGF treated and lesioned control animals was most pronounced at intermediate antero-posterior levels of the hippocampus (corresponding to the level of the habenular nuclei). At this level, staining intensity on lesioned sides of NGF treated rats was similar to that observed in unlesioned hippocampus, whereas strong reductions were seen on lesioned sides of rats treated with a control protein.

AChE is considered a specific marker for cholinergic neurons in the septal area (Levey et al., 1983). This fact and reductions after lesions suggest that AChE is a marker for hippocampal cholinergic fibers. However, intraventricular injections in rats with septal lesions result in growth of sympathetic noradrenergic fibers into the hippocampus (Crutcher and Davis, 1981). These neurons also express AChE. Therefore, to ascertain that the increase in hippocampal AChE staining intensity in NGF treated animals indeed reflected growth of cholinergic fibers, it was necessary to use a more selective marker for cholinergic fibers. We chose hemicholinium-3 binding site autoradiography, a method earlier shown to be a reliable marker for cholinergic axons and terminals in the central nervous system (Quirion et al., 1985; Rainbow et al., 1984, Vickroy et al., 1985). Furthermore, using this method it was possible to obtain a quantitative parameter reflecting the density of cholinergic fibers. In rats with unilateral partial fimbrial transections treated for 22 weeks with NGF, the number of [3H]-hemicholinium-3 binding sites on lesioned sides was higher than on lesioned sides of animals treated with a control protein (figure 2). In NGF treated rats, the number of binding sites on lesioned sides reached levels similar or higher than those measured on unlesioned sides of control animals. Furthermore, the number of binding sites on unlesioned sides of NGF treated animals was higher than that on unlesioned sides of control animals. These findings indicate that chronic long-term treatment promotes the regrowth of cholinergic fibers into the hippocampus denervated after fimbrial transections. Furthermore, long-term NGF treatment apparently is able to induce growth of cholinergic fibers in an intact hippocampus.

CONCLUSIONS

Our studies on rats with experimental lesions show that exogenously administered NGF is able to counteract lesion-induced degenerative changes of forebrain cholinergic neurons. Chronic intraventricular injections of NGF prevent the degeneration of cholinergic neurons in the septum and promote the regrowth of cholinergic fibers into the denervated hippocampus. NGF seems to affect cholinergic neurons not only after axonal transections as used in the present study but also after other types of lesions. Intraventricular NGF administration was reported to attenuate the reductiom of ChAT activity in the cortex induced by ibotenic acid-induced lesions in the nucleus basalis (Haroutunian et al., 1986). These findings suggest that application of NGF to the human brain might retard the age-related or disease-related degenerative changes of these cells. Cholinergic neurons are involved in functions related to memory and the forebrain cholinergic neurons have been implicated in the pathophysiology of Alzheimer's disease. The relationship between NGF, cholinergic neurons, and Alzheimer's disease was subject of a recent review (Hefti and Weiner, 1986).

Our findings not only show the effects of exogenously administered NGF but are also compatible with a role for endogenous NGF in the maintenance of the forebrain cholinergic neurons. According to this concept, adult cholinergic neurons are dependent upon the continuous supply of NGF provided by cells in their target areas. By depriving them of NGF, axonal transections result in retrograde degeneration of the cholinergic cells. This degeneration is prevented by exogenous NGF. Furthermore, by inducing regrowth of cholinergic axons into the hippocampus, NGF administration enables the severed cells to re-establish contact to their natural target cells. When the target is reached and sufficient quantities of endogenous NGF become again available, the cholinergic neurons survive independent of the exogenous source of the trophic factor.

REFERENCES

Crutcher KA, Davis JN (1981) Sympathetic noradrenergic sprouting in response to central cholinergic denervations. Trends Neurosci 4:70-72.
Gähwiler BH, Enz A, Hefti F, (1987) Nerve growth factor promotes development of the rat septo-hippocampal cholinergic projection in vitro. Neurosci Lett 75:6-10.
Gnahn H, Hefti F, Heumann R, Schwab M, Thoenen H (1983) NGF mediated increase of choline acetylgransferase (ChAT) in the neonatal forebrain; evidence for a physiological role of NGF in the brain? Dev Brain Res 9:45-52.
Haroutunian V, Kanof PD, Davis KL (1986) Partial reversal of lesion-induced deficits in cortical cholinergic markers by nerve growth factor. Brain Res 386:397-399.
Hefti F (1986) Nerve growth factor promotes survival of septal cholinergic neurons after fimbrial transections. J Neurosci 6:2155-2162.
Hefti F, Weiner WJ (1986) Nerve growth factor and Alzheimer's disease. Ann Neurol 20:275-281.
Hefti F, Dravid A, Hartikka J (1984) Chronic intraventricular injections of nerve growth factor elevate hippocampal choline acetyltransferase activity in adult rats with partial septo-hippocampal lesions. Brain Res 293:305-309.
Hefti F, Hartikka J, Eckenstein F, Gnahn H, Heumann R, Schwab M (1985) Nerve growth factor (NGF) increases choline acetyltransferase but not survival of fiber growth of cultured septal cholinergic neurons. Neuroscience 14:55-68.
Hefti F, Hartikka J, Salvatierra A, Weiner WJ Mash DC (1986) Localization of nerve growth factor receptors in cholinergic neurons of the human basal forebrain. Neurosci Lett 69:37-41.
Honegger P, Lenoir D (1982) Nerve growth factor (NGF) stimulation of cholinergic telencephalic neurons in aggregating cell cultures. Dev Brain Res 3:229-238.

Johnson EM, Taniuchi M, Clark HB, Springer JE, Koh S, Tayren MW, Loy R (1987) Demonstration of the retrograde transport of nerve growth factor in the peripheral and central nervous system. J Neurosci 7:923-929.

Koenig JFR, Klippel RA (1963) "The Rat Brain", Baltimore: Williams and Wilkins.

Korsching S, Auburger S, Heumann R, Scott J, Thoenen H (1985) Levels of nerve growth factor and its mRNA in the central nervous system of the rat correlate with cholinergic innervation. EMBO J 4:1389-1393.

Kromer LF (1986) Nerve growth factor treatment after brain injury prevents neuronal death. Science 235:214-216.

Large TH, Bodary SC, Legg DO, Weskamp G, Otten U, Reichardt LF (1986) Nerve growth factor gene expression in the developing rat brain. Science 234:352-355.

Levey AI, Wainer BH, Mufson EJ, Mesulam MM (1983) Co-localization of acetylcholinesterase and choline acetyltransferase in the rat cerebrum. Neuroscience 9:9-22.

Mesulam MM, Mufson EJ, Wainer BH, Levey AI (1983) Central cholinergic pathways in the rat: an overview based on an alternative momenclature (Ch1-Ch6). Neuroscience 10:1185-1201.

Mobley WC, Rutkowski JL, Tennekoon GI, Buchanan K, Johnston MV (1985) Choline acetyltransferase activity in striatum of neonatal rats increased by nerve growth factor. Science 229:284-286.

Quirion R (1985) Comparative localization of putative pre- and postsynaptic markers of muscarinic cholinergic nerve terminals in rat brain. Europ J Pharmacol 111:287-289.

Rainbow TC, Parsons B, Wieczorek CM (1984) Quantitative autoradiography of [3H] hemicholinium binding sites in rat brain. Europ J Pharmacol 102:195-196.

Richardson PM, Verge Issa VMK, Riopelle RJ (1986) Distribution of neuronal receptors for nerve growth factor in the rat. J Neurosci 6:2312-2321.

Shelton DL, Reichardt LF (1986) Studies on the expression of the β nerve growth factor (NGF) gene in the central nervous system: level and regional distribution of NGF mRNA suggest that NGF functions as a trophic factor for several distinct populations of neurons. Proc Natl Acad Sci USA 83:2714-2718.

Springer JE, Koh S, Tayrien MW, Loy R (1987) Basal forebrain magnocellular neurons stain for nerve growth factor receptor: correlation with cholinergic cell bodies and effects of axotomy. J Neurosci Res 17:11-118.

Vickroy TW, Roeske WR, Gehlert DR, Wamsley JK, Yamamura HI

(1985) Quantitative light microscopic autoradiography of [3H]hemicholinium binding sites in the rat central nervous system: a novel biochemical marker for mapping the distribution of cholinergic nerve terminals. Brain Res 329:368-373.
Whittemore SR, Ebendal T, Larkfors L, Olson L, Seiger A, Sromberg I, Persson H (1986) Developmental and regional expression of β nerve growth factor mRNA and protein in the rat central nervous system. Proc Natl Acad Sci USA 83:817-821.
Will B, Hefti F (1985) Behavioral and neurochemical effects of chronic intraventricular injections of nerve growth factor in adult rats with fimbria lesions. Behav Brain Res 17:17-24.
Williams LR, Varon S, Peterson GM, Wictorin K, Fischer W, Bjorklund A, Gage FH (1986) Continuous infusion of nerve growth factor prevents basal forebrain neuronal death after fimbria fornix transection. Proc Natl Acad Sci USA 83:9231-9235.

Acknowledgments. The study was supported by NIH grant NS22933 and grants from the Alzheimer's Disease and Related Disorders Association, Chicago IL (P-85-004) and the National Parkinson Foundation, Miami, FL.

EXTRACELLULAR MATRIX AND CELL SURFACE INTERACTIONS

EXTRACELLULAR MATRIX AND CELL SURFACE INTERACTIONS

Louis F. Reichardt

Department of Physiology and
Howard Hughes Medical Institute
University of California, U426
San Francisco, California 94143-0724

After axotomy, regeneration in the central nervous system (CNS) is minimal. Instead, axons grow for only short distances; axotomized neurons often die; and there is little or no recovery of function. In contrast, the consequences of nerve transection in the peripheral nervous system (PNS) are much more reversible. Axotomized neurons receive trophic support that enables them to survive during the time span that they lack contact with their targets. The neurons can also regenerate for long distances with significant or total recovery of target contacts and function. Many of the differences between regeneration in the CNS and PNS appear to reflect differences in the tissue microenvironment in which neurons regenerate, not differences between central and peripheral neurons (Aguayo et al., 1987). First, axotomized central neurons can extend axons for long distances in living grafts of peripheral nerve. Second, the axons of peripheral neurons invade peripheral, but not central nerve explants (Caroni and Schwab, 1988). Successful regeneration in the PNS has been attributed to the presence of trophic factors and favorable substrates for axonal growth. The failure of regeneration in the CNS may reflect, in part, absence of trophic factors or favorable substrates. It also appears to reflect unfavorable consequences of reactive gliosis (Reier et al., 1983; Houle and Reier, 1988; Smith et al., 1986; Whittemore et al., 1985) and the presence in the CNS of oligodendrocyte-derived glycoproteins that inhibit axonal growth (Schwab and Caroni, 1988). Reports in this section focus on the surface and secreted molecules of non-neuronal cells in the PNS that enable neurons to survive and regenerate after nerve injury.

Work in the past few years has suggested that efficient regeneration in peripheral nerves reflects a number of responses by non-neuronal cells that act synergistically to promote regeneration. Non-neural cells in peripheral nerve have been shown to respond to denervation with dramatic increases in synthesis of Nerve Growth Factor (NGF). Most of this increase requires

Subfamilies:

β_1

β_1
(110/130 kD)
NR/R

CSAT Band 3
FNR β
PC12 120 kD
Platelet IIa
VLA β

		Heterodimer Common Name
α_1 (200/210 kD) NR/R		VLA1
α_2 (150/165 kD) NR/R		VLA2 platelet Ia/IIa
α_3 (150/135 kD) NR/R		VLA3 CSAT Bands 2/3
α_4 (140/150 kD) NR/R		VLA4
α_5 (150/135 kD) NR/R		VLA5 FNR

β_2

β_2
(95 kD)

	Heterodimer Common Name
α_6 (170 kD)	LFA-1 (mouse) OKM-1 (human)
α_7 (180 kD)	Mac-1 (mouse) Mo-1 (human)
α_8 (150 kD)	p150/95 (mouse)

β_3

β_3
(95/110 kD)
NR/R

Platelet IIIa

	Heterodimer Common Name
α_9 (136/125, 23 kD) NR/R	Platelet IIb/IIIa
α_{10} (150/125, 25 kD) NR/R	Human VNR

Other: Drosophila Position-Specific Antigens (PSA)

Figure 1. Integrin family of adhesive protein receptor heterodimers. Each receptor consists of two non-covalently associated subunits - one α one β. The β subunits (β_1, β_2 and β_3) define different subfamilies. Within these subfamilies, ligand specificity depends on the particular α subunit which is associated with a given β subunit. Receptors in the β_1 subfamily mediate attachment to laminin, fibronectin, and collagen IV (Hall et al., 1987). Figure is adapted from Hynes (1987).

Extracellular and Surface Interactions / 121

infiltration of macrophages and is caused by secretion of interleukin-1 (Lindholm et al., 1987). As living cells are required in peripheral nerve grafts for efficient regeneration (Anderson and Turmaine, 1986), this suggests that increased trophic factor synthesis in peripheral nerves acts to promote neuronal survival, which is a prerequisite for successful regeneration. In this section, Johnson and colleagues present their interesting observations on the synthesis of the NGF receptor by Schwann cells in culture and in denervated peripheral nerve in vivo. Denervation is shown to induce synthesis of a low affinity form of the NGF receptor whose major role may be to bind NGF for subsequent use by neurons. The affinity of NGF for the Schwann cell NGF receptor is low compared to its affinity for high affinity NGF receptor that is present on neurons. Thus, NGF bound on the surface of Schwann cells is expected to be accessible to regenerating growth cones. Neurons that are not dependent on NGF also regenerate successfully in peripheral nerves. This suggests that Schwann cells may also synthesize other trophic factors and their receptors. In turn, these would act to promote survival and regeneration of non-NGF-dependent neurons by similar mechanisms.

Growth cones in regenerating peripheral nerves contact both Schwann cell surfaces and the surrounding channels of basal lamina, which contain laminin, a potent promoter of neuritic outgrowth. Axonal growth over Schwann cell surfaces has been shown to depend on interactions with both basal lamina glycoproteins and Schwann cell surface-associated cell adhesion molecules (Tomaselli et al., 1986; Bixby et al., 1988; Seilheimer and Schachner, 1988). In particular, laminin has been identified as a significant promoter of regeneration in vivo (Sandrock and Matthew, 1987). In this section, Letourneau and colleagues present the most direct evidence implying that the major receptor for laminin that promotes growth cone motility is a member of the family of integrin class extracellular matrix receptors (see Fig. 1). The function of this class of heterodimeric glycoprotein receptors has previously been shown to be required for virtually all adhesive interactions between neurons and the extracellular matrix (see Fig. 2; Tomaselli et al., 1986; Hall et al., 1987; Ruoslahti and Pierschbacher, 1987). Carbonetto and colleagues discuss the isolation from brain of several putative non-integrin class receptors for laminin. They present convincing evidence that at least one of these receptors with an Mr of 180-200k functions to promote neurite outgrowth on laminin (see also Kleinman et al., 1988). The cell adhesion molecules L1/NgCAM, N-cadherin, and N-CAM are present on both neurons and Schwann cells. They have important roles in promoting growth cone motility on Schwann cell surfaces in vitro (see Fig. 3) and are consequently strong candidates to promote regeneration in peripheral nerves in vivo (Bixby et al., 1988; Seilheimer and Schachner, 1988). The roles of individual cell adhesion molecules is discussed by Schachner and colleagues in a separate section of this book (see also Jessell, 1988, for review of cell adhesion molecules).

During regeneration, growth cones must penetrate tissues and one reason for the failure of regeneration in the CNS may be the establishment of physical barriers, including basal lamina proteins, during reactive gliosis (Smith et al., 1986). Cultured neurons release proteases which probably facilitate the invasion of growth cones into tissues (Pittman, 1985). In addition, glia have been shown to secrete protease nexins (Rosenblatt et al., 1987), which probably regulate the activities of these proteases. Proteases and their nexins are likely to have important influences on the abilities of neuronal growth cones to penetrate extracellular matrices, glial scars, and other environments encountered by neurons during regeneration. In this section, Monard and colleagues discuss their fascinating results on a glial derived neurite promoting factor, which has been shown to be a potent serine protease, viz., nexin. They suggest a relationship between the distribution of this nexin and ability of particular nerves, such as the olfactory nerve, to be favorable substrates for regeneration.

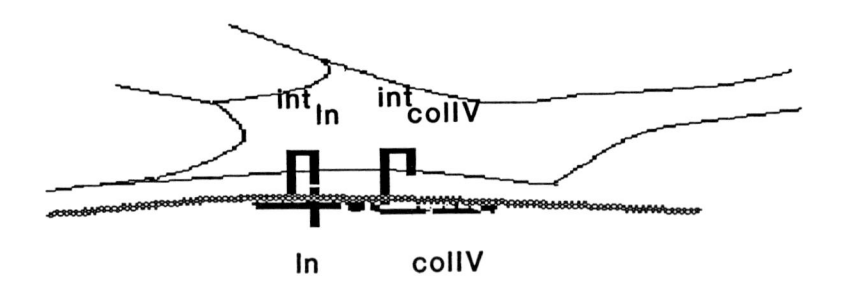

e8 CG on extracellular matrix

Figure 2. Model for growth cone interactions with an extracellular matrix. Different integrin heterodimers present on embryonic day 8 ciliary ganglion neurons (e8 CG) are shown mediating attachment to different extracellular matrix glycoproteins.

Successful regeneration requires re-establishment of synaptic contacts with targets. The model system for identifying molecules important in directing synapse formation has been the neuromuscular junction (e.g., Nitkin et al., 1987). In this section, Yao and colleagues describe their very interesting findings that have resulted in the identification of a glycoprotein that appears to be synthesized by motoneurons and secreted at nerve terminals, where it may induce the accumulation of acetylcholine receptor and acetylcholinesterase in the muscle plasmalemma and synaptic basal lamina.

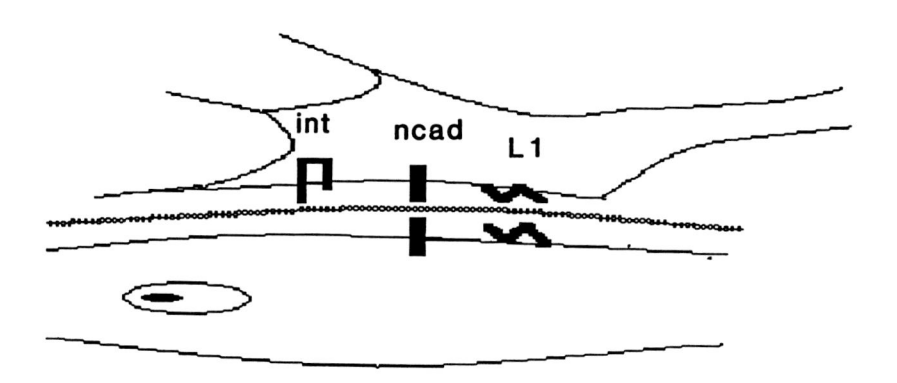

e8 CG / Schwann Cell

Figure 3. Model for growth cone interactions with Schwann cells. A growth cone of an embryonic day 8 ciliary ganglion neuron (e8 CG) is shown with receptors that bind independently to proteins in the extracellular matrix and on the cell surface. Neuronal integrin class receptors (int) are shown binding to the basal lamina secreted by Schwann cells (known constituents include laminin and collagen IV). Two neuronal cell adhesion molecules, N-cadherin (Ncad) and L1, are shown binding to homologues on the Schwann cell plasma membrane. Adapted from Bixby et al, (1988).

While there has been dramatic progress in identifying molecules that are candidates to direct initial development and regeneration of the nervous system, it is not yet clear how their influences yield the final pattern of any individual neuron or nerve tract. The most promising systems for doing this are found in invertebrates, such as nematodes, insects and leeches, and in at least one vertebrate, the zebra fish (White, 1985; Lefcort and Bentley, 1987; Westerfield and Eisen, 1988). Illustrating one of these, Nardi describes development of the normal neural pattern in an insect wing--an elegant preparation where a variety of perturbation techniques can be applied to test specific hypotheses.

ACKNOWLEDGMENTS

I thank Kevin Tomaselli for contributing Figure 1. I thank Kevin Tomaselli, Deborah Hall, John Bixby, Mike Ignatius, Karla Neugebauer, and Heidi Gaspary for stimulating conversations that contributed to this article. I am an investigator of the Howard Hughes Medical Institute.

REFERENCES

Aguayo AJ, Vidal-Sanz M, Villegas-Perez MP, Bray GM (1987). Growth and connectivity of axotomized retinal neurons in adult rats with optic nerves substituted by PNS grafts linking the eye and midbrain. Ann NY Acad Sci 495:1-9.

Anderson P, Turmaine M (1986). Peripheral nerve regeneration through grafts of living and freeze-dried CNS. Neuropath and Appl Neurobiol 12:389-399.

Bixby JL, Lilien J, Reichardt LF (1988). Identification of the major proteins that promote neuronal process outgrowth on Schwann cells in vitro. J Cell Biol, In Press.

Caroni P, Schwab E (1988). Antibody against myelin-derived, membrane-bound inhibitor of neurite growth neutralized CNS white matter non-permissive substrate properties. Neuron 1:85-96.

Hall DE, Neugebauer KM, Reichardt LF (1987). Embryonic neural retinal cell response to extracellular matrix proteins: developmental changes and effects of the cell substratum attachment antibody (CSAT). J Cell Biol 104:623-634.

Houle JD, Reier PJ (1988). Transplantation of fetal spinal cord tissue into the chronically injured adult rat spinal cord. J Comp Neurol 269:535-547.

Hynes RO (1987). Integrins: a family of cell surface receptors. Cell 48:549-554.

Jessell TM (1988). Adhesion molecules and the hierarchy of neural development. Neuron 1:3-13.

Kleinman HK, Ogle RL, Cannon FB, Little CD, Sweeny TM, Luckenbill-Edds L (1988). Laminin receptors for neurite formation. Proc Natl Acad Sci USA 85:1282-1286.

Lefcort F, Bentley D (1987). Pathfinding by pioneer neurons isolated, opened and mesoderm-free limb buds of embryonic grasshoppers. Develop Biol 119:466-480.

Lindholm D, Heumann R, Meyer M, Thoenen H (1987). Interleukin-1 regulated Nerve Growth Factor (NGF) synthesis in the non-neuronal cells of the rat sciatic nerve. Nature (Lond.) 330:658-659.

Nitkin RM, Smith MA, Magill C, Fallon JR, Yao Y-MM, Wallace BG, McMahan UJ (1987). Identification of agrin, a synaptic organizing protein from Torpedo electric organ. J Cell Biol 105:2471-2478.

Pittman RN (1985). Release of plasminogen activator and a calcium-dependent metalloprotease from cultured sympathetic and sensory neurons. Develop Biol 110:91-101.

Reier PJ, Stensaas LJ, Guth L (1983). The astrocytic scar as an impediment to regeneration in the central nervous system. In Kao CC, Bunge RP, Reier PJ (eds): "Spinal Cord Reconstruction." New York: Raven Press, pp 163-196.

Rosenblatt DE, Cotman CW, Nieto-Sampedro M, Rowe JW, Knauer DJ (1987). Identification of a protease inhibitor produced by astrocytes that is structurally and functionally homologous to human protease nexin I. Brain Res 415:40-48.

Ruoslahti E, Pierschbacher MD (1987). New perspectives in cell adhesion: RGD and integrins. Science 238:491-497.

Sandrock AW, Matthew WD (1987). An in vitro neurite-promoting antigen functions in axonal regeneration in vivo. Science 237:1605-1608.

Schwab ME, Caroni P (1988). Oligodendrocytes and CNS myelin are non-permissive substrates for neurite growth and fibroblast spreading in vitro. J Neurosci, In Press.

Seilheimer B, Schachner M (1988). Studies of adhesion molecules mediating interactions between cells of peripheral nervous system indicate a major role for L1 in mediating sensory neuron growth on Schwann cells. J Cell Biol, In Press.

Smith G, Miller R, Silver J (1986). Changing role of forebrain astrocytes during development, regenerative failure and induced regeneration upon transplantation. J Comp Neurol 251:23-43.

Tomaselli KJ, Reichardt LF, Bixby JL (1986). Distinct molecular interactions mediate neuronal process outgrowth on extracellular matrices and non-neuronal cell surfaces. J Cell Biol 103:2659-2672.

Westerfield M, Eisen JS (1988). Neuromuscular specificity: pathfinding by identified motor growth cones in a vertebrate embryo. TINS 11:18-22.

White JG (1985). Neuronal connectivity in Caenorhabditis elegans. TINS 8:277-283.

Whittmore S, Nieto-Sampedro M, Needeles D, Cotman C (1985). Neuronotrophic factors for mammalian brain neurons: injury induction in neonatal, adult and aged rat brain. Develop Brain Res 20:169-178.

ESTABLISHMENT OF A TWO-DIMENSIONAL NEURAL NETWORK IN AN
INSECT WING

James B. Nardi

Department of Entomology
University of Illinois
Urbana, Illinois 61801

INTRODUCTION

   The neurons in the wing of an insect form a two-
dimensional network nestled in the space between two epithelial monolayers. All these neurons are sensory, and
their axons grow in a distal to proximal direction over
the basal surface of the upper epithelial monolayer. Certain
properties of the pathways for axonal growth in the insect
wing have suggested that the epithelial substratum may
guide this well-defined directionality of axonal growth.
To impart directional information to axons, each of these
pathways must have an asymmetry to which axons can respond.

ORGANIZATION OF THE SUBSTRATUM FOR AXONAL GROWTH

   Information about the organization of the epithelial
substratum traversed by sensory neurons in the wing of the
insect, Manduca sexta, first came from a series of trans-
positions of epithelial squares. On the apical surface of
the pupal wing, a stiff cuticle is secreted that provides
a rigid support for transposition of small populations of
cells from the upper epithelial monolayer. The interaction of transposed cells with new environments along the
length of the wing has suggested that certain properties
of wing epithelial cells are not uniformly distributed
within the wing: the greater the distance separating host
and graft cell populations along the proximodistal (PD)
axis of the wing, the more circular and constricted the
interface between graft and host cells. This observation

prompted the hypothesis that the surfaces of epithelial cells have graded, position-specific differences in their affinities for one another. As differences in affinity increase, the extent of cellular contact between graft and host decreases, resulting in the epithelial configurations that are observed (Fig. 1A). (Nardi and Kafatos, 1976 a,b).

Two additional experiments support the hypothesis that the graded response of wing epithelial squares to transposition along the PD axis of the wing arises from graded differences in cellular affinity.

In one of these experiments, three different epithelial populations were simultaneously juxtaposed (Fig. 1B). From the configurations that resulted, two possible hierarchies of affinity could be infered: either Ip > IVa > VIIa or VIIa > IVa > Ip.

In the other experiment, binary combinations of the same three epithelial populations were transposed to leg epithelium (Fig. 1C). In this host environment, the square pieces of wing epithelium are not miscible with leg cells. The wing monolayers eliminate their free edges by forming hollow vesicles. Two grafts from the same wing region always join to form a single vesicle without any obvious discontinuity at their interface. Although two grafts from different wing regions always join to form a single vesicle, a marked constriction forms at the interface of the two grafts. The width of this constriction decreases as the distance separating the two grafts along the PD axis increases.

While results from all these sets of experiments imply that cell surface properties are graded along the length of the wing, from none of these experiments (Fig. 1) can a choice be made between the two possible affinity hierarchies: Ip > IVa > VIIa or VIIa > IVa > Ip.

However, the behavior of cells within Ip and VIIa grafts following their exchange suggests that the former hierarchy is the correct one. The peripheries of both grafts circularize in their new environments; but only Ip grafts show rearrangement of cells from the proximalmost periphery to the interior, as expected if the affinity hierarchy is proximalmost Ip > distal Ip > VIIa. Neither the proximalmost nor distalmost cells of the VIIa graft undergo such a rearrangement (Nardi and Kafatos, 1976b).

A. Pupal Transposition — Adult Phenotype — Conclusion

Ip control
IVa control
VIIa control

Ip ↔ IVa

The response to transposition is graded. Homotypic contacts among cells increase at the expense of heterotypic contacts as grafts are further displaced from their original sites.

Ip ↔ VIIa

B.

Ip and VIIa at IVa

Ip and IVa at VIIa

IVa and VIIa at Ip

Region IVa engulfs Ip and VIIa: but neither Ip nor VIIa engulf each other. The affinity hierarchy is either: Ip>IVa>VIIa or VIIa>IVa>Ip.

C.

Six binary combinations of Ip, IVa, VIIa

leg

Ip-Ip   Ip-VIIa
IVa-IVa Ip-IVa
VIIa-VIIa IVa-VIIa

Differences in cell affinities for two regions increase with distance separating them on the proximodistal axis.

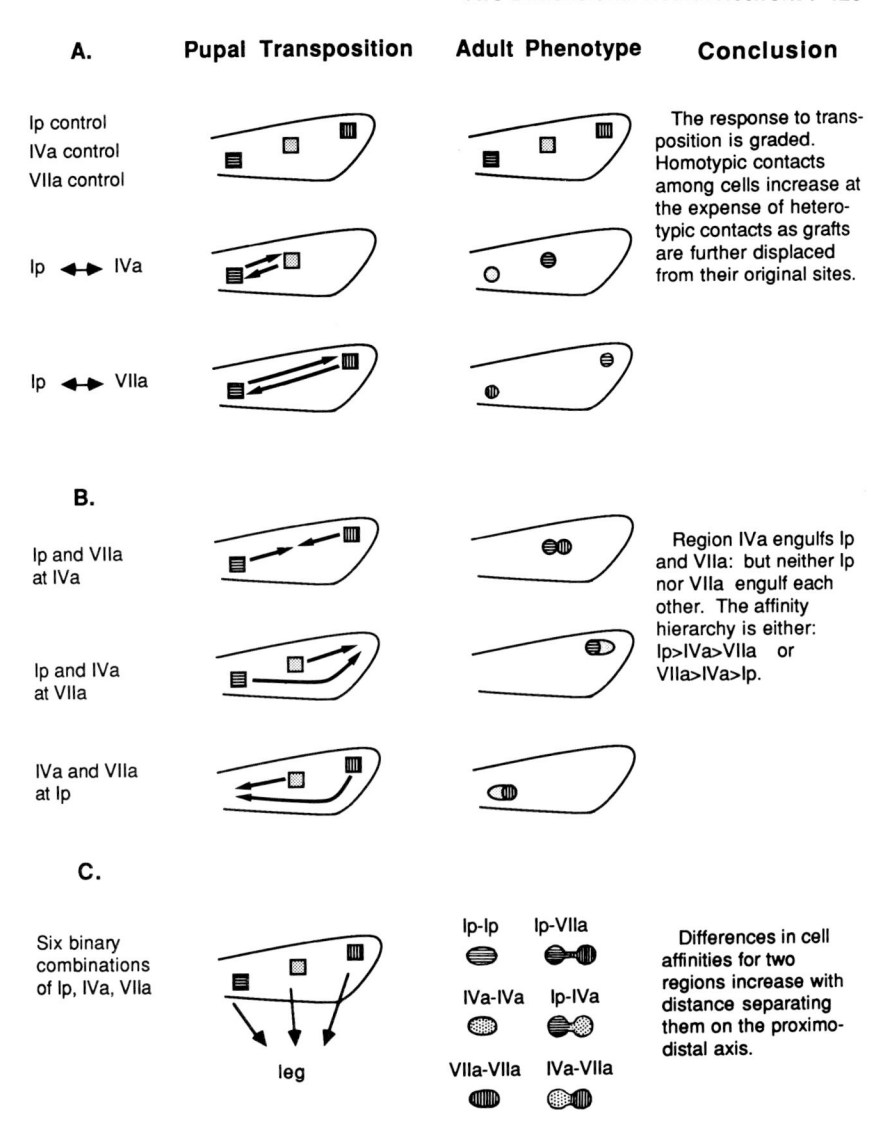

Figure 1. Schematic representation of three grafting experiments (A,B,C) with pupal wing epithelium which support the hypothesis that cellular affinities are graded along the PD axis of the wing. Grafts (Ip, IVa, VIIa) are indicated respectively with horizontal lines, stippling, and vertical lines. Wings are not drawn to scale; adult wings are larger than pupal wings.

RESPONSE OF REGENERATING AXONS TO CHANGES IN THEIR EPITHELIAL SUBSTRATUM

With this knowledge about the adhesive organization of the epithelial substratum for axonal growth, experiments were planned to test how regenerating axons respond to changes in the affinity of the terrain over which they move. Work with neurons and other cells in vitro had shown that cells move from less adhesive substrata to more adhesive substrata (Letourneau, 1982), but similar cellular behavior had been difficult to demonstrate in situ.

Grafts of epithelial cells were removed and transposed to ectopic locations in the upper monolayer of the pupal wing. Regeneration of cut axons at the distal edge of each graft-host interface was then examined in wing whole mounts stained with methylene blue. Axonal outgrowth not only proceeded in the normal distal to proximal direction across control grafts but also across grafts that had been transposed distally. Only upon encountering grafts that had been transposed proximally did regenerating axons halt in their outgrowth or bypass the ectopic graft (Nardi, 1983).

This asymmetric response of regenerating axons to perturbation of their substratum implies that some feature(s) of the epithelial substratum is also asymmetric. Not only is a feature(s) of the epithelial substratum asymmetric but the same or another feature is also graded, as has already been suggested by other experiments (Fig. 1). The graded, axial differences in cellular affinity may be the epithelial asymmetry to which regenerating axons respond.

Regenerating axons are always closely apposed to the basal lamina of the upper epithelial monolayer. Examination of the wing's basal lamina with scanning electron microscopy reveals that components of the basal lamina are not only oriented along the PD axis but are also graded along this axis (Nardi, 1983). Both this graded distribution of extracellular matrix as well as graded affinity properties on surfaces of epithelial cells could provide directional cues for regenerating axons.

GUIDANCE OF PIONEERING NEURONS

The gradients associated with the epithelial monolayer--

cellular as well as extracellular--may both guide regenerating axons along the PD axis of the moth wing; but only one of these factors is evidently involved in guiding the initial outgrowth of pioneering neurons at an earlier stage of development. A basal lamina is absent from the epithelial monolayer of the wing at the time that pioneering neurons first appear on day 5 of the last larval stadium (i.e., 4 days before the regeneration of axons was studied); this environment for pioneering neurons is qualitatively different from the environment encountered by regenerating axons (Nardi et al., 1985).

Pioneering neurons of the wing imaginal disc grow along preestablished, relatively wide (~100µm) channels known as lacunae (Figs. 2 and 3) between days 5 and 6 of the last larval stadium. Most lacunae are occupied by a few guidepost neurons during axonal growth; however, no guidepost neurons exist along the entire length (800µm) of the lacuna (IVa5) that has been most extensively examined in this study. Obviously, guidepost neurons do not provide critical guidance cues for axons of this lacuna.

Between day 5 and day 6, numerous cellular events in addition to neuronal growth occur within the lacunae of this very dynamic tissue. Tracheole cells move through the lacunae of the wing in a proximal to distal direction--exactly the opposite direction in which pioneering axons move. Epithelial cells extend basal processes into the lacunae; and it appears that these processes exert traction on tracheole cells and control their final distribution within wing tissue. In contrast to the active movement of axons, the movement of tracheoles is passive and is nearing completion as axonal growth is beginning (Nardi et al., 1985).

By separating the two epithelial monolayers during the period of axonal and tracheolar migration, the surfaces of entire neuronal pathways can be examined for asymmetries in physical cues as well as molecular cues. During the surgical separation of monolayers, tracheae and tracheoles segregate with the lower monolayer while neurons segregate with the upper monolayer.

Between days 4 and 5 before neurons are observed in the wing, the basal surface of the upper monolayer is densely and uniformly covered with long basal processes (Fig. 4).

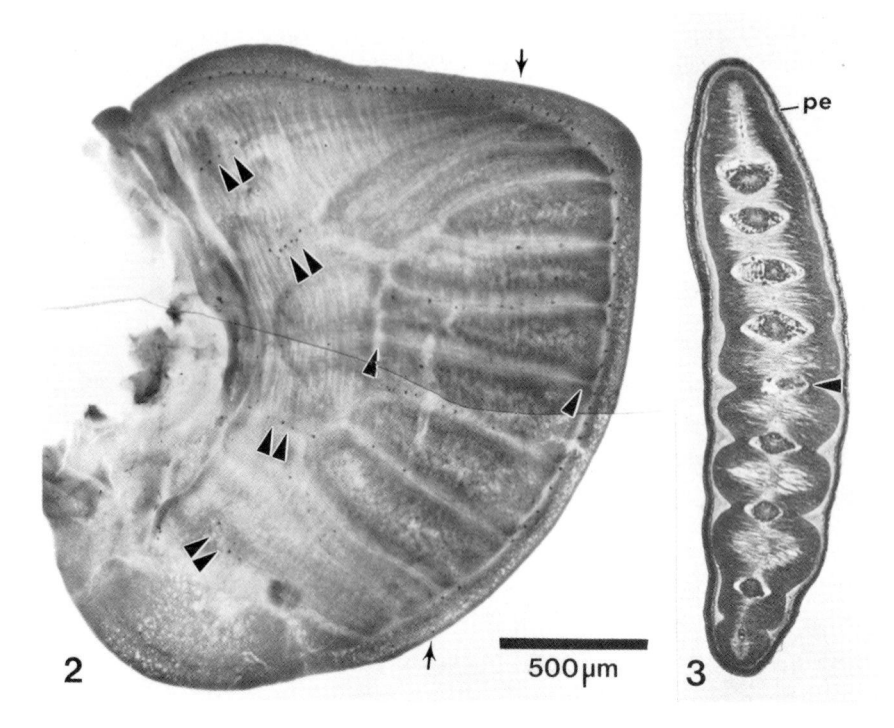

Figure 2. Whole mount of a day 5 + 6 hr wing disc in which an antibody to horseradish peroxidase has been used to mark sensory neurons (Jan and Jan, 1982). Most of the approximately 90 pioneering neurons are located along the periphery of the disc, but a few are located in interior positions, such as those marked by double arrowheads. Pathfinding of peripheral neurons was most extensively examined along lacunar channel IVa5, whose proximal and distal extremes are indicated with single arrowheads. Proximal is to left; anterior is at top. Dorsal surface is up.

Figure 3. Section of day 5 + 6 hr wing disc cut along the plane indicated by arrows in Fig. 2. Lacuna IVa5 is marked with an arrowhead. At this developmental stage the wing blade is enveloped by a peripodial epithelium (pe). Dorsal is to right; anterior is at top. Magnification is same as that for Fig. 2.

These processes shorten as tracheole migration concludes and as neurons begin to appear after day 5. From an examination of over 200 wing discs between day 5 and day 6, some general features of axonal growth have been noted. As axons grow proximally, the density of basal processes decreases in their wake and a basal lamina is laid down in a distal to proximal wave shortly after the axons have passed. At the advancing end of the axon, growth is evidently oriented by a channel formed by basal processes (Fig. 5). Between days 5 and 6 as axons traverse the wing, a graded distribution of epithelial processes is evident along the PD axes of neural pathways that only hours earlier showed no such asymmetry (Figs. 6-9). By day 6 a basal lamina has been laid down along the entire length of each pathway.

While directional cues seem to reside in the epithelial monolayer of the wing, these cues may take one or more forms. The physical configuration of the epithelial substratum has a graded organization that alone could be responsible for the directional growth of pioneering axons. In addition to, or in place of, topographic cues, the distribution of molecules on the basal surface of the epithelium may impart directional information to pioneering growth cones. This latter possibility is currently being investigated using an immunological approach.

GENERALITY OF AXONAL GUIDANCE BY BASAL SURFACES OF EPITHELIAL CELLS

Lefcourt and Bentley (1987) have shown that growth cones of pioneering neurons in limb buds of grasshopper embryos also seem to be guided by a proximally increasing gradient of affinity. The neuronal substratum in embryonic limbs of grasshoppers consists of both mesodermal and epidermal epithelial cells. By eliminating the mesodermal component from cultured limbs, these authors demonstrated that growth cones can still extend with the proper directionality. If a proximally increasing gradient of affinity is crucial for neuronal guidance, then this gradient apparently resides in the limb epithelium.

In *Drosophila* and *Manduca* wing discs where mesodermal cells are not present, neuronal guidance also occurs independently of mesodermal cells.

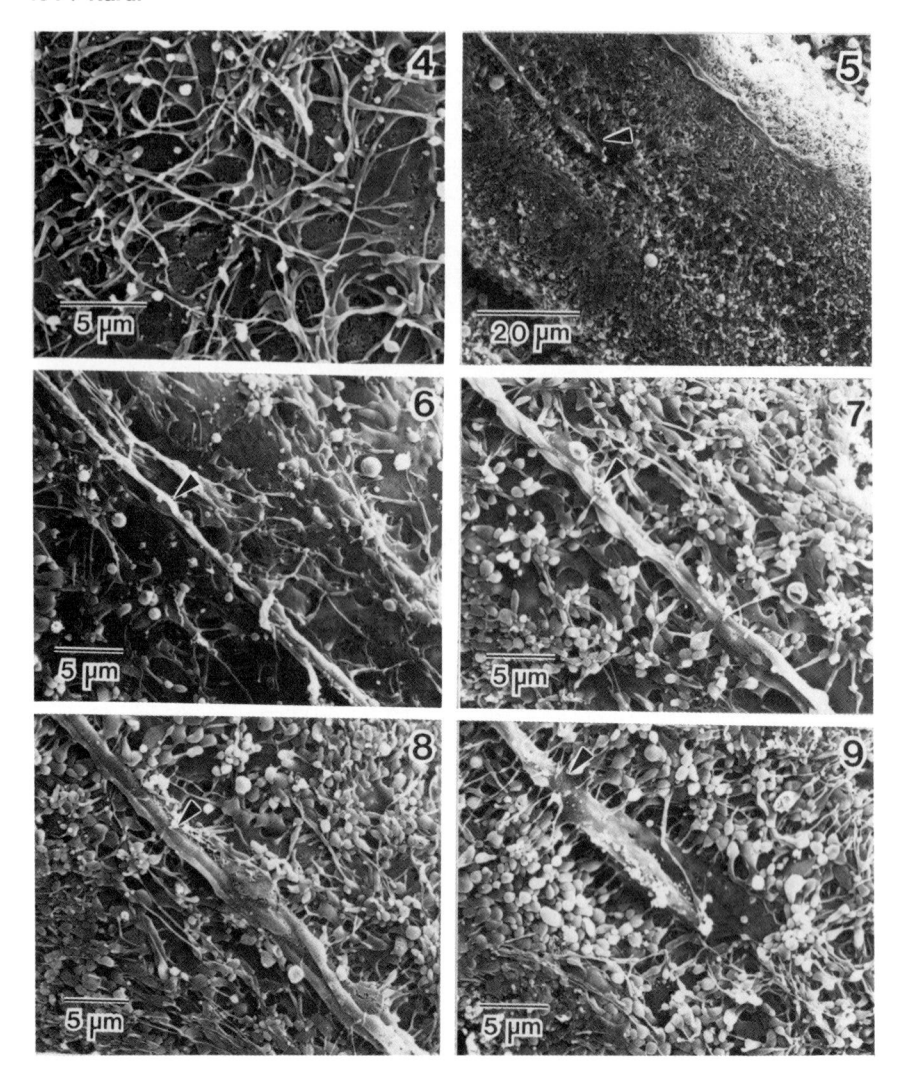

Figures 4–9. Surface views of epithelial substratum traversed by pioneering axons in lacuna IVa5. Arrowheads indicate axons in each figure. Distal to proximal = upper left to lower right. Figure 4 shows basal processes on day 5 before axonal outgrowth. Figure 5 shows a growth cone (arrowhead) on day 5 + 12 hr and the terrain proximal to it. Figures 6–9 represent a distal to proximal progression along the axon of this growth cone with 30 µm intervals separating consecutive figures.

Additional support for the claim that pathfinding cues reside in epidermal epithelia of insect appendages comes from a consideration of the role of other possible guidance factors such as guidepost neurons, diffusion gradients established by localized sources, and axial electrical fields. By eliminating these factors in cultures of embryonic insect limbs and wing discs, these cues have been demonstrated to be nonessential for guiding the growth of pioneering neurons (Blair et al., 1985; Palka, 1986; Lefcourt and Bentley, 1987).

Likewise, guidance cues for vertebrate growth cones seem to be localized on endfeet of epithelial cells. Pioneering growth cones in the embryonic fish spinal cord contact cell bodies of other neurons as well as basal processes of neuroepithelial cells; but ablation of the other neurons does not alter the route followed by pioneering neurons. Guidance by other neuronal surfaces is not critical for these pioneering neurons; whatever guidance cues are essential for them apparently are provided by endfeet of neuroepithelial cells (Kuwada, 1986). During regeneration as well as embryonic development, primary axons in the newt spinal cord move through spaces formed by the endfeet of neuroepithelial cells (Singer et al., 1979). These epithelial endfeet may provide not only mechanical guidance for axons but molecular guidance as well (Silver and Rutishauser, 1984).

Cues for orienting the growth of both vertebrate and invertebrate neurons seem to reside on the basal surfaces of epithelial cells. Although such cues can orient neurons along particular pathways, it is not always evident how these cues specify the directionality of axonal growth. Perhaps it is a graded arrangement of epithelial endfeet that plays an important role in guiding this directional growth, as suggested from examination of neuronal pathways in the Manduca wing.

ACKNOWLEDGMENTS

The author acknowledges the skillful secretarial assistance of Jacqueline Smith. Facilities for electron microscopy were provided by the Center for Electron Microscopy at the University of Illinois. Funding was provided by NSF grant BNS 83-15538.

REFERENCES

Blair SS, Murray MA, Palka J (1985). Axon guidance in cultured epithelial fragments of the Drosophila wing. Nature 315:406-409.

Jan LY, Jan YN (1982). Antibodies to horseradish peroxidase as specific neuronal markers in Drosophila and in grasshopper embryos. Proc Natl Acad Sci USA 79:2700-2704.

Kuwada JY (1986). Cell recognition by neuronal growth cones in a simple vertebrate embryo. Science 233:740-746.

Lefcourt F, Bentley D (1987). Pathfinding by pioneer neurons in isolated, opened and mesoderm-free limb buds of embryonic grasshoppers. Dev Biol 119:466-480.

Letourneau PC (1982). Nerve fiber growth and its regulation by extrinsic factors. In Spitzer NC (ed): "Neuronal Development," New York:Plenum, p. 213.

Nardi JB, Kafatos FC (1976a). Polarity and gradients in lepidopteran wing epidermis. I. Changes in graft polarity, form and cell density accompanying transposition and reorientation. J Embryol Exp Morphol 36:469-487.

Nardi JB, Kafatos FC (1976b). Polarity and gradients in lepidopteran wing epidermis. II. The differential adhesiveness model: Gradient of a non-diffusible cell surface parameter. J Embryol Exp Morph 36:489-512.

Nardi JB (1983). Neuronal pathfinding in developing wings of the moth Manduca sexta. Dev Biol 95:163-174.

Nardi JB, Hardt TA, Magee-Adams SM, Osterbur DL (1985). Morphogenesis in wing imaginal discs: Its relationship to changes in the extracellular matrix. Tissue & Cell 17:473-490.

Palka J (1986). Epithelial axon guidance in Drosophila. J Neurobiol 17:581-584.

Silver J, Rutishauser U (1984). Guidance of optic axons in vivo by a preformed adhesive pathway on neuroepithelial endfeet. Dev Biol 106:485-499.

Singer M, Nordlander RH, Egar M (1979). Axonal guidance during embryogenesis and regeneration in the spinal cord of the newt: The blueprint hypothesis of neuronal pathway patterning. J Comp Neurol 185:1-22.

CELLULAR BIOLOGY OF NEURONAL INTERACTIONS WITH FIBRONECTIN AND LAMININ

Paul Letourneau[1], Sherry Rogers[2], Irene Pech[1], Sally Palm[3], James McCarthy[3], and Leo Furcht[3], Departments of Cell Biology and Neuroanatomy[1], Anatomy[2], and Laboratory Medicine and Pathology[3], University of Minnesota, Minneapolis, MN 55455[1,3], University of New Mexico, Albuquerque, NM 87131[2]

INTRODUCTION

Successful regeneration of damaged or severed axons depends on factors both intrinsic and extrinsic to responding neurons. Large differences in extracellular milieu may be a key element in differences in axonal regeneration in the peripheral vs the central nervous system of higher vertebrates. Schwann cell sheaths and other connective tissues contain adhesive glycoproteins like fibronectin and laminin (Bignami et al, 1984; Cornbrooks et al, 1983; Palm and Furcht, 1983; Rogers et al, 1986a), that mediate adhesion to extracellular surfaces and promote growth of peripheral axons. Although fibronectin and laminin are present in the developing CNS, where they may also promote axonal elongation (Chun et al, 1986; Hatten et al, 1982; Hynes et al, 1986; Letourneau et al, 1987; Stewart and Pearlman, 1987), these two molecules are absent from axonal pathways of the adult CNS. Perhaps, poor axonal regeneration in the CNS is related to lack of extracellular spaces with adhesive substrata.

In addition, equal significance must be placed on the ability of growing axons to detect and respond to specific ligands. The growth cone at the tip of an axon contains multiple surface receptors for soluble and bound molecules. These receptors provide sensory information that permits growth cones to choose among several pathways for axonal growth. Thus, increased information about the molecular basis of neuronal interaction with adhesive ligands may help understand why some axons do not regenerate and indicate ways to improve axonal regeneration in the central nervous system.

For several years we have collaborated on studies of the interactions of chick embryo neurons with the glycoproteins fibronectin and laminin. These experiments will be described here, and because of limitations to the length of this article, a reader must refer to published papers for relevant figures and tables. Neurons interact with at least two domains of fibronectin (Rogers et al, 1985, 1987), and evidence also indicates that neurons interact with several portions of laminin (Rogers et al, 1986b). Using cell cultures prepared from the central and peripheral nervous systems of chick embryos, we found that neurons of different types possess different surface molecules that mediate adhesion to extracellular surfaces (Rogers et al, 1987). Recently, synthetic polypeptides have helped to further probe interactions with fibronectin and laminin. We expect this approach to yield new information about the interactions of neurons with extracellular surfaces.

Although fibronectin and laminin are widely distributed in connective tissues, a critical factor has been the ability to purify these proteins in large amounts from unusually rich sources (Hynes and Yamada, 1982; Timpl et al, 1983). Fibronectin is soluble in blood at concentrations of several hundred µg/ml, and laminin is copiously secreted by a tumor line. Apparently, multiple variants of these molecules are synthesized in different tissues (Hynes, 1985). Only the most available forms have been studied in depth, and any functional differences will have to be defined later.

PNS AND CNS AXONAL GROWTH IN VITRO

Neurons from chick embryo dorsal root ganglia attach to and readily extend axons on culture dishes coated with fibronectin or laminin (Rogers et al, 1983). This behavior involves neuronal interaction with the added glycoproteins, because cell attachment and neurite elongation is specifically blocked by antibodies to the glycoprotein used for coating the substratum. Laminin also promotes cell attachment and axon growth from spinal cord neurons, but fibronectin is much less effective at supporting axon growth from these neurons.Similar results were achieved with sympathetic and retinal neurons, and these initial experiments indicated that peripheral and central neurons interact differently with fibronectin and laminin.

Interactions with different fibronectin domains

Fibronectin and laminin contain multiple domains that bind to several molecules (Edgar et al, 1984; Hynes, 1985; McCarthy et al, 1986, 1987; Timpl et al, 1983). Fibronectin has been thoroughly characterized, and it is known to form specific associations with collagens, heparin, hyaluronic acid, fibrin, thrombospondin, and several components of cell surfaces. These diverse interactions involve distinct domains that comprise a series of tightly folded globular units, each specialized for binding to a particular molecular configuration (Hynes, 1985).We cultured sensory and spinal cord neurons on a series of fibronectin fragments, generated by proteolysis and affinity binding (McCarthy et al, 1986; Rogers et al, 1985). Only two of five fragments supported neuronal attachment and axonal growth. One fragment from the central region contains a tetrapeptide sequence, arg-gly-asn-ser (RGDS), that is recognized by a class of putative receptors for extracellular matrix molecules that is present on several cell types (Hynes, 1987; Pierschbacher and Ruoslahti, 1984a, b; Ruoslahti and Pierschbacher, 1986), and the other active fragment is a 33 kD sequence from the carboxyl end that binds heparin strongly, but have a higher level of interaction with the chymotrypsin fragment than spinal cord neurons. These data indicate that laminin, like fibronectin, has multiple domains that interact with neurons via binding sites that are differentially expressed.

Axonal growth on synthetic peptides

In order to gain more detailed knowledge of how neurons interact with fibronectin and laminin, we are examining cell attachment and neurite elongation on substrata coated with synthetic polypeptides from the sequences of these adhesive glycoproteins. Areas of interest are those with a low hydropathy index, as well as those which are rich in cationic residues, such as lys and arg. Preliminary experiments have examined neurite outgrowth by spinal cord and sensory neurons on substrata treated with four peptides based on the primary sequence of fibronectin. Three of these bind heparin and are from the 33 kD heparin-binding fragment, and one is an RGDS-like peptide. One of the heparin-binding peptides promotes strong attachment and neurite outgrowth from spinal cord neurons, but has only a slight effect on sensory neurons. Two other peptides from the 33 kD fragment were not as effective. The RGDS-like peptide had a small effect on sensory neurons, but none on spinal cord neurons. Again, it is interesting that sensory and spinal cord neurons interact differently with these peptides from the fibronectin sequence. This supports the notion that these neuronal types differ in receptors for extracellular components.

These peptides are powerful tools for studying neuronal interaction with fibronectin. However, *in vitro* data does not necessarily mean that neurons interact with these same sequences in intact fibronectin. Future studies will develop polyclonal antibodies to these peptides that block neurite elongation on substrata treated with a particular peptide. Finding that these antibodies also interfere with neurite elongation on intact fibronectin or on the heparin-binding fragment would increase our confidence that neurons do interact with a particular sequence in the fibronectin molecule. Additional evidence would come from finding that soluble peptides block neuronal interaction with fibronectin, as shown for the RGDS tetrapeptide. Once neuronal interactions with specific domains are characterized *in vitro*, *in vivo* studies can begin. The peptides can be injected into particular regions of embryos, and the embryos allowed to survive for some time before sacrifice and examination for perturbations of the CNS or PNS. Similar *in vivo* studies can be performed using polyclonal antibodies to the peptides.

Another avenue will be to use these peptides to identify neuronal surface binding sites or receptors for active domains of fibronectin and laminin. Membrane fractions can be prepared in large amounts from cultures of neuroblastoma or pheochromocytoma cells, and membrane receptors can be isolated by affinity chromatography, using the synthetic peptides or isolated fragments of the glycoproteins. Further characterization of receptors will determine binding to soluble peptides and fragments, and can be used to prepare antibodies to the surface receptors that block neuronal interactions with fibronectin or laminin *in vitro* and *in vivo*.

Conclusions

These studies will help to understand the mechanisms of neuronal interactions with extracellular matrices. Cell culture and molecular approaches can reveal the domains of fibronectin and laminin to which neurons bind and can identify cell surface components mediating neuronal adhesion to these specific ligands. The relationship between growth cone binding to specific extracellular species and axonal elongation or neuronal metabolism can indicate which interactions are most relevant to axonal development and regeneration. Temporal and neuron specific differences in receptors and adhesive ligands can indicate whether these components are related to defective axonal regeneration in the central nervous system. It is particularly critical to have information about the functions of these components during *in vivo* growth and regeneration of axons. Because fibronectin and laminin can be purified in large amounts, these two glycoproteins have been the focus of studies of neuronal interactions with the extracellular matrix. However, this work can help elucidate other interactions. The putative fibronectin receptor, integrin, is one of a family of surface receptors that may share important properties. In addition, adhesive domains that are recognized by surface receptors may be similar in different extracellular components. Even if adult central nervous system neurons do not interact with fibronectin, growth cones may be able to gain adhesive support for axonal growth by binding to similar sites in other matrix components.

References

Akiyama SK, Yamada SS, Yamada KM (1986). Characterization of a 140-kD avian cell surface antigen as a fibronectin-binding molecule. J Cell Biol 102:442-448.

Bignami A, Chi HN, Dahl D (1984). First appearance of laminin in peripheral nerve, cerebral blood vessels and skeletal muscle of the rat embryo. Immunofluorescence study with laminin and neurofilament antisera. Int J Dev Neurosci 2:367-376.

Bozyczko D, Horwitz AF (1986). The participation of a putative cell surface receptor for laminin and fibronectin in peripheral neurite extension. J Neurosci 6:1241-1251.

Cohen J, Burne JF, Winter J, Bartlett P (1986). Retinal ganglion cells lose response to laminin with maturation. Nature (Lond.) 322:465-467.

Cornbrooks CJ, Carey DJ, McDonald JA, Timpl R, Bunge RP (1983). In vivo and in vitro observations on laminin production by Schwann cells. Proc Natl Acad Sci USA 80:3850-3854.

Chun JJM, Nakamura MJ, Shatz CJ (1986). Transient fibronectin-like immunostaining in the subplate during development of the cat's telencephalon. Soc Neurosci Abst 12:502.

Edgar D, Timpl R, Thoenen H (1984). The heparin binding domain of laminin is responsible for its

effects on neurite outgrowth and neuronal survival. EMBO J 3:1463-1468.
Hatten ME, Furie MB, Rifkin DB (1982). Binding of developing mouse cerebellar cells to fibronectin; a possible mechanism for the formation of the external granule layer. J Neurosci 2:1195-1206.
Horwitz AF, Duggan K, Greggs R, Decker C, Buck C (1985). The cell substrate attachment (CSAT) antigen has properties of a receptor for laminin and fibronectin. J Cell Biol 101:2134-2144.
Hynes RO (1985). Molecular biology of fibronectin. Ann Rev Cell Biol 1:67-90.
Hynes RO (1987). Integrins: A family of cell surface receptors. Cell 48:549-554.
Hynes RO, Patel R, Miller RH (1986). Migration of neuroblasts along preexisting axonal tracts during prenatal cerebellar development. J Neurosci 6:867-876.
Hynes RO, Yamada KM (1982). Fibronectins: multifunctional modular glycoproteins. J Cell Biol 95:369-378.
Letourneau PC, Madsen AM, Palm SL, Furcht LT (1987). Immunoreactivity for laminin in the developing ventral longitudinal pathway of the brain. Dev Biol in press.
Letourneau PC, Pech IV, Rogers SL, Palm SL, McCarthy JB, Furcht LT. Growth cone migration across extracellular matrix components depends on integrin, but migration across glioma cells does not. Submitted.
McCarthy JB, Chelberg MK, Mickelson DJ, Furcht LT (1987). Localization of unique melanoma adhesion domains in fibronectin with heparin binding activity. Bioc in press.
McCarthy JB, Hagen ST, and Furcht LT (1986). Human fibronectin contains distinct adhesion- and motility-promoting domains for metastatic melanoma cells. J Cell Biol 102:179-188.
Palm SL, Furcht LT (1983). The production of laminin and fibronectin by Schwannoma cells: cell-protein interactions in vitro and protein localization in peripheral nerve in vivo. J Cell Biol 96:1218-1226.
Palm SL, Furcht LT (1985). Alternate model for the internal structure of laminin. Bioc 24:7753-7760.

Pierschbacher MD, Ruoslahti E (1984a). Cell attachment activity of fibronectin can be duplicated by small synthetic fragments of the molecule. Nature (Lond.) 309:30-33.

Pierschbacher MD, Ruoslahti E (1984b). Variants of the cell recognition site of fibronectin that retain attachment promoting activity. Proc Natl Acad Sci USA 81:5985-5988.

Rogers SL, Edson KJ, Letourneau PC, McLoon SC (1986a). Distribution of laminin in the developing nervous system of the chick. Dev Biol 113:429-435.

Rogers SL, Letourneau PC, Palm SL, McCarthy JB, Furcht LT (1983).Neurite extension by peripheral and central nervous system neurons in response to substratum-bound fibronectin and laminin. Dev Biol 98:212-220.

Rogers SL, Letourneau PC, Peterson BA, Furcht LT, McCarthy JB (1987). Selective interaction of peripheral and central nervous system cells with two distinct cell binding domains of fibronectin. J Cell Biol 105:1435-1442.

Rogers SL, McCarthy JB, Palm SL, Furcht LT, Letourneau PC (1985). Neuron-specific interactions with two neurite-promoting fragments of fibronectin. J Neurosci 5:369-378.

Rogers SL, Palm SL, McCarthy JB, Furcht LT, Hanlon K, Letourneau PC (1986b). Interaction of central and peripheral neurons with proteolytic fragments of laminin. Soc Neurosci Abst 12:1113.

Ruoslahti E, Piersbacher MD (1986). Arg-Gly-Asp: a versatile cell recognition signal. Cell 44:517-518.

Stewart GR, Pearlman AL (1987). Fibronectin-like immunoreactivity in the developing cerebral cortex. J Neurosci 7:3325-3333.

Timpl R, Engel J, Martin GR (1983). Laminin- a multifunctional protein of basement membranes. Trends Biochem Sci 8:207-209.

Tomaselli KJ, Reichardt LF, Bixby JL (1987). Distinct molecular interactions mediate neuronal process outgrowth on non-neuronal cell surfaces and extracellular matrices. J Cell Biol 103:2659-2672.

LAMININ, FIBRONECTIN, COLLAGEN AND THEIR RECEPTORS IN NERVE FIBER GROWTH.

S. Carbonetto, P. Douville, W. Harvey and D.C. Turner
Neuroscience Unit, Montreal General Hospital Research Inst. McGill University, Montreal, Canada and Dept. of Biochemistry and Molecular Biology, SUNY Medical Center at Syracuse, Syracuse, N.Y. 13210 (D.C.T)

INTRODUCTION

How neurons connect with their targets has been a major question of neurobiology. The experiments of Sperry and his coworkers led to one of the earliest and clearest statements of the problem (Sperry, 1963). To account for the remarkable regeneration of retinal ganglionic axons to their correct locations in the frog tectum, Sperry advanced his now famous chemoaffinity hypothesis that neurons must have chemical "identification tags" enabling them to form specific connections with their targets.

While we are still far from understanding the cellular and molecular mechanisms responsible for the extraordinary specificity of neuronal connections, recent research has revealed two classes of neuronal cell surface molecules that appear to have important contributions. Here we focus on receptors for components of the extracellular matrix (ECM), which mediate cell-to-matrix adhesion and allow neurons to respond to molecular cues in the ECM by extension of nerve fibers. Molecules of the second class, designated CAMs (for cell adhesion molecules), are involved in cell-to-cell adhesion; they are the subject of the papers by M. Schachner, E. Bock, and U. Rutishauser in this volume.

The notion that cell-to-matrix interactions regulate nerve fiber growth comes from direct observations of neurons in culture on substrata coated with purified ECM proteins. Laminin, fibronectin (see Letourneau, this volume), and collagen have been shown to be particularly effective in eliciting fiber growth in culture; one of these, laminin, uniquely stimulates nerve fiber growth by dorsal root ganglion neurons which otherwise require nerve growth factor (NGF; Lander et al., 1982; Edgar et al., 1984; Davis et al., 1985). Moreover, oriented deposits of purified ECM proteins can guide nerve fiber extension in vitro (Turner and Carbonetto, 1984; Hammarback et al., 1985).

Several findings suggest that the ECM may similarly influence nerve regeneration in vivo. Most impressively, McMahan and coworkers (Marshall et al., 1977) have shown that muscle fiber "ghosts", consisting of the basement membranes surrounding degenerated muscle fibers, support ingrowth of regenerating axons to their original synaptic sites and differentiation of these axons into nerve terminals. Regenerating nerve fibers in the peripheral nervous system (PNS) can be seen to follow tubes of basement membranes vacated by degenerated axons of damaged peripheral nerves (Ide et al., 1983). Similar growth in contact with basement membranes can be achieved by adult mammalian central nervous system (CNS) neurons regenerating into peripheral nerve grafts (Aguayo et al., 1986). These and other data have prompted much interest in the distribution and regulation, during neuronal regeneration and development, of the various ECM proteins and of their receptors.

Several years ago one of us presented a model, drawn from the work of many laboratories, that described a sequence of cellular events in growth cone motility and focused on the function of neuron-substratum adhesion in nerve fiber growth (Carbonetto, 1984). A key feature of this model was that growth cones, known to be the motile organelle of the extending nerve fiber, must have on their surfaces specific receptors for ECM proteins. Binding of these receptors to the ECM would lead to a stable association of the ECM-receptor complexes with the cytoskeleton of the growth cone which consists mainly of actin-containing microfilaments. Ultimately this interaction would trigger contractile events responsible for generating forces that extend the axon. We now briefly update this model with newer data from our laboratory, while taking into account observations by others, especially with regard to the several receptors for ECM proteins that have been identified on neural cells.

ECM PROTEINS:

The best studied ECM adhesive proteins are laminin, fibronectin, collagens and entactin (nidogen). All of these are found in or near the basement membranes surrounding axon-Schwann cell units in the PNS (Bunge and Bunge, 1983). Laminin (Liesi, 1984; Carbonetto et al., 1987) and possibly fibronectin (Hatten et al., 1982; Stewart and Pearlman, 1987; c.f. Hynes et al., 1986) are found within the developing CNS in diffuse or punctate deposits, outside the basement membranes that line meninges and blood vessels, where they may be involved in neuroblast migration and differentiation.

Laminin and fibronectin are multi-functional glycoproteins (reviewed in Yamada, 1983). Each contains multiple sites for binding to other ECM components (eg. collagen, heparin) as well as at least two sites for binding to cells. Laminin, for example, has one region to which several types of nonneural cells attach and a distinct site that mediates nerve fiber outgrowth (Edgar et al., 1984). Despite the obvious progress in understanding these two molecules, however, the ECM of the nervous system is only beginning to be characterized biochemically. New adhesive proteins continue to be identified. The ECM also contains glycosaminoglycans and proteoglycans which may inhibit adhesion of neurons to ECM proteins (Carbonetto et al., 1983).

RECEPTORS FOR ECM PROTEINS:

Figure 1 shows several putative receptors for ECM proteins that have been identified on neural cells. These include: integrins, heterodimeric receptors with relatively low affinities for fibronectin, laminin and collagen; a 67kDa, high-affinity, laminin receptor; the 3A3 antigen, which mediates nerve fiber growth on laminin and collagen and which may be a subunit of an integrin ; and a 120 KDa membrane protein that is a major laminin-binding protein on several cell types including neurons.

Integrins: These receptors were first identified by precipitation with antibodies that detached myoblasts and fibroblasts from fibronectin (reviewed in Buck and Horwitz, 1987). It is now clear that the inhibitory antibodies react with a 120 kDa glycoprotein species that is the common β-subunit of several related receptors. The mammalian fibronectin receptor of this class (α = 140kDa, β = 120 kDa) has little or no affinity for laminin. Antibodies against integrin β-chains inhibit attachment of chick cells to fibronectin, laminin and some collagens. They also precipitate, besides the 120-kDa β-chain, two additional bands (140 kDa and 160 kDa). These may be the α-chains of distinct fibronectin and laminin receptors. Recently, cDNAs for the chick β-subunit have been cloned (Tamkun et al., 1986); the cDNA sequences reveal extensive homology with subunits found in a number of other previously identified heterodimeric membrane proteins that are now collectively referred to as the integrin family (reviewed in Hynes, 1987). Family members are present on a wide variety of cell types. Many, but not all, integrins recognize a sequence of 3 amino acids (Arg-Gly-Asp) in their respective ligands (reviewed by Ruoslahti and Pierschbacher, 1987).

Integrin has been identified in cultured peripheral neurons (Bozyczko and Horwitz, 1986; Tomaselli et al., 1986), CNS (retinal ganglion) neurons (Cohen et al., 1986) and PC12 cells (Tomaselli et al., 1987) and shown to be involved in nerve fiber growth on fibronectin and laminin. Interestingly, nerve fiber growth by retinal ganglion neurons becomes refractory to laminin at a developmental age when the neurons continue to express integrin and are capable of extending fibers on astrocytes (Cohen et al., 1986; Tomaselli et al., 1986).

67KDa laminin receptor: A laminin receptor has been isolated from muscle and several other sources by chromatography on laminin affinity columns (reviewed in von der Mark and Kühl, 1985; Liotta et al., 1986). This receptor binds laminin with a Kd of $\simeq 10^{-9}$M i.e. with approximately 1000-fold higher affinity than the laminin-binding integrin. Our recent studies indicate that a receptor similar and possibly identical to the muscle receptor is present on chicken CNS neurons (Douville et al., 1987). Graf et al. (1987) have shown that a 67-kDa receptor is present on a neuroblastoma-glioma cell line NG 108, where it apparently mediates attachment to one of the short arms of the cruciform laminin molecule. These workers have identified a critical pentapeptide (Tyr-Ile-Gly-Ser-Arg) within the sequence of the cell attachment region of laminin that is recognized by this receptor. When bound to the substratum, synthetic peptides containing this sequence promote cell attachment. However, addition of the same peptides to the culture medium blocks attachment to laminin, presumably by competing with substratum-bound laminin for binding to the 67 KDa receptor.

The 67kDa receptor from mammary tumor cells is not homologous to the integrins; also, because it has no obvious membrane-spanning domain, it is probably not an integral membrane protein but instead anchored to the membrane by one or more "docking" proteins that span the lipid bilayer.

3A3 antigen: We have shown that PC12 cells extend nerve fibers on laminin and collagen substrata, to which they adhere by a Mg^{2+}-dependent mechanism, but fail to extend fibers on polylysine, to which they adhere in the absence of divalent cations (Turner et al., 1987a). Recently, we have obtained a monoclonal antibody, 3A3, that is directed against a cell surface antigen on PC12 cells and that inhibits PC12 nerve fiber growth on laminin and collagen, but not on polylysine (Turner et al., 1987b). 3A3 also inhibits nerve fiber growth by rat DRG neurons on laminin and collagen. 3A3 immunoprecipitates a protein of ≈185 kDa that we believe is a functional part of a dual laminin-collagen receptor. The relationship of this antigen to other ECM receptors is at present a matter of conjecture. One intriguing possibility is that the 3A3 antigen is the α-chain of a novel member of the integrin family. It may be that the binding of 3A3 to an α-subunit promotes dissociation of the β-subunit, so that a prominent β band is not detected in immunoprecipitates. Interestingly, Tomaselli et al (1987) have shown that an integrin α-subunit of about the same size is precipitable from PC12 extracts by polyclonal antibodies against an integrin β-subunit.

120 KDa: Binding studies with radioiodinated laminin following SDS-PAGE and electroblotting

of membrane proteins led to the identification of a ≃120-kDa molecule as the most prominent laminin-binding protein; this integral membrane protein has been called cranin (Smalheiser and Schwartz, 1987). We have identified a similar or identical laminin-binding protein by these same methods in cultures highly enriched for neurons (Douville et al., 1987). By indirect criteria, the 120-kDa protein appears not to be an integrin subunit. For example, it binds laminin with a much higher affinity than integrin, is more protease-sensitive and its laminin binding is not inhibited by antibodies to integrin (Douville et al., 1987).

In future work, it will be necessary to determine the relationships, if any, among the putative receptors described above and, in each case, whether the molecule functions in cell- substratum adhesion or in other processes such as ECM assembly.

CONCLUDING REMARKS

Although studies of the ECM of the nervous system are still in their infancy, several interesting generalizations have emerged. First, the composition of the ECM of the CNS changes dramatically with development, from one that contains ECM proteins necessary for cell motility and nerve fiber growth to one devoid of these proteins. These same adhesive proteins do persist within the basement membranes of the PNS where they facilitate nerve regeneration (Sandrock and Matthew, 1987). Second, neural cells have multiple ECM receptors, and some of these may recognize multiple ECM components. Finally, there is evidence that, like ECM proteins, ECM receptors are developmentally regulated.

Why do cells of the nervous system have multiple receptors for ECM adhesive proteins? First, even though different receptors may be unequally distributed on the various cell types (neurons, astroglia, etc.) there is evidence that a single type of neuron can have multiple receptors (Douville et al., 1987). These multiple receptors may be necessary if the three dimensional ECM of the nervous system is to guide neuroblasts or nerve fibers. In the studies of Sandrock and Matthew (1987) a monoclonal antibody that potently inhibits nerve fiber growth on relatively simple culture substrata is much more modest in its inhibition of nerve regeneration in vivo consistent with the notion that fibers extending on a complex substratum may utilize multiple adhesive mechanisms.

Perhaps the most interesting aspect of work in this area is that it is now possible to begin to model, at a molecular level, the interrelationship of cell-substratum adhesion and cytoskeletal dynamics in nerve fiber growth. The tension generated along the growing axon and the effect of the microfilament-disrupting drug cytochalasin B on growth cone motility have been taken to indicate that cell-substratum adhesion is somehow coupled to microfilament-dependent contractile events (discussed in Carbonetto, 1984). Recent studies show that the β subunit of the integrin fibronectin receptor spans the plasma membrane (Tamkun et al., 1986) and is capable of binding both fibronectin and the cytoskeletal accessory protein talin (Horwitz et al., 1986). Vinculin, another cytoskeletal accessory protein, binds to fibronectin receptor-talin complexes (Horwitz et al., 1986). Thus, one can imagine a cascade of events beginning with an ECM molecule binding to its receptor, leading through cytoskeletal accessory proteins to assembly and/or rearrangement of actin filaments, (Fig. 1) and ultimately to growth cone movement.

MATRIX RECEPTORS ON NEURAL CELLS

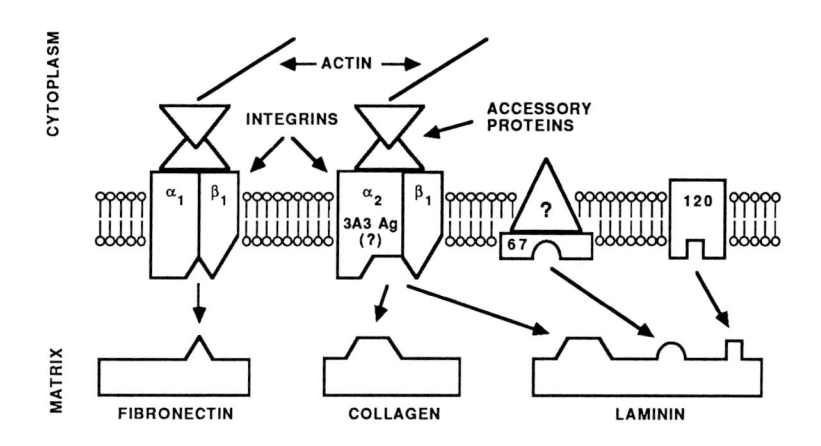

Figure 1: Four possible neural cell receptors for the ECM proteins fibronectin, laminin and collagen. In this scheme, one integrin is shown as a fibronectin receptor, the 3A3 antigen is shown hypothetically as an α-subunit of a second integrin which binds to collagen and laminin. The 67kDa protein is a peripheral membrane protein anchored to the membrane via unidentified molecules; it binds to laminin at a site distinct from that recognized by the laminin-binding integrin. A non-integrin 120-kDa protein also binds to laminin. This model is drawn from available data on neural ECM receptors, but some details are speculative (see text).

REFERENCES

Aguayo AJ, Vidal-Sanz M, Villegas-Perez M, Keirstead S, Rasminsky M, Bray GM (1986). Axonal regrowth and connectivity from neurons in the adult retina. In Agardh A, Ehinger B (eds): "Retinal Signal Systems Degeneration and Transplants" Elsevier, p 257.

Bozyczko D, Horwitz AF (1986). The partici-

pation of a putative cell surface receptor for laminin and fibronectin in peripheral neurite extension. J Neurosci 6: 1241.
Buck CA, Horwitz AF (1987). Cell surface receptors for extracellular matrix molecules. Ann Rev Cell Biol 3: 179.
Bunge RP, Bunge MB (1983). Interrelationship between Schwann cell function and extracellular matrix production. Trends in Neurosci 6: 499.
Carbonetto S, Gruver MM, Turner DC (1983). Nerve fiber growth in culture on fibronectin collagen and glycosaminoglycan substrates. J Neurosci 3: 2324.
Carbonetto S (1984). The extracellular matrix of the nervous system. Trends in Neurosci 7: 382.
Carbonetto S, Evans D, Cochard P (1987). Nerve fiber growth in culture on tissue substrata from central and peripheral nervous system. J Neurosci 7: 610.
Cohen J, Burne JF, Winter J, Bartlett P (1986). Retinal ganglion cells lose response to laminin with maturation. Nature 322: 465.
Davis GE, Manthorpe M, Engvall E, Varon S (1985). Isolation and characterization of rat Schwannoma neurite-promoting factor: Evidence that the factor contains laminin. J Neurosci 5: 2662.
Douville PJ, Harvey WJ, Carbonetto S (1987). Identification and purification of a high affinity laminin receptor from embryonic chick brain: evidence for developmental regulation. Soc Neurosci Abs 13: 1982.
Edgar D, Timpl R, Thoenen H (1984). The heparin binding domain of laminin is responsible for its effects on neurite outgrowth and neuronal survival. EMBO J 3: 1463
Graf J, Iwamoto Y, Sasaki M, Martin GR, Kleinman HK, Robey FA, Yamada Y (1987). Identification of an amino acid sequence in laminin mediating cell attachment chemotaxis and receptor binding. Cell 48: 989.
Hammarback JA, Palm SL, Furcht LT, Letourneau

PC (1985). Guidance of neurite outgrowth by pathways of substratum-adsorbed laminin. J Neurosci Res 13: 213.

Hatten MW, Furie MB, Rifkin DB (1982). Binding of developing mouse cerebellar cells to fibronectin: A possible mechanism for the formation of the external granule layer. J Neurosci 2: 1195.

Horwitz A, Duggan K, Buck C, Beckerle MC, Burridge K (1986). Interaction of a plasma membrane fibronectin receptor with talin- a transmembrane linkage. Nature 320: 531.

Hynes RO (1987). Integrins: A family of cell surface receptors. Cell 48: 549.

Hynes RO, Patel R, Miller RH (1986). Migration of neuroblasts along preexisting axonal tracts during prenatal cerebellar developments. J Neurosci 6: 867.

Ide C, Tohyama K, Yokota R, Nitatori T, Onodera S (1983). Schwann cell basal lamina and nerve regeneration. Brain Res 288: 61.

Lander AD, Fujii DK, Gospodarowicz D, Reichardt LF (1982). Characterization of a factor that promotes neurite outgrowth: Evidence linking activity to a heparan sulfate proteoglycan. J Cell Biol 94: 574.

Liesi P (1984). Laminin and fibronectin in normal and malignant neuroectodermal cells. Med Biol 61: 163.

Liotta LA, Nageswara Rao C, Wewer UM (1986). Biochemical interactions of tumor cells with the basement membrane. Ann Rev Biochem 55: 1037.

Marshall LM, Sanes JR, McMahan UJ (1977). Reinnervation of original synaptic sites on muscle fiber basement membrane after disruption of muscle cells. Proc Natl Acad Sci (USA) 74: 3073.

Ruoslahti F, Piersbacher MD (1987). New perspectives in cell adhesion: RGD and integrins. Science 238: 491.

Sandrock AW, Matthew WD (1987). An in vitro neurite-promoting antigen functions in axonal regeneration in vivo. Science 237: 1605.

Smalheiser NR, Schwartz NB (1987). Cranin: A laminin binding protein of cell membranes. Proc Natl Acad Sci (USA) 84: in press.

Sperry RW (1963). Chemoaffinity in the orderly growth of nerve fiber patterns and connections. Proc Natl Acad Sci (USA) 50: 703.

Stewart GR, Pearlman AL (1987). Fibronectin-like immunoreactivity in the developing cerebral cortex. J Neurosci 7: 3325.

Tamkun JW, DeSimone DW, Fonda D, Patel RS, Buck C, Horwitz AF, Hynes RO (1986). Structure of integrin a glycoprotein involved in transmembrane linkage between fibronectin and actin. Cell 46: 271.

Tomaselli KJ, Damsky CH, Reichardt LF (1987). Interactions of a neuronal cell line (PC12) with laminin collagen IV and fibronectin: Identification of integrin-related glycoproteins involved in attachment and process outgrowth. J Cell Biol 105: 2347.

Tomaselli KJ, Reichardt LF, and Bixby JL (1986). Distinct molecular interactions mediate neuronal process outgrowth on non-neuronal cell surfaces and extracellular matrices. J Cell Biol 103: 2659.

Turner DC, Carbonetto ST (1984). Model systems for studying the functions of extracellular matrix molecules in muscle development. Exptl Biol Med 9: 72.

Turner DC, Flier LA, Carbonetto ST (1987a). Magnesium-dependent attachment and neurite outgrowth by PC12 cells on collagen and laminin substrata. Dev Biol 121: 510.

Turner DC, Flier LA, Carbonetto ST (1987b). Identification of a protein involved in adhesion of PC12 cells to collagen and laminin. J Cell Biol 105: 137a

von der Mark K, Kühl U (1985). Laminin and its receptor. Biochem Biophys Acta 823: 147.

Yamada KM (1983). Cell surface interactions with extracellular materials. Ann Rev Biochem 52: 761.

GLIA-DERIVED NEXINS AND NEURITE OUTGROWTH

Denis Monard

Friedrich Miescher Institut, P.O. Box 2543
CH-4002 BASEL, Switzerland

The rate of neurite outgrowth determines the success or failure in the regeneration phenomena. Even neurons of the central nervous system have the ability to regenerate neurites if provided with a permissive environment (Benfey and Aguayo, 1982). The identification of the biochemical events which modulate the rate of neurite outgrowth could thus increase our chances of influencing the regeneration of functional connections.

Neurite outgrowth is obviously a complex phenomenon where multiple interactions between the growth cone, the growing neuritic membrane and some components of the extracellular matrix are required. The molecular mechanisms triggering these interactions are difficult to approach in vivo. The use of in vitro models provides opportunities to detect and characterize some of the molecules involved.

Cultured glial cells, including glioma cells, release a macromolecular factor which induces a dose-dependent neurite outgrowth in neuroblastoma cells (Monard et al., 1973). This neurite promoting activity is also detected in the medium conditioned by rat brain primary cultures if they are established at or after a critical developmental stage at which the burst of glial cell proliferation takes place (Schuerch-Rathgeb and Monard, 1978). This glia-derived neurite promoting factor is distinct from the well-studied nerve growth factor (NGF) (Monard et al., 1975).

During the purification of this glia-derived protein, it was realized that fractions with neurite promoting activity also contained a very potent inhibitory activity for serine proteases such as thrombin, urokinase or plasminogen activator (Monard et al., 1983). Preparative gel electrophoresis demonstrated that the 43 Kd protein purified has both neurite promoting activity and protease inhibitory activity (Guenther et al., 1985).

The cDNAs coding for the human and the rat glia-derived neurite promoting factors have now been cloned and sequenced (Gloor et al., 1986; Sommer et al., 1987). The correct identity of the cDNA coding for the rat protein has been confirmed by the sequence of many tryptic peptides derived from the purified protein. These glia-derived protease inhibitors belong to the serpins, a family of serine protease inhibitors. The aminoterminal sequence of the human glia-derived protein is identical with the first 28 amino acid residues presently identified in protease nexin I, a serine inhibitor released by cultured human foreskin fibroblasts (Scott et al., 1985). The biochemical properties of the rat glia-derived protein are similar to those of protease nexin I (Stone et al., 1987). The cloning and sequencing of protease nexin I presently in progress should assess the similarity, possibly the identity of these two proteins. In any case the glia-derived neurite promoting factor can be considered as a glia-derived nexin (GDN).

Rat GDN has 397 amino acids including a putative signal peptide of 19 amino acids. Native rat GDN being a glycoprotein (Guenther et al., 1985), its molecular weight calculated from the amino acid sequence (41752 daltons) is lower than the one estimated by SDS-polyacrylamide gel electrophoresis. Two different sequences have been established for human GDN; one coding for Arg, the other for Thr-Gly at position 329. The sequence with the Thr-Gly at position 329 (human GDNα) indicates a protein with 398 amino acids and a molecular weight of 41867 daltons. The human GDNβ sequence (Arg in position 329) matches exactly with the rat GDN sequence at this position and leads to a protein with 397 amino acids having a molecular weight of 41865 daltons. There is a 84% homology between rat GDN and the corresponding protein from human glioma cells. The alignment of rat GDN, human GDNs, human endothelial-cell-type plasminogen activator inhibitor (Ny et al., 1986; Pannekoek et al., 1986), and human α-1 protease inhibitor (Kurachi et al., 1981) indicates a homology of 84%, 41%, 32% and 25% respectively. This alignment suggests $Arg^{364}-Ser^{365}$ to be at the reactive center ($P_1-P'_1$) of rat GDN and human

GDNβ. Correspondingly, Arg^{365}-Ser^{366} can be considered as the reactive center of human GDNα. All the GDNs have a glutamic acid in position P_{17} and a lysine in position P_{69}. The position of these two residues is conserved in many serpins (Carell and Travis, 1985). They have been reported to be involved in the formation of a salt bridge which stabilizes the three-dimensional structure of α-1 proteinase inhibitor (Loebermann at al., 1984). The fact that the distance between the reactive center (P_1) and the P_{17} and the P_{69} is as well maintained in all GDNs is an additional indication of the proper identification of the reactive center of the GDNs.

Rat GDN has two, human GDN three putative glycosylation sites (Asn-X-Thr/Ser). The position of the two putative glycosylation sites in the rat protein have been conserved in the human GDNs. Three Cys residues are found in both rat and human GDNs. Two of these Cys are at the same position in all GDNs. The importance of these conserved Cys positions for the properties of GDNs remains to be demonstrated.

Rat GDN forms SDS-resistant complexes with proteases such as tissue plasminogen activator, urokinase or thrombin (Guenther et al., 1985). Recent results have demonstrated that elastase cleaves GDN between the P_1 and P_2 residues. The elastase cleaved GDN has lost both its protease inhibitory activity and its neurite promoting activity.

Recent experiments have shown that purified rat GDN promotes neurite outgrowth in chick sympathetic neurons (Zurn et al., 1988). GDN does also potentiate in a dose-dependent manner the neurite outgrowth induced by nerve growth factor (NGF) in those cells. Rat GDN inhibits the migration of granule neurons monitored in cultured explants from early postnatal mouse cerebellum (Lindner et al., 1986). Hirudin and synthetic tripeptides with anti-thrombin activity mimic GDN effect in neuroblastoma cells but not in the primary cultures mentioned above. Taken together with the lack of activity of elastase treated GDN, these results suggest that the inhibition of proteolytic activity is necessary but not sufficient to explain the neurite promoting activity of GDN. The formation of the stable high molecular weight complex with a protease seems therefore important for the biological activity. It is tempting to speculate that GDN (or the protease) has to undergo a conformational change during the formation of the protease/protease inhibitor complex and that newly exposed epitopes are required for GDN biological activity on primary neurons.

The importance of the function of proteases and protease inhibitors in neurite outgrowth remains to be demonstrated. The unexpected discovery that glia-derived serine protease inhibitors (GDNs) promote neurite extension does only allow speculations which should stimulate new experimental approaches.

Cell-associated proteases are involved in the mechanisms triggering migrating or invasive cells (Unkeless et al., 1973). The demonstration of plasminogen activator activity at the level of the growth cone suggests that proteolytic enzymes could as well be involved in the motility and the invasive properties characterizing this subcellular structure at the tip of the neurite (Krystosek and Seeds, 1981). One can envisage that the presence of GDN in the vicinity of the growth cone would lead to the formation of stable complexes with some of the growth cone associated proteases. The resulting reduction in proteolytic activity would contribute to the stabilization of zones located just at the origin of the growth cone, thus allowing a net increase in neurite length. Alternatively, such complexes might form at discrete locations in the area explored by the microspikes. Such localized decrease in proteolytic activity would reduce the deadhesion phases characterizing microspike activity, and thus establish new zones of preferential adhesion. This, in turn, could trigger the "immobilization" of certain microspikes which, as mentioned above, seem to drag the growth cone forward (Bray and Chapman, 1985).

If the sensitivity of the assay available has permitted the localization of plasminogen activator at the growth cone, kinetic studies indicate that GDN has a 10 times higher affinity for thrombin than for plasminogen activator (Stone et al., 1987). One has therefore to consider that GDN would react much more efficiently with an yet unknown growth cone associated serine protease with thrombin-like specificity. A calcium-dependent protease activity has also been recently localized at the level of the growth cone (Pittman, 1985). These facts suggest that different types of proteases can trigger the motility of the growth cone. Conversely, their specific inhibitors might, like GDN, contribute to a localized stabilization that sustains neurite outgrowth. Of course, if the balance between distinct proteases and their respective inhibitors has an influence, it is not necessary to assume that each of them will always have the same importance. The impact of each protease/protease inhibitor balance will depend of the availability of their substrates in different locations. The concentration (or density) of distinct extracellular substrates in the vicinity of the incoming growth cone could thus determine which protease/protease inhibitor system becomes rate limiting.

Further investigations should establish if the balance between proteases and protease inhibitors could regulate the amount and the quality of some components of the extracellular matrix known to promote neurite outgrowth. The turnover of cell surface receptors or of cell adhesion molecules involved in neurite extension could as well be influenced by the local balance between proteases and their inhibitors.

The role of proteases in the degenerative and regenerative processes taking place in the nervous system remain to be elucidated. The use of in vitro experimental models will certainly allow to answer some of the questions. The in vivo localization and quantification of proteases and of inhibitors such as GDNs will, however, be necessary to study their relevance. Preliminary experiments indicate that GDN or GDN-like proteins able to complex iodinated urokinase are detected following lesions in the peripheral nervous system where regeneration is possible. This does not seem to be the case following lesions in the central nervous system where the environment is not able to support fiber regeneration (Patterson, 1985). Grafting experiments demonstrate that the non-neuronal environment determines the success or the failure in regenerative processes (Benfey and Aguayo, 1982). The existence of glia-derived nexins is compatible with those facts. Further studies should therefore aim at the identification of the mechanisms regulating the synthesis and release of GDNs or GDN-like substances.

The identification, cloning and sequencing of GDNs represent an important step providing the molecular biological tools necessary to estimate the role of proteases and protease inhibitors in neurite outgrowth during development or regeneration.

REFERENCES

Benfey M, Aguayo AJ (1982). Extensive elongation of axons from rat brain into peripheral nerve grafts. Nature 296:150-152.
Bray D, Chapman K (1985). Analysis of microspike movements on the neuronal growth cone. J Neurosci 5:3204-3213.
Carell R, Travis J (1985). α_1-Antitrypsin and the serpins: variation and countervariation. TIBS 10:20-24.
Gloor S, Odink K, Guenther J, Nick H, Monard D (1986). A glia-derived neurite promoting factor with protease inhibitory activity belongs to the protease nexins. Cell 47:687-693.
Guenther J, Nick H, Monard D (1985). A glia-derived neurite-promoting factor with protease inhibitory activity. EMBO J 4:1463-1468.
Krystosek A, Seeds NW (1981). Plasminogen activator release at the neuronal growth cone. Science 213:1532-1534.
Kurachi K, Chandra T, Friezner Degen SJ, White TT, Marchioro TL, Woo SLC, Davie EW (1981). Cloning and sequence of cDNA coding for α_1-antitrypsin. Proc Natl Acad Sci USA 78:6826-6830.
Lindner J, Guenther J, Nick H, Zinser G, Antonicek H, Schachner M, Monard (1986). Modulation of granule cell migration by a glia-derived protein. Proc Natl Acad Sci USA 83:4568-4571.
Loebermann H, Tokuoka R, Deisenhofer J, Huber R (1984). Human α_1-proteinase inhibitor. J Mol Biol 177:531-556.
Monard D, Solomon F, Rentsch M, Gysin R (1973). Glia-induced morphological differentiation in neuroblastoma cells. Proc. Natl Acad Sci USA 70:1894-1897.
Monard D, Stockel K, Goodman R, Thoenen H (1975) Distinction between nerve growth factor and glial factor. Nature 258:444-445.
Monard D, Niday E, Limat A, Solomon F (1983). Inhibition of protease activity can lead to neurite extension in neuroblastoma cells. Prog Brain Res 58:359-364.
Ny T, Sawday M, Lawrence D, Millan JL, Loskutoff DJ (1986). Cloning and sequence of a cDNA coding for the human β-migrating endothelial-cell-type plasminogen activator inhibitor. Proc Natl Acad Sci USA 83:6776-6780.

Pannekoek H, Veerman H, Lambers H, Diergaarde P, Verweij CL, van Zonnefeld AJ, van Mourik, JA (1986). Endothelial plasminogen activator inhibitor (PAI): a new member of the Serpin gene family. EMBO J 5:2539-2544.

Patterson PJ (1985). On the role of proteases, their inhibitors and the extracellular matrix in promoting neurite outgrowth. J Physiol Paris 80:207-211.

Pittman RN (1985). Release of plasminogen activator and a calcium-dependent metalloprotease from cultured sympathetic and sensory neurons. Dev Biol 110:91-101.

Schuerch-Rathgeb Y, Monard D (1978). Brain development influences the appearance of glial factor-like activity in rat brain primary cultures. Nature 273:308-309.

Sommer J, Gloor SM, Rovelli GF, Hofsteenge J, Nick H, Meier R, Monard D (1987). cDNA sequence coding for a rat glia-derived nexin and its homology to members of the serpin superfamily. Biochemistry 26:6407-6410.

Scott RW, Bergman BL, Bajpai A, Hersch RT, Rodriguez H, Jones BN, Barreda C, Watts, S., Baker JB (1985). Protease nexin. J Biol Chem 260:7029-7034.

Stone S, Nick H, Hofsteenge J, Monard D (1987). Glia-derived neurite-promoting factor is a slow-binding inhibitor of trypsin, thrombin and urokinase. Arch Biochem Biophys 252:237-244.

Unkeless JC, Tobia A, Ossowski L, Quigley JP, Rifkin DB, Reich E (1973). An enzymatic function associated with transformation of fibroblasts by oncogenic viruses. J exp Med 137:85-111.

Zurn AD, Nick H, Monard D (1988). A glia-derived nexin promotes neurite outgrowth in cultured chick sympathetic neurons. Dev Neuroscience, in press.

MAINTENANCE OF AXON TERMINALS AT SYNAPTIC SITES IN THE
ABSENCE OF MUSCLE FIBERS

Yung-mae M. Yao
Department of Neurobiology
Stanford University School of Medicine
Stanford, California 94305

INTRODUCTION

The structure of the neuromuscular junction in skeletal muscles of the frog is simple and orderly. As the motor axon approaches the muscle fiber, it branches giving rise to an arborization of terminal branches which lie in close apposition to the muscle fiber. Each terminal branch runs longitudinally along the basal lamina sheath of the muscle fiber for up to a few hundred micrometers and releases the transmitter, acetylcholine. At approximately 1 micron intervals along the length of the terminal there are "active zones" (Couteaux and Pechot-Dechavassine, 1970) which are involved in the release of transmitter; the active zones are situated precisely opposite junctional folds in the muscle fiber surface. Moreover, each terminal branch is capped by a Schwann cell which, at widely separated points, sends narrow processes through the synaptic cleft to belt the terminal. A collagen-rich basal lamina surrounds each muscle fiber and sends a finger into each of the junctional folds (eg. Sanes et al. 1978; Sanes, 1982).

For normal muscles, the paucity of junctional folds unapposed by axon terminals and of immature, developing terminal branches makes it seem likely that the overall structural plan changes little over months to years. In the study presented here, I examined the role of the muscle fiber in the maintenance of the structure of the terminal arborization. Specifically, I removed muscle fibers from their basal lamina sheaths without damaging axon terminals and examined (a) the extent of the arborization, (b) the size of the axon terminals, and (c) the axon terminal's fine structure. I found that changes did occur but they were detectable only after several months. Even after 1 year, the arborization was still intact, vesicles and active zones were present, and the average size of the axon terminals was similar to control values. Schwann cell belts were also present but they covered a greater percentage of the length of the axon terminal arborization. I conclude that muscle fibers provide factors required for the maintenance of terminals at synaptic sites and that either the factors are maintained in the muscle fiber basal lamina or their effect is long-lasting.

RESULTS

Removal of muscle fibers

My experiments were carried out on the cutaneous pectoris muscle of the adult frog. In order to assess the role of muscle fibers on maintenance of axon terminals at synaptic sites, muscle fibers were caused to degenerate without damaging the innervating axons, the axon's Schwann cells or the synaptic basal lamina (Fig. 1). Following surgical damage, the muscle fibers retracted and degenerated, leaving behind their basal lamina sheaths. Within 2 weeks, the basal lamina sheaths were almost completely empty of debris and fragments of plasma membrane. The empty muscle fiber basal lamina sheaths remained intact for at least 12 months. Muscle fiber regeneration was successfully prevented by x-irradiation of the frogs for the first 3 days after muscle fiber damage (irradiation procedure: Philips 250 kV 15 mA X-ray unit, 0.35 mm Cu filter, total dose/day = 3900 rads).

There was little evidence of damage to the innervating axons, their axon terminals or the axon's Schwann cells as a result of the surgical procedure used to remove muscle fibers. Preparations were examined 1-3 days after muscle fiber damage in the electron microscope, the period during which terminals of deliberately severed axons in the cutaneous pectoris muscle are known to degenerate (Letinsky et al., 1976). Less than 5 % of the axon terminals examined showed evidence of degeneration including: vesicle clumping, mitochondrial swelling, or increased cytoplasmic density (Birks et al. 1960). The terminal Schwann cells maintained their normal position, simply capping the axon terminals during this initial period after muscle fiber damage. Moreover, no evidence of axonal damage or disruption of myelin in the intramuscular branches was observed indicating that damage resulting from the surgical procedure was localized to axon terminal regions.

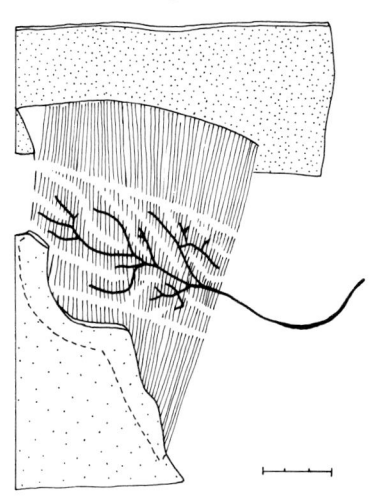

Fig. 1. The surgical procedure on the cutaneous pectoris muscle that causes degeneration and phagocytosis of muscle fibers while leaving the innervated region of muscle fiber basal lamina and motor axons intact. In order to cause complete degeneration of severed muscle fiber segments in frog, the segments can be no greater than 1-2 mm. The junctional region of the cutaneous pectoris muscle is 3-5 mm wide, but within this region, the junctions, which occupy less than a 1 mm stretch along a muscle fiber, are arranged in groups where those on adjacent fibers are nearly in register (Connor and McMahan, 1987). Because the muscle is thin and transparent, nerve bundles leading to these groups of neuromuscular junctions are clearly seen *in vivo* with a dissecting microscope. First I cut across the muscle on each side of the junctional region and removed and discarded the extrajunctional regions. Next I cut the muscles between the nerve branches leading to the groups of neuromuscular junctions taking care not to come any closer to a nerve bundle than 0.5-1.0 mm in order to avoid damage to the axons and their terminals. Bar, 3 mm.

Maintenance of terminals of intact motor axons at synaptic sites on empty basal lamina sheaths.

To identify the synaptic sites following muscle degeneration, whole mounts of muscle were stained for cholinesterase which remains associated with the synaptic basal lamina for several months even after the removal of all cellular components, including muscle fibers, axon terminals and Schwann cells (McMahan and Slater, 1984; Anglister and McMahan, 1985). Similarly, in the present study, light microscopic examination of whole mounted material revealed that the pattern of cholinesterase staining was similar to controls up to 12 months after muscle fiber damage.

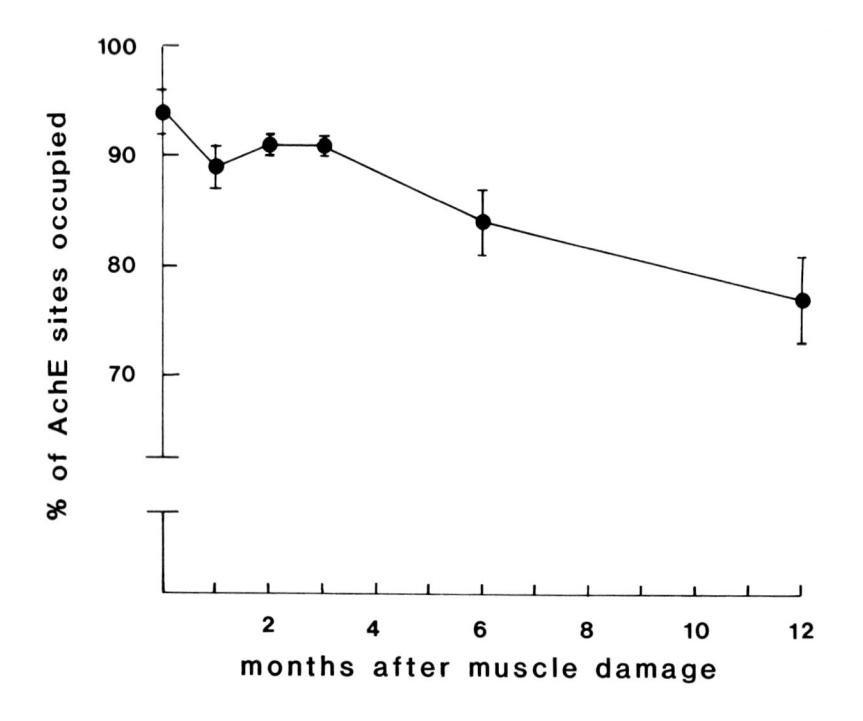

Fig. 2. Percent of synaptic sites, marked by cholinesterase stain, that are apposed by axon terminals after muscle fiber damage only. Terminals of intact axons are maintained at synaptic sites on the empty muscle fiber basal lamina sheath. Each point represents the mean ± SEM from 5 muscles, 50 synaptic sites from each muscle.

Axon terminals persisted at synaptic sites on empty basal sheaths for at least 12 months (Fig. 2). Preparations were examined in the electron microscope and the number of vacant and occupied synaptic sites after the removal of muscle fibers was counted to determine the percentage of synaptic sites occupied by axon terminals. Controls consisted of muscles that were not damaged or received x-irradiation treatment only. One, 2 and 3 months after selective muscle fiber damage, the percentage of synaptic sites apposed by axon terminals did not differ from the control value of 94 ± 2 %. A small percentage of axon terminals began to vacate some of the synaptic sites after the prolonged absence of muscle; however, 78 ± 4 % of the junctional sites remained apposed by axon terminals 12 months after muscle fiber damage. Thus, in the absence of muscle, most of the synaptic sites remain apposed by axon terminals of intact motor axons. However, the presence of muscle is clearly required for prolonged maintenance of terminals at synaptic sites.

Fine structure of the axon terminals after muscle fiber removal.

The fine structure of the terminals at synaptic sites on the empty basal lamina sheaths is similar to mature axon terminals up to 12 months after the removal of muscle fibers. That is, the axon terminals contained accumulations of synaptic vesicles some of which were focused at active zones. The active zones remained positioned directly opposite the fingers of the synaptic basal lamina that formerly extended into junctional folds (Fig. 3).

The structure of the active zones was studied in greater detail using freeze-fracture techniques in combination with electron microscopy. In freeze-fracture replicas of adult frog neuromuscular junctions, active zones are characterized by the presence of two double rows of large particles on the protoplasmic (P) face of the fractured axon terminal (Dreyer et al. 1973; Peper et al. 1974). As shown in Fig. 4, six months after the removal of muscle the P-face of the axon terminal contained two double rows of particles characteristic of normal active zones. In general, these double rows of particles were oriented perpendicular to the long axis of the axon terminal arborization characteristic of active zones at normal neuromuscular junctions. No examples of the widespread disruption, fragmentation or loss of active zone regions observed following denervation (Ko, 1981) were seen after muscle fiber damage.

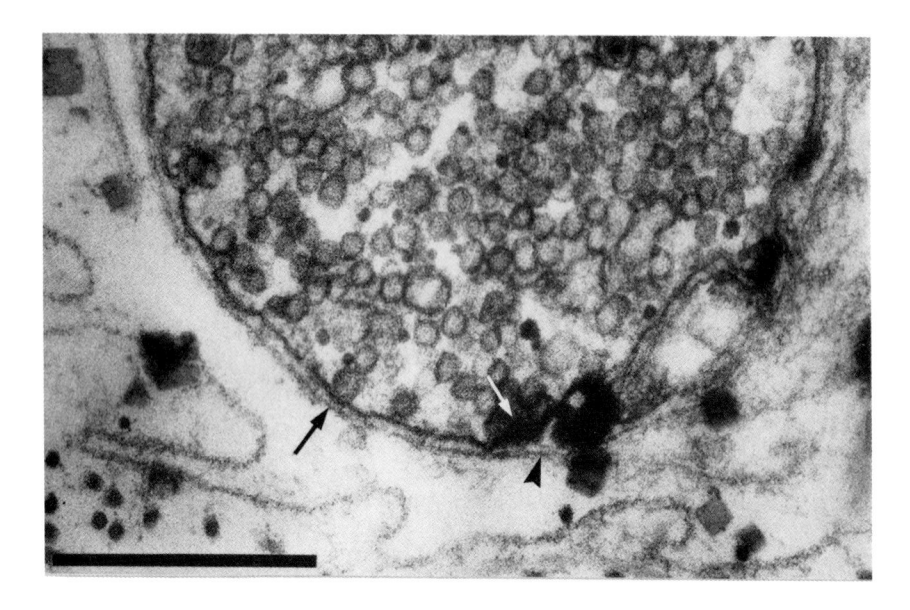

Fig. 3. Synaptic site on a muscle fiber basal lamina (black arrow) in a muscle damaged and x-irradiated 4 months previously. Electron dense crystals are cholinesterase stain. The axon terminal contains numerous synaptic vesicles some of which are focused on an active zone (white arrow). The active zone lies opposite the intersection (arrowhead) of junctional fold and synaptic cleft basal lamina which is characteristic of active zones in normal muscles (Couteaux and Pechot-Dechavassine, 1973). Bar, 0.5 microns. (From Yao 1987).

Cross-sectional area of the axon terminals after muscle fiber removal.

Cross-sectional area was determined as a measure of axon terminal size. Up to 12 months after the removal of muscle fibers the average cross-sectional area did not differ from the control value of 1.4 um^2. Thus, the average value of cross-sectional areas of the terminals of the undamaged axons was not altered after muscle fiber removal.

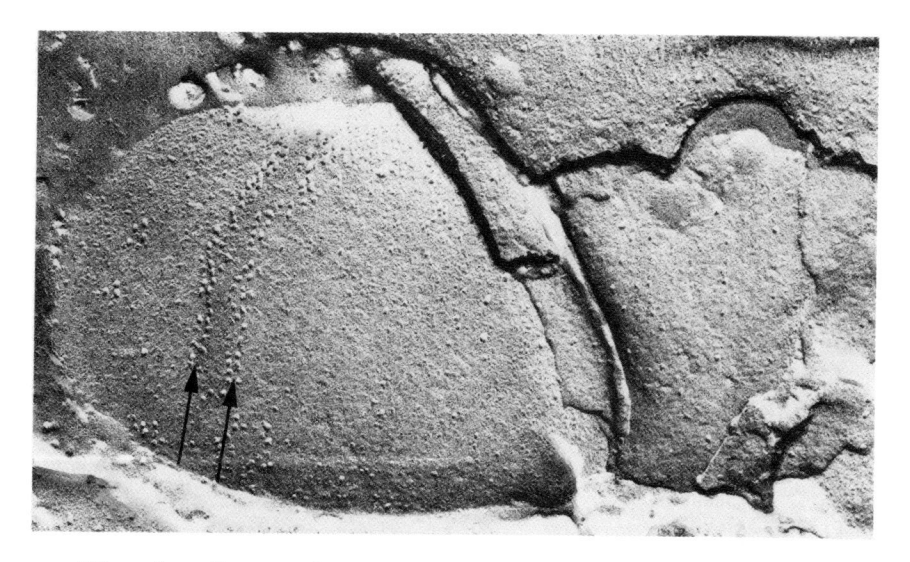

Fig. 4. Freeze-fracture replica of a frog neuromuscular junction 6 months after muscle fiber damage. Double rows of particles characteristic of normal active zones are shown at the arrows.

Altered relationship between terminal Schwann cell and axon terminal.

Normally, the terminal Schwann cells simply cap the axon terminal sending their processes completely around the axon terminal at 1-2 micron intervals along its length (McMahan et al., 1972). Accordingly, when the axon terminal arborization is serially cross-sectioned, a small percentage of the axon terminals observed are completely enwrapped by Schwann cell processes.

I have found that the normal relationship between the axon terminal and Schwann cell is altered after the removal of muscle fibers. Figure 5 summarizes my findings demonstrating that a greater percentage of axon terminal profiles are enwrapped by Schwann cell processes in the absence of muscle. Up to 2 months following the removal of muscle fibers, the percentage of axon terminal profiles enwrapped by Schwann cell processes did not differ from our control value of 4 ± 1 %. However, between 2 and 12 months, the percentage of terminals enwrapped increased significantly to a value of 42 ± 2 % at 12 months after muscle fiber damage. These findings are consistent with those of Duchen and collegues (1974) and Jirmanova (1975) who found that after pharmacological damage of muscle fibers, Schwann cell processes envelop apparently undamaged axon terminals. These results show that muscle fibers play a role in the maintenance of the normal relationship between the axon terminal and the overlying Schwann cells.

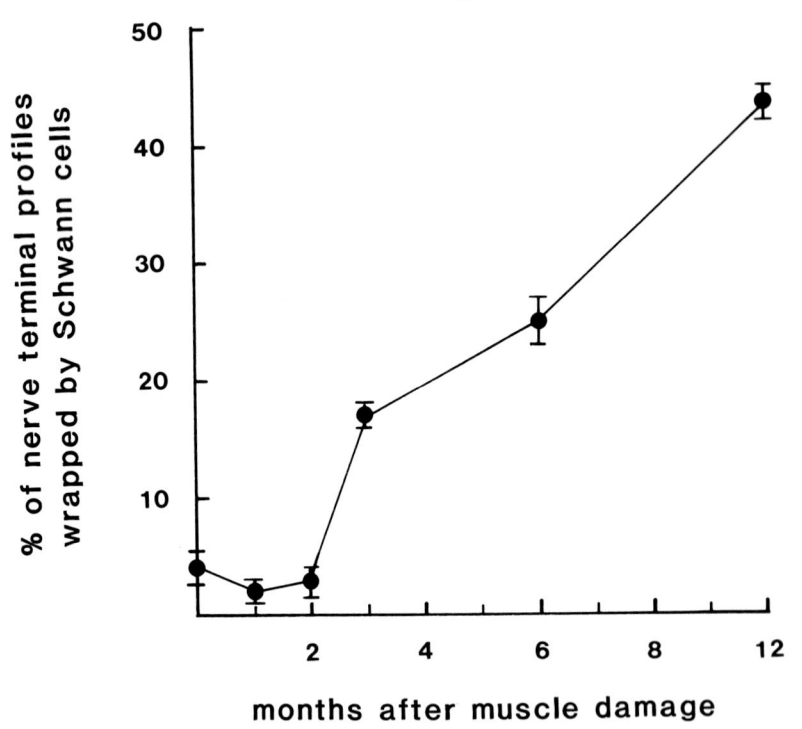

Fig. 5. Percent of axon terminal profiles enwrapped by Schwann cell processes after muscle damage. Each point represents the mean ± SEM for 5 muscles, 50 axon terminals per muscle. Within 3 months the percentage of axon terminal profiles enwrapped by Schwann cell processes was significantly greater than the mean value from control muscles by Student's t-test ($p < 0.01$).

CONCLUDING REMARKS

Several lines of evidence have shown that developing motor neurons require the presence of and/or connections with skeletal muscle. For example, if muscles are removed before they are innervated, all corresponding motor neurons and their growing axons degenerate (Hamburger, 1958, 1975; see Grinnell and Herrera, 1981). Such findings raise the possibility that trophic factors are provided by muscle fibers (Giller et al., 1977; Godfrey et al., 1980; Calof & Reichardt, 1984; 1985; Nurcombe et al. 1984; Kaufman et al., 1985; Smith et al., 1985). Moreover, recent studies have demonstrated that mature neurons may differ from developing ones with regard to their dependency on such trophic factors. For example, when axons are not allowed contact with muscle, immature motor neurons die (Hamburger, 1958; Kashihara et al. 1987) while mature ones persist for extended periods of time (Carlson et al. 1979; Habgood et al. 1984). Thus, it appears that motor neurons become less dependent on their target muscle for survival as they mature. However, it remains unclear whether adult motor neurons survive indefinitely; Kawamura and Dyck (1981) found reduced numbers of motor neurons in adult humans several years after total amputation of a lower limb. Similarly, in a previous study I have demonstrated that regenerating motor neurons, in contrast, to undamaged adult motor neurons are highly dependent upon the presence of muscle for maintenance of their axon terminals at synaptic sites (Yao, 1987). Here, I have presented evidence that intact, adult axon terminals persist at synaptic sites and maintain their mature structure for at least one year after removal of muscle fibers from their basal lamina sheaths. Two possible explanations for my findings are that 1) normal axon terminals may be much less dependent on muscle released factors than embryonic ones or that 2) the terminals are still highly dependent on trophic factors provided by the muscle fibers but such trophic factors are stably bound to the adult basal lamina. This latter proposal is supported by recent findings demonstrating that molecules which are provided, at least in part, by muscle such as the enzyme acetylcholinesterase are stably maintained in the synaptic basal lamina after the removal of muscle (eg. Anglister and McMahan, 1985).

Acknowledgments

This study was supported by a National Institutes of Health (NIH) grant 14506. Y.M. Yao was supported by a NIH National Research Service Award (NS 07089), a National Amyotrophic Lateral Sclerosis postdoctoral fellowship and a gift from L. Harvey, A. Levien and K. Linden.

REFERENCES

Anglister L, McMahan UJ (1985). Basal lamina directs acetylcholinesterase accumulation at synaptic sites in regenerating muscle. J Cell Biol 101:735-743.

Birks RI, Katz B, Miledi R (1960). Physiological and structural changes at the amphibian myoneural junction, in the course of nerve degeneration. J Physiol 150:145-168.

Calof AL, Reichardt LF (1984). Motoneurons purified by cell sorting respond to two distinct activities in myotube-conditioned medium. Dev Biol 106:194-210.

Calof AL, Reichardt, LF (1985). Response of purified chick motoneurons to myotube conditioned medium: laminin is essential for the substratum-binding, neurite outgrowth-promoting activity. Neurosci Lett 59:183-189.

Carlson J, Lais AC, Dyck PJ (1979). Axonal atrophy from permanent peripheral axotomy in adult cat. J Neuropathol Exp Neurol 38:579-585.

Connor EA, McMahan UJ (1987). Cell accumulation in the junctional region of denervated muscle. J Cell Biol 104:109-120.

Couteaux R, Pechot-Dechavassine, M (1970). Vesicules synaptiques et poches au niveau des "zones active" de la jonction neuromusculaire. C R Acad Sci (Paris) D 271: 2346-2349.

Couteaux R, Pechot-Dechavassine, M (1973) Donnees ultrastructurales et cytochimiques sur le mecanisme de liberation de l'acetylcholine dans la transmission synaptique. Arch ital Biol 3:231-262.

Dreyer FK, Peper,K, Akert K, Sandri C, Moor H (1973). Ultrastructure of the 'active zone' in the frog neuromuscular junctions. Brain Res 62:47-55.

Duchen LW, Excell BJ, Patel R, Smith B (1974). Changes in motor end-plates resulting from muscle fibre necrosis and regeneration. A light and electron microscopic study of the effects of the depolarizing fraction (cardiotoxin) of Dendroaspis jamesoni venom. J Neurol Sci 21:391-417.

Giller EL, Neale JH, Bullock PN, Schrier BK, Nelson, PG (1977). Choline acetyltransferase activity of spinal cord cell cultures increased by co-culture with muscle and by muscle-conditioned medium. J Cell Biol 74:16-28.

Godfrey EW, Schrier BK, Nelson PG (1980). Source and target cell specificities of a conditioned medium factor that increases choline acetyltransferase activity in cultured spinal cord cells. Dev Biol 77:403-418.

Grinnell AP, Herrera AA (1981). Specificity and plasticity of neuromuscular connections: Long-term regulation of motoneuron function. Progr Neurobiol 17:203-282.

Habgood MD, Hopkins WG, Slack JR (1984). Muscle size and motor unit survival in mice. J. Physiol. 356:303-314.

Hamburger V (1958). Regression versus peripheral control of differentiation in motor hypoplasia. Am J Anat 102:365-410.

Hamburger V (1975). Cell death in the development of the lateral motor column of the chick embryo. J Comp Neurol 160:535-546.

Jirmanova I (1975). Ultrastructure of motor end-plates during pharmacologically-induced degeneration and subsequent regeneration of skeletal muscle. J Neurocytol 4:141-155.

Kashihara Y, Kuno M, Miyata Y (1987). Cell death of axotomized motoneurons in neonatal rats, and its prevention by peripheral reinnervation. J Physiol 386:135-148.

Kaufman LM, Barry SR, Barrett JN (1985). Characterization of tissue-derived macromolecules affecting transmitter synthesis in rat spinal cord neurons. J Neurosci 5:160-166.

Kawamura Y, Dyck PJ (1981). Permanent axotomy by amputation results in loss of motor neurons in man. J Neuropathology and Experimental Neurology 40:658-666.

Ko CP (1981). Electrophysiological and freeze-fracture studies of changes following denervation at frog neuromuscular junctions. J Physiol 321: 627-639.

Letinsky MS, Fischbeck KH, McMahan UJ (1976). Precision of reinnervation of original postsynaptic sites in frog muscle after a nerve crush. J Neurocytol 5:691-718.

McMahan UJ, Slater CR (1984). The influence of basal lamina on the accumulation of acetycholine receptors at synaptic sites in regenerating muscle. J Cell Biol 98:1453-1473.

McMahan UJ, Spitzer NC, Peper, K (1972). Visual identification of nerve terminals in living isolated skeletal muscle. Proc R Soc B 177:485-508.

Nurcombe V, Hill MA, Eagleson KL, Bennett MR (1984). Motor neuron survival and neuritic extension from spinal cord explants induced by factors released from denervated muscle. Brain Res 291:19-28.

Peper K, Dreyer F, Sandri C, Akert K (1974). Structure and ultrastructure of the frog motor end-plate. A freeze-etching study. Cell Tiss Res 149:437-455.

Sanes JR (1982). Laminin, fibronectin, and collagen in synaptic and extrasynaptic portions of muscle fiber basement membrane. J Cell Biol 93:442-451.

Sanes JR, Marshall LM, McMahan UJ (1978). Reinnervation of muscle fiber basal lamina after removal of myofibers. J Cell Biol 78:176-198.

Smith RG, McManaman J, Appel SH (1985). Trophic effects of skeletal muscle extracts on ventral spinal cord neurons in vitro: separation of a protein with morphologic activity from proteins with cholinergic activity. J Cell Biol 101:1608-1621.

Yao YM (1987). Factors that influence the maintenance of normal and regenerating axon terminals. In Gordon T, Stein RB, Smith PA (eds): "The Current Status of Peripheral Nerve Regeneration," New York: Alan R. Liss, pp 235-246.

EXPRESSION OF NERVE GROWTH FACTOR RECEPTORS ON SCHWANN CELLS AFTER AXONAL INJURY

Eugene M. Johnson, Jr.[1], H. Brent Clark[2], John B. Schweitzer[3] and Megumi Taniuchi[1]

Department of Pharmacology, Washington University School of Medicine, St. Louis, MO 63110 (E.M.J., M.T.); Department of Laboratory Medicine, Memorial Medical Center Springfield, IL 62781 (H.B.C.); and Division of Neuropathology, Department of Pathology, University of Tennessee, Memphis, TN 38163 (J.B.S.)

Nerve growth factor (NGF) is a neurotrophic factor required for the survival of sympathetic and neural crest-derived sensory neurons (for review, see Thoenen and Barde, 1980). Recent data suggest a similar role in some populations of central nervous system (CNS) neurons (for review, see Whittemore and Seiger 1987). The sequence of events by which NGF normally exerts its effects on responsive neurons includes elaboration of the factor by the target, NGF binding to specific receptors on nerve termini, and subsequent retrograde transport of NGF and its receptor to the cell soma.

Although the precise molecular mechanism(s) of NGF action are not resolved, it is clear that the first step involves interaction with specific receptors (see Sutter et al., 1979). Equilibrium binding studies on sympathetic or sensory neurons have demonstrated two kinetically distinct binding entities. A high-affinity ($K_d \approx 10^{-10}$-10^{-11}M) receptor is generally associated with NGF internalization and biological action on neuronal and PC12 cells (Bernd and Greene, 1984). A second, low-affinity ($K_d \approx 10^{-9}$M) receptor or binding site is also found on these responsive cells.

We have recently (Taniuchi et al., 1986b) reported that in response to axotomy of peripheral nerve, Schwann cells distal, but not proximal, to the lesion express NGF receptor. NGF receptor increased approximately 20 fold as measured by a cross-link/immunoprecipatation assay using a monoclonal antibody, 192-IgG against the rat NGF receptor (Chandler et al., 1984). Similar increases were seen in other structures (muscle, skin) distal to the lesion. This increase in receptors was immunohistochemically localized to the nerves within these tissues. Based this observation, and on reports of Schwann cell production of NGF after nerve injury (Rush, 1984), we proposed

(Taniuchi et al., 1986b) that disruption of the normal interaction between axons and Schwann cells induces the Schwann cell to produce both NGF and NGF receptor. The NGF binds to the Schwann cell surface receptors and becomes concentrated upon the substratum over which regenerating axons grow. The surface-bound NGF molecules supply trophic support and haptotactic guidance (chemotactic activity over a surface) for sympathetic and sensory axons regenerating through the bands of Bungner.

In this paper we address several issues raised by our initial observations. For example, where are NGF receptors located at the ultrastructural level? What is the effect of axonal regeneration on the expression of NGF receptors by Schwann cells? Is the ability to induce NGF receptor expression restricted to the subpopulation of Schwann cells ensheathing NGF-responsive neurons, or is it a general phenomenon? Do central neuroglial cells behave similarly and produce NGF receptors after axonal injury? A more detailed description of these experiments is provided in Taniuchi et al., 1988.

Ultrastructural localization of NGF receptors

The ultrastructural location of the receptor was determined in distal sciatic nerve seven days after lesion by using electron-microscopic immunohistochemistry with 192-IgG, the monoclonal against the rat NGF receptor. Immunoreactivity was restricted to cells and cell processes identifiable as Schwann cells by their ultrastructural morphology and by their investment with basal lamina. Immunoreactivity was most pronounced on the surfaces of the cell processes, indicating that the receptors were located on Schwann cell plasmalemma. Occasionally staining was also observed in Schwann cell cytoplasm, presumably representing recently synthesized receptor molecules. No nuclear staining was observed. The only cells within the nerve which were stained were enclosed within a basal lamina (i.e., Schwann cells).

Reversibility of receptor expression

The effect of regeneration on the expression of NGF receptors on Schwann cells was determined by comparing distal nerve after either a transection (preventing regeneration) or a crush (permitting regeneration). Both biochemical and immunohistochemical examinations were done on nerve and skeletal muscle for up to 10 weeks after lesion. For example, the data in Fig. 1 are the NGF receptor levels, measured by a crosslink/immunoprecipitation assay (Taniuchi et al, 1986b) the tibialis anterior muscle after sciatic nerve transection or crush. After either lesion, NGF receptor increased approximately 10 fold during the first two weeks. In the transected nerve, receptor density remained elevated for the 10-week period examined. In contrast, receptor density decreased in the crushed nerve after two weeks and returned to the level of uninjured nerve after 10 weeks. In the transected nerves, there was intense immunostaining of Schwann cells throughout the 10-week period. In the crushed nerves staining of Schwann cells decreased in distal sciatic nerve and subsequently in the nerve within the tibialis anterior muscle.

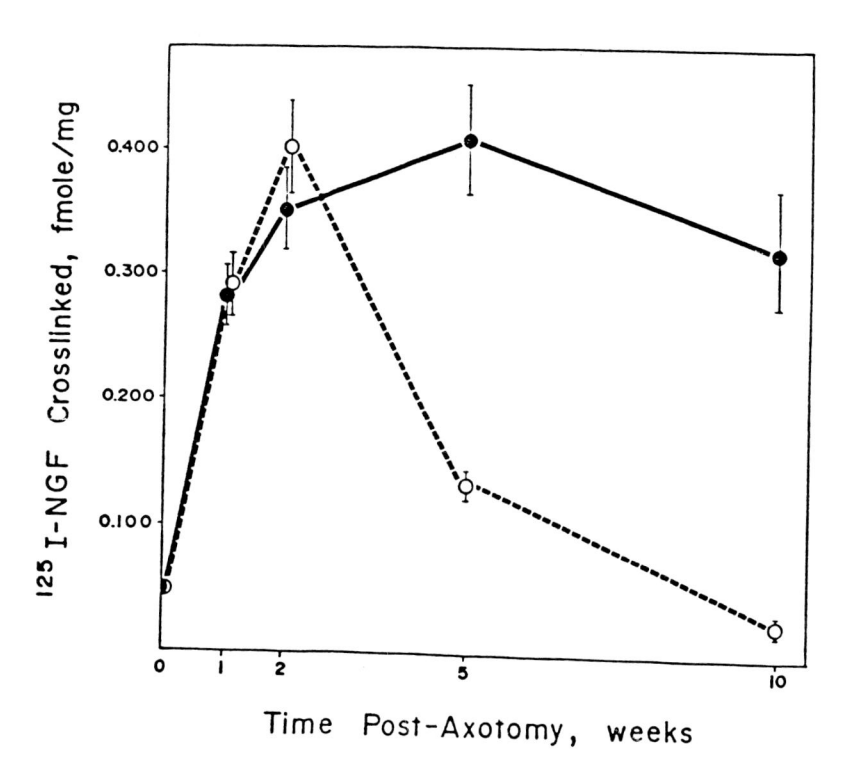

Fig. 1. NGF receptor density in tibialis anterior muscle after sciatic nerve transection or crush. Muscles from 6 rats were pooled, homogenized, and centrifuged to obtain an S_2 fraction (Taniuchi et al., 1986b). The protein content of the S_2 samples was determined, and 500 µg of each sample assayed in triplicate with the ^{125}I-NGF crosslinking/192-IgG immunoprecipitation assay (Taniuchi et al., 1986a). The values plotted represent the mean ± SEM from muscle homogenates of rats that initially received transection (closed circles) or nerve crush (open circles).

It was possible to determine more precisely the relationship of regenerating fibers to receptor expression on Schwann cells. Ultrastructural examination of the regeneration zone revealed a decrease or loss of NGF receptors in Schwann cells making contact with elongating axonal processes. These results strongly suggest that NGF receptor expression by Schwann cells is negatively regulated by interaction with axons. The loss of the normal Schwann cell-axon relationship causes an induction in NGF receptor production by Schwann cells, and reestablishment of this interaction by axonal regeneration suppresses receptor expression.

Do Schwann cells which do not ensheathe NGF-responsive axons induce receptors?

The question of whether all Schwanns cells, or only those ensheathing axons of NGF-dependent neurons, would express NGF receptors upon loss of axonal contact was addressed in several ways. And, indeed, all Schwann cells do express NGF receptors. A particularly informative paradigm involved lesioning the motoneurons of the sciatic nerve by performing ventral rhizotomies. If only NGF-responsive neurons can generate the inducing agent, then there should be no induction on any Schwann cells following axotomy of NGF-independent motoneurons. If all Schwann cells are capable of "inducing" receptor following degeneration of the axons they ensheathe, then ablation of motor axons should cause receptor induction. If a diffusible signal is generated, then those Schwann cells ensheathing the degenerated axons and at least some Schwann cells in the vicinity, but not ensheathing dying axons, should be induced. The results of the immunohistochemistry of the sciatic nerve after L_5 ventral rhizotomy showed that Schwann cells surrounding degenerating motoneuron axons were positively stained with 192-IgG. In contrast, Schwann cells ensheathing intact axons (primarily sensory fibers) showed no immunostaining at the light or EM level.

Interestingly, sciatic nerves from control, uninjured animals occasionally contained spontaneously degenerating fibers. In those cases, the bands of Bungner associated with the degenerating axons stained for 192-IgG. Again, neighboring, intact Schwann cell/axon units were devoid of stain. These results strongly suggest that the signal to induce NGF receptors is the loss of contact with viable axons, not elaboration of a soluble factor.

Kinetic properties of induced receptors in injured nerve

We have examined the kinetic properties of receptors induced on the Schwann cells after axonal injury. Equilibrium binding experiments were done on membranes prepared from either superior cervical ganglia (SCG) or from intact or injured sciatic nerve. The resulting Scatchard plots are shown in Fig. 2. SCG membranes demonstrate a biphasic curve of ^{125}I-NGF binding and yield a K_d of approximately 10 pM and 1.8 nM. Membranes from injured sciatic nerves, in contrast, show a single binding site with a K_d of 1.5 nM. Thus sciatic nerves distal to an injury appear to express only the low-affinity form of the NGF receptor. Consistent with the equilibrium binding experiments, membranes of SCG show a significant component of slow dissociation, whereas distal nerve membranes do not (Fig. 2, inset). The in vivo results are consistent with previous data showing only the presence of low-affinity NGF receptors on cultured ganglionic nonneuronal cells (Sutter et al., 1979; Carbonetto and Stach, 1982; Zimmerman and Sutter, 1983) and on cultured Schwann cells from newborn rat peripheral nerve (DiStefano and Johnson, 1988).

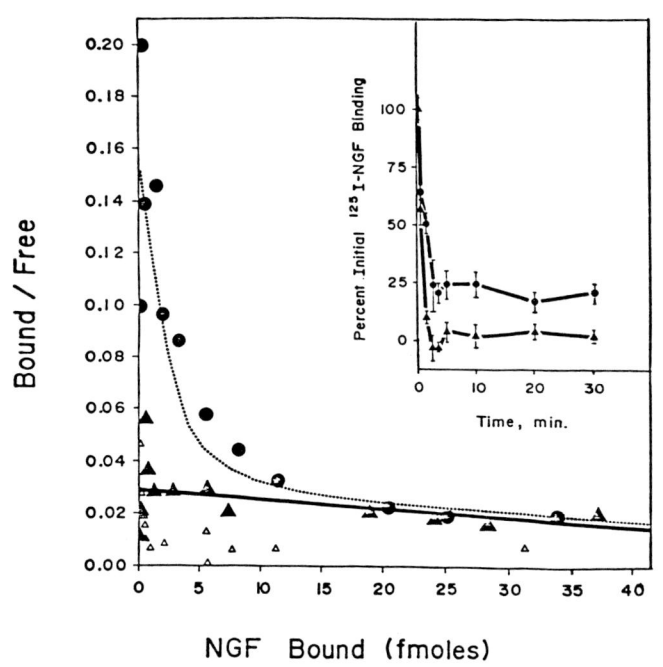

Fig. 2. Comparison of the equilibrium binding of ^{125}I-NGF on Schwann cell NGF receptors to sympathetic neuronal NGF receptors. Radiolabeled NGF at concentrations ranging from 20 pm to 50 nm were combined with 40 μg of S_2 protein prepared from distal sciatic nerve at 14-day posttransection (closed triangles), S_2 from SCG (closed circles), or S_2 from control sciatic nerve (open triangles). After 1.5 hr incubation at 22°C, the free ^{125}I-NGF was removed by filtration through Millipore membrane disks. Nonsaturable binding was determined by parallel incubations in the presence of 1 μM nonlabeled NGF. All

determinations were in triplicate. A Scatchard analysis of the data is shown. The curve was fitted to the data from SCG homogenate in accordance with a quadratic equation describing the binding of a single ligand to 2 independent sites. The line was determined by linear regression to the data from the transected sciatic nerve homogenate. Inset: Dissociation of ^{125}I-NGF from Schwann cell receptors and from sympathetic neuronal receptors. Radiolabeled NGF at 50 pm was incubated with 40 µg of S_2 protein from transected sciatic nerve (triangles) or from SCG (circles) and allowed to reach equilibrium. Dissociation at 0.4°C was initiated by the addition of nonlabeled NGF to a final concentration of 500 nm. At the various times, aliquots were filtered through Millipore disks. The data were normalized to the amount of initial binding; the means ± SEM of triplicate determinations are plotted.

Are NGF receptors induced in the CNS? NGF and NGF receptors are widely distributed in the CNS (Shelton and Reichard, 1984; Korsching et al., 1985, Taniuchi et al., 1986a). Because the CNS is clearly much less conducive to axonal regeneration than is peripheral nerve, we wished to determine whether part of the reason might be because of a failure of CNS glial elements to express NGF receptor in a manner analogous to peripheral nerve after injury. To address this issue, we examined tracts of neurons known to bear NGF receptors: The dorsal column fibers of the spinal cord (which contain central processes of DRG neurons) and the fornix-fimbria tract of the medial septal neurons projecting to the hippocampus. We also examined lesioned optic nerve. Tissues were removed from animals up to two weeks after lesion, and NGF receptors assessed by the crosslink/immunoprecipatation assay (Taniuchi et al., 1986a). None of injured tissue had induced NGF receptors. Consistent with these biochemical results, CNS injury is not associated with immunohistochemical evidence of NGF receptors after injury. Similarly we have failed to observe NGF receptors on cultured rat astrocytes (DiStefano and Johnson, 1988) or on oligodendroglia (unpublished).

In summary, we find that loss of axonal contact results in the expression on all Schwann cells of low-affinity NGF receptors. The receptors are located on the plasmalemma of Schwann cells and we could find no evidence that a diffusible factor has a role in their induction. Rather, intimate axonal contact is the critical factor. Reestablishment of axonal contact with regeneration suppresses the receptor expression. CNS glial do not appear to express NGF receptors in response to loss of axonal contact.

Based on these data, we have proposed a working hypothesis whereby axotomy causes degeneration of neuronal fibers distal to the injury, thereby depriving the neuron cell body of target-derived trophic support. The loss of axolemma induces Schwann cells to express low-affinity NGF receptors on their surface and to produce and release NGF (Heumann et al., 1987). The NGF binds to and becomes concentrated on Schwann cells. As regenerating sympathetic and sensory fibers enter the distal nerve, they are guided haptotactically along the Schwann cell substratum by the NGF bound to the receptors. The close apposition of regenerating axolemma (which contains high-affinity NGF receptors) and the Schwann cell plasmalemma would facilitate the receptor-mediated, intercellular transfer of NGF. The high-affinity neuronal receptors internalize the NGF, which is subsequently retrogradely transported to the neuronal cell body. The Schwann cell-derived trophic support temporarily replaces the target-derived trophic support. Concurrently, axonal contact suppresses NGF receptor and NGF protein production by the Schwann cells. Thus, activated Schwann cells are always located distally to the growing fiber. When the neuronal fibers reinnervate the target, these tissues again become the primary source of NGF and the Schwann cell becomes quiescent. We speculate that NGF and NGF receptors are but one of a repertoire of possible trophic factors and receptors made by Schwann cells in response to axotomy.

References

Bernd, P., Greene, L.A. (1984) Association of ^{125}I-nerve growth factor with PC12 pheochromocytoma cells. Evidence for the internalization via high-affinity receptors only and long-term regulation by nerve growth factor of both high- and low-affinity receptors. J. Biol. Chem. 259:15509-15516.

Carbonetto, S., Stach, R.W. (1982) Localization of nerve growth factor bound to neurons growing nerve fibers in culture. Dev. Brain Res. 3:463-473.

Chandler, C.E., Parsons, L.M., Hosang, M., and Shooter, E.M. (1984) A monoclonal antibody modulates the interaction of nerve growth factor with PC12 cells. J. Biol. Chem. 259:6882-6889.

DiStefano, P.S., Johnson, E.M., Jr. (1988) Nerve growth factor receptors on cultured rat Schwann cells. J. Neurosci. 8:231-241.

Heumann, R., Korsching, S., Bandtlow, C., Thoenen, H. (1987) Changes in nerve growth factor synthesis in nonneuronal cells in response to sciatic nerve transection. J. Cell Biol. 104:1623-1631.

Korsching, S.I., Auberger, G., Heumann, R., Scott, J., Thoenen, H. (1985) Levels of nerve growth factor and its mRNA in the central nervous system of the rat correlate with cholinergic innervation. EMBO J. 4:1389-1393.

Rush, R.A. (1984) Immunohistochemical localization of endogenous nerve growth factor. Nature 312:364-367.

Shelton, D.L., Reichardt, L.F. (1984) Expression of the β-nerve growth factor gene correlates with the density of sympathetic innervation in effector organs. Proc. Natl. Acad. Sci. USA 81:7951-7955.

Sutter, A.R., Riopelle, R.J., Harris-Warwick, R.M., Shooter, E.M. (1979) Nerve growth factor receptors. Characterization of two distinct classes of binding sites on chick embryo sensory ganglia cells. J. Biol. Chem. 254:5972-5982.

Taniuchi, M., Schweitzer, J.B., Johnson, E.M., Jr. (1986a) Nerve growth factor receptor molecules in rat brain. Proc. Natl. Acad. Sci. USA 83:1950-1954.

Taniuchi, M., Clark, H.B., and Johnson, E.M., Jr. (1986b) Induction of nerve growth factor receptor in Schwann cells after axotomy. Proc. Natl. Acad. Sci. USA 83:4094-4098.

Taniuchi, M., Clark, H.B., Schweitzer, J.B., Johnson, E.M., Jr. (1988) Expression of nerve growth factor receptors by Schwann cells of axotomized peripheral nerves: ultrastructural location, suppression by axonal contact, and binding properties. J. Neuroscience, in press.

Thoenen, H., Barde, Y.-A. (1980) Physiology of nerve growth factor. Physiol. Rev. 60:1284-1335.

Whittemore, S.R., Seiger, A. (1987) The expression, localization and functional significance of β-nerve growth factor in the central nervous system. Brain Res. Rev. 12:439-464.

Zimmerman, A., Sutter, A. (1983) β-nerve growth factor (βNGF) receptors on glial cells. Cell-cell interaction between neurones and Schwann cells in cultures of chick sensory ganglia. EMBO J. 2:879-885.

NEURONAL SURFACE MOLECULES

STRUCTURAL PROPERTIES OF NEURONAL SURFACE MACROMOLECULES

Richard U. Margolis

Department of Pharmacology, New York University Medical Center, New York, NY 10016

Most of the putative cell adhesion and recognition molecules undergo post-translational modification, especially glycosylation, but also sulfation, phosphorylation, and acylation. This introduction will briefly outline some aspects of the biochemistry of these neural cell surface macromolecules, particularly insofar as such information may be pertinent to their localization, developmental changes, and functional roles.

GLYCOPROTEINS

Many of these proteins are glycosylated and occur in the form of glycoproteins or proteoglycans. Nervous tissue glycoproteins contain predominantly "complex" tri- and tetraantennary oligosaccharides (i.e., having three or four peripheral branches) which are linked to asparagine residues in the protein moiety. They also contain a small proportion of high mannose and biantennary oligosaccharides, as well as O-glycosidic oligosaccharides which are linked via N-acetylgalactosamine to the hydroxyl groups of serine and threonine residues.

A few structural features of nervous tissue glycoproteins deserve particular attention. The first of these is the presence of polysialosyl chains (Fig. 1) in embryonic forms of N-CAM (for a review, see Finne, 1985). Polysialic acid may not occur in other brain glycoproteins, but it has been detected in neuroblastoma and PC12 pheochromocytoma cells, in the voltage-sensitive sodium channel from <u>Electrophorus electricus</u>, as well as in embryonic kidney (Margolis and Margolis, 1983; Roth et al., 1987; James and Agnew, 1987). While this structure is therefore not unique to N-CAM or nervous tissue, it nonetheless has a rather limited distribution.

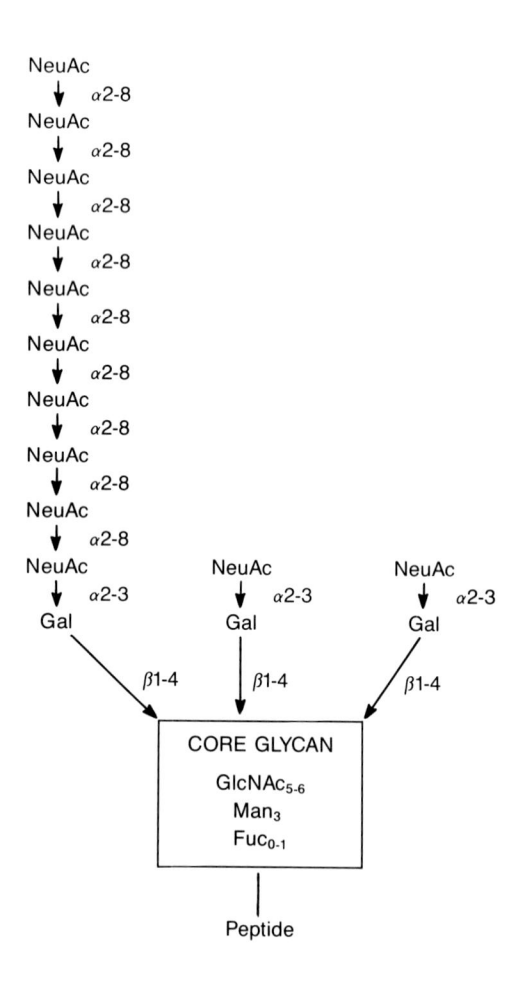

```
NeuAc
  ↓ α2-8
NeuAc
  ↓ α2-8
NeuAc
  ↓ α2-8
NeuAc
  ↓ α2-8
NeuAc
  ↓ α2-8
NeuAc
  ↓ α2-8
NeuAc
  ↓ α2-8
NeuAc
  ↓ α2-8
NeuAc
  ↓ α2-8
NeuAc          NeuAc          NeuAc
  ↓ α2-3         ↓ α2-3         ↓ α2-3
 Gal            Gal            Gal
    ↘ β1-4     ↓ β1-4      ↙ β1-4
      ┌─────────────────────┐
      │   CORE GLYCAN       │
      │   GlcNAc₅₋₆         │
      │   Man₃              │
      │   Fuc₀₋₁            │
      └─────────────────────┘
               │
            Peptide
```

Fig. 1. Structural model of a tri- or tetraantennary asparagine-linked oligosaccharide containing polysialic acid. The polysialosyl chain is of variable length, containing up to 12 or more sialic acid residues (Finne and Mäkelä, 1985).

Another type of oligosaccharide whose structure has been found to be developmentally regulated in certain tissues is the poly(N-acetyllactosaminyl) glycan, which contains -galactose(ß1-4)N-acetylglucosamine(ß1-3)- disaccharide repeating units. The degree of branching and the substitution of this basic structure with sulfate or fucose residues has been shown to be under developmental control, especially in certain blood cells (for a review, see Fukuda, 1985). It is present to only a limited extent in brain, where it may be confined to its sulfated form (as keratan sulfate chains) in the chondroitin sulfate proteoglycan (Krusius et al., 1986, 1987), but poly(N-acetyllactosaminyl) units are also found in sympathetic neurons, neuroblastoma cells, and in a considerable number of PC12 cell glycoproteins, some of which are affected by nerve growth factor-induced differentiation and neurite outgrowth (Margolis et al., 1986; Spillmann and Finne, 1987). A prominent example of these is the NILE glycoprotein (also known as the L1 antigen or Ng-CAM), in which the major (or possibly only) difference of the larger PC12 cell form from that in brain is the presence in PC12 cells of poly(N-acetyllactosaminyl) oligosaccharides, some of which appear to be sulfated (Margolis et al., 1986; and unpublished results).

Finally, with regard to interesting glycoprotein structures, I should mention glucuronic acid 3-sulfate, which is the epitope recognized by the HNK-1 monoclonal antibody to a human lymphocyte antigen. This epitope was later detected in certain acidic glycolipids present in peripheral nerve and embryonic central nervous tissue, as well as in a number of brain glycoproteins thought to be involved in cell-cell interactions, such as N-CAM, the myelin associated glycoprotein, and the L1 and J1 antigens. We have recently shown a much wider distribution of the HNK-1 epitope in brain and PC12 cell glycoproteins, chromaffin granule membranes, and proteoglycans, especially the chondroitin sulfate (but not the heparan sulfate) proteoglycan of brain (Margolis et al., 1987a). The biological significance of this structure, which is shared by both the nervous and immune systems as well as connective tissue proteoglycans and at least one bacterial enzyme (chondroitinase ABC) remains to be determined.

PROTEOGLYCANS

Nervous tissue also contains chondroitin sulfate and heparan sulfate proteoglycans. Chondroitin sulfate is composed of disaccharide repeating units consisting of glucuronic acid and N-acetytgalactosamine 4- or 6-sulfate. Most of the chondroitin sulfate proteoglycans of brain occur in an easily extractable form, and have an average molecular size of approximately 300,000 Da as determined by gel filtration. They appear to contain a number of core proteins (which may be specific to particular cell types), to which three or four 18,000-19,000 Da chondroitin sulfate chains and a wide variety of N- and O-glycosidically linked oligosaccharides are attached (Krusius et al., 1986, 1987). A portion of the chondroitin sulfate proteoglycans occurs in the form of aggregates with hyaluronic acid and a link protein, as indicated by similar localizations and coordinate developmental changes of chondroitin sulfate proteoglycan, hyaluronic acid, link protein, and the hyaluronic acid-binding region of the chondroitin sulfate proteoglycan subunits (Ripellino et al., 1988). Chondroitin sulfate proteoglycans are primarily present extracellularly in the early postnatal period, after which they gradually assume an intracellular (cytoplasmic and axoplasmic) localization in neurons and astrocytes of mature brain (Aquino et al., 1984a,b). However, it is also possible that a small portion of the chondroitin sulfate proteoglycans of brain may have a different localization, such as being associated with plasma membranes.

Studies of cerebellar cultures and PC12 cells, utilizing antibodies to the chondroitin sulfate proteoglycan and ß-xyloside inhibition of proteoglycan biosynthesis, have demonstrated significant effects on cell morphology and adhesion. These findings support other evidence indicating that chondroitin sulfate proteoglycans are involved in cell surface events during nervous tissue development and differentiation.

In contrast to the chondroitin sulfate proteoglycans, the heparan sulfate proteoglycans of PC12 cells and brain are mostly membrane-associated. Like the other glycosaminoglycans, heparan sulfate has a disaccharide repeating unit composed of a uronic acid (D-glucuronic acid and L-iduronic acid) and an amino sugar (N-acetyl- and N-sulfo-D-glucosamine). However, there is a large degree of structural variation in heparan sulfates which is beyond the scope of this presentation.

The heparan sulfate proteoglycans of brain, with molecular sizes of approximately 220,000 Da, have glycosaminoglycan chains of 14,000-15,000 Da together with N- and O-glycosidically-linked oligosaccharides (Klinger et al., 1985). In PC12 cells the heparan sulfate proteoglycans are present in several pools, in which the heparan sulfate chains have different structural properties. We have found that nerve growth factor-induced differentiation and neurite outgrowth in PC12 cells are accompanied by significant alterations in the charge, size, and sulfation pattern of PC12 cell heparan sulfate (Margolis et al., 1987b). These results are consistent with a number of other studies which indicate a role of heparan sulfate proteoglycans in neuronal surface events.

However, it should be emphasized in this connection that the heparan sulfate proteoglycans present in plasma membranes (such as those of PC12 cells or brain) frequently have quite different structural properties from their counterparts in basement membranes of peripheral nerve and other tissues. One must therefore be cautious in the interpretation of results obtained from using an antibody to a basement membrane heparan sulfate proteoglycan in studies of brain, to give just one example.

PHOSPHATIDYLINOSITOL MEMBRANE PROTEIN ANCHORS

Most integral membrane proteins are anchored by a balance of interactions between relatively hydrophobic and polar polypeptide domains with the hydrophobic core of the lipid bilayer and the surrounding medium, respectively. However, it has recently been recognized that an extremely diverse group of proteins is anchored to the plasma membrane through a covalently attached glycosyl-phosphatidylinositol moiety. These include various enzymes, a number of lymphocyte antigens including the Thy-1 glycoprotein, decay accelerating factor (a complement regulatory protein), the trypanosomal variant surface glycoprotein, the smallest (120 kDa) component of the neural cell adhesion molecule, and a rat liver heparan sulfate proteoglycan (for a review, see Low, 1987).

Based on those proteins for which detailed information is available, the anchoring structure generally consists of a phosphatidylinositol molecule whose 1,2-diacylglycerol moiety is embedded in the membrane bilayer and is responsible for anchoring, and an oligosaccharide of variable structure and composition. The oligosaccharide is linked to the membrane phosphatidylinositol via a glycosidic linkage with a glucosamine that has a free amino group, and via a non-reducing terminal mannose-6-phosphate to the hydroxyl of an ethanolamine residue, which is amide-linked via its amino group to the α-carboxyl of the C-terminal amino acid (Fig. 2).

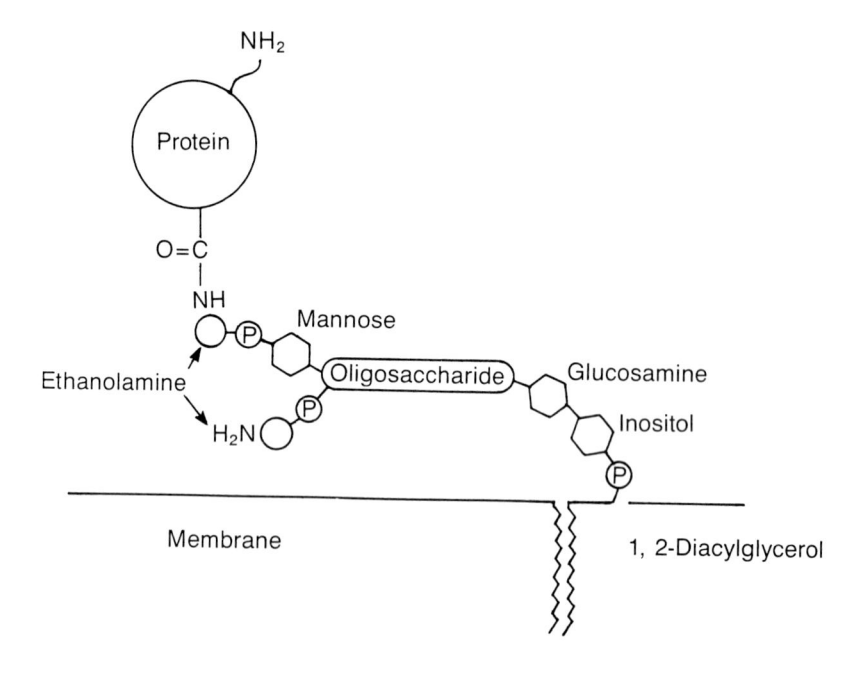

Fig. 2. Schematic representation of the phosphatidylinositol membrane protein anchor (Low, 1987). In certain cases there is only a single ethanolamine, and other sugars may be present in the oligosaccharide (e.g., mannose, 1-2 mol/mol; galactose, 1-8 mol/mol; and galactosamine, 1 mol/mol).

In an attempt to evaluate the extent to which this novel membrane anchoring mechanism is employed in nervous tissue, we have used biosynthetic labeling with [^{3}H]ethanolamine and a phosphatidylinositol-specific phospholipase C (PIPLC) to study the prevalence of this structure in cultures of early postnatal rat cerebellum, and in a homogeneous population of rat PC12 cells. We have found that in PC12 cells there are at least four proteins which appear to be anchored to the plasma membrane by a glycosyl-phosphatidylinositol linkage. The major component is Thy-1. This is accompanied by two proteins having apparent molecular sizes of 46 and 48 kDa and which are not released by PIPLC although they are biosynthetically labeled with [^{3}H]ethanolamine, and by a PIPLC-released 158 kDa glycoprotein which is soluble in chloroform-methanol and contains fucosylated poly(N-acetyllactosaminyl) oligosaccharides. None of these latter three components can be identified with previously investigated proteins having known functional roles, and the biological significance of Thy-1 in nervous tissue also remains unclear. In comparison with PC12 cells, we found a significantly greater number of phosphatidylinositol-anchored glycoproteins in cultures of early postnatal rat cerebellum, including five major sulfated glycoproteins ranging in size from 21 to 155 kDa. Two of these phosphatidylinositol-anchored proteins may be common to both PC12 cells and brain (Margolis et al., 1988).

The physiological functions of the phosphatidylinositol membrane protein anchor are likely to be different (when functionally relevant at all) among many of the highly diverse proteins which employ this linkage mechanism. However, it is reasonable to assume that a glycosyl-phosphatidylinositol anchor would confer a greater degree of lateral mobility within the outer leaflet of the membrane bilayer, and would also facilitate the selective release and/or uptake of certain enzymes, cell adhesion molecules, or other proteins having a role in cell-surface events. The generation at the cell surface by specific phospholipases C of 1,2-diacylglycerol (an activator of protein kinase C) and of glycosylinositol phosphates also suggests that these products may serve as second messengers, which could be delivered to their intracellular target sites by diffusion across the lipid bilayer or by receptor-mediated endocytosis, respectively. The presence of at least four phosphatidylinositol-anchored proteins on the plasma membrane of a single cell type suggests that this novel linkage mechanism is probably widely employed to serve a number of biological functions in nervous and other tissues.

REFERENCES

Aquino DA, Margolis RU, Margolis RK (1984a) Immunocytochemical localization of a chondroitin sulfate proteoglycan in nervous tissue. I. Adult brain, retina, and peripheral nerve. J Cell Biol 99:1117.

Aquino DA, Margolis RU, Margolis RK (1984b) Immunocytochemical localization of a chondroitin sulfate proteoglycan in nervous tissue. II. Studies in developing brain. J Cell Biol 99:1130.

Finne J (1985). Polysialic acid - a glycoprotein carbohydrate involved in neural adhesion and bacterial meningitis. Trends Biochem Sci 10:129.

Finne J, Mäkelä PH (1985). Cleavage of the polysialosyl units of brain glycoproteins by a bacteriophage endosialidase. J Biol Chem 260:1265.

Fukuda M (1985). Cell surface glycoconjugates as onco-differentiation markers in hematopoietic cells. Biochim Biophys Acta 780:119.

James WM, Agnew WS (1987). Multiple oligosaccharide chains in the voltage-sensitive Na channel from Electrophorus electricus: Evidence for α-2,8-linked polysialic acid. Biochem Biophys Res Commun 148:817.

Klinger MM, Margolis RU, Margolis RK (1985). Isolation and characterization of the heparan sulfate proteoglycans of brain. J Biol Chem 260:4082.

Krusius T, Finne J, Margolis RK, Margolis RU (1986) Identification of an O-glycosidic mannose-linked sialylated tetrasaccharide and keratan sulfate oligosaccharides in the chondroitin sulfate proteoglycan of brain. J Biol Chem 261:8237.

Krusius T, Reinhold VN, Margolis RK, Margolis RU (1987). Structural studies on sialylated and sulphated O-glycosidic mannose-linked oligosaccharides in the chondroitin sulphate proteoglycan of brain. Biochem J 245:229.

Low MG (1987). Biochemistry of the glycosyl-
phosphatidylinositol membrane protein anchors. Biochem
J 244:1.
Margolis RK, Margolis RU (1983). Distribution and
characteristics of polysialosyl oligosaccharides in
nervous tissue glycoproteins. Biochem Biophys Res
Commun 116:889.
Margolis RK, Greene LA, Margolis RU (1986).
Poly(N-acetyllactosaminyl) oligosaccharides in
glycoproteins of PC12 pheochromocytoma cells and
sympathetic neurons. Biochemistry 25:3463.
Margolis RK, Ripellino JA, Goossen B, Steinbrich R,
Margolis RU (1987a). Occurrence of the HNK-1 epitope
(3-sulfoglucuronic acid) in PC12 pheochromocytoma cells,
chromaffin granule membranes, and chondroitin sulfate
proteoglycans. Biochem Biophys Res Commun 145:1142.
Margolis RK, Salton SRJ, Margolis RU (1987b). Effects of
nerve growth factor-induced differentiation on the
heparan sulfate of PC12 pheochromocytoma cells and
comparison with developing brain. Arch Biochem Biophys
257:107.
Margolis RK, Goossen B, Margolis RU (1988). Phosphatidylinositol-anchored glycoproteins of PC12 pheochromocytoma
cells and brain. Biochemistry, in press.
Ripellino JA, Bailo M, Margolis RU, Margolis RK (1988).
Light and electron microscopic studies on the
localization of hyaluronic acid in developing rat
cerebellum. J Cell Biol, in press.
Roth J, Taatjes DJ, Bitter-Suermann D, Finne J (1987).
Polysialic acid units are spatially and temporally
expressed in developing postnatal rat kidney. Proc Natl
Acad Sci 84:1969.
Spillmann D, Finne J (1987). Poly-N-acetyllactosamine
glycans of cellular glycoproteins: Predominance of
linear chains in mouse neuroblastoma and rat
pheochromocytoma cell lines. J. Neurochem 49:874.

REGULATORY MECHANISMS IN NERVE GROWTH CONES

Karl H. Pfenninger

Department of Cellular and Structural Biology
University of Colorado School of Medicine
Denver, Colorado 80262

INTRODUCTION

The nerve growth cone is the terminal enlargement, i.e., the leading edge of the growing neurite. It is capable of finding its path to the appropriate target area and of recognizing specific target cells for synaptogenesis. At the time of synapse formation the nerve growth cone is replaced by a presynaptic terminal. Therefore, the nerve growth cone is a developmentally regulated structure and is likely to contain a number of functionally important, developmentally regulated molecules. As shown by Hughes in 1953, nerve growth cones severed from the perikaryon continue to advance for some time. This relative autonomy is also indicated by the observation of Gundersen and Barrett (1980) that growth cones of peripheral neurons respond rapidly to a gradient of nerve growth factor and display chemotactic behavior. Thus, the nerve growth cone appears to be equipped with all the structural and regulatory elements necessary for directed locomotion.

Detailed biochemical analysis of nerve growth cones was not possible until the successful fractionation of homogenates of developing brain had been achieved. Pfenninger et al. (1983) and Gordon-Weeks and Lockerbie (1984) have independently developed protocols that result in subcellular fractions highly enriched in sheared-off fragments of nerve growth cones. We call these structures growth cone particles (GCPs). GCPs contain the organelles characteristic of nerve growth cones, and radiolabeled growth cones microdissected from cultures co-purify with GCPs. Furthermore, a number of growth-regulated proteins are enriched in this fraction (Simkowitz and Pfenninger, 1983; Ellis et al., 1985; Greenberger and Pfenninger, 1986; Meiri et al., 1986; Skene et al., 1986; Simkowitz et al., 1988). It appears, therefore, that the major characteristics of the GCP fraction are representative of those of nerve growth cones of the central nervous system (see also Pfenninger, 1986).

One of the striking features of the GCPs is the relative simplicity of the electrophoretic patterns of major proteins and phosphoproteins. Particularly prominent are three major substrates of calcium-kinases. The regulation of these kinase activities, probably by a novel peptide factor, is the major topic of this chapter.

SUBSTRATES OF CALCIUM/CALMODULILN- AND CALCIUM/PHOSPHOLIPID-DEPENDENT PROTEIN KINASES.

The GCPs used for our studies are prepared from 17- or 18-day-gestation rat brain. If these GCPs are permeabilized and incubated with ^{32}P-labeled ATP and calcium one finds a series of prominent phosphoproteins (Hyman and Pfenninger, 1985) even though the level of phosphoproteins in the fetal brain homogenate, from which GCPs are prepared, are very low (Katz et al., 1985). More specificially, radioautograms of two-dimensional gels reveal three major polypeptide species plus a small group of spots (at approximately 52 kDa) presumably representing tubulin (Katz et al., 1985). The three major polypeptides have molecular masses of 80, 46, and 40 kDa. One of these, the 46-kDa species (pp46), is the only major target of a calcium/calmodulin-dependent kinase in GCPs. Protein pp46 has an acidic isoelectric point (4.3) and co-migrates with a major, developmentally regulated membrane protein of the GCPs (Ellis et al., 1985; Simkowitz et al., 1988). A number of results (Meiri et al., 1986; Skene et al., 1986) suggest that pp46 is identical to the growth-associated protein GAP 43 (e.g., Skene and Willard, 1981; cf. Pfenninger, 1986; Benowitz and Routtenberg, 1987). It should be stressed that this protein is a bona-fide membrane protein as indicated by its resistance to salt extraction from the membrane and its behavior in the detergent Triton X-114 (Dosemeci and Rodnight, 1987; Simkowitz et al., 1988). Phosphorylation of growth cone proteins in the presence of the phorbol ester 12-0-tetradecanoylphorbol 13-acetate (TPA), an activator of the calcium/phospholipid-dependent protein kinase C (e.g., Nishizuka, 1984), also increases the phosphorylation of pp46 relative to controls. Thus, pp46 appears to be the substrate not only of a calcium/calmodulin-dependent protein kinase but also of protein kinase C, at least in vitro (Hyman and Pfenninger, 1987). Experiments with TPA also reveal stimulated phosphorylation of the 80- and 40-kDa proteins (pp80ac and pp40), which have isoelectric points near 4.0. Both of these proteins can be found associated with the membrane as well as in the cytosol, and pp80ac appears to be identical to a phosphoprotein described initially in the adult brain by Wu et al. (1982). This protein also seems to be present in fibroblasts, where its phosphorylation is stimulated by fibroblast growth factor (Rozengurt et al., 1983; Blackshear et al., 1985, 1986). Overall, protein kinase C has three major substrates in GCPs, pp40, pp46 and pp80ac. The apparent prevalence of this protein kinase activity in growth cones is consistent with the particularly high density of TPA receptors observed in nervous system structures rich in growing axons (Murphy et al., 1983). However upon maturation, these substrates and, presumably, protein kinase C activity decrease substantially as shown by the comparison of GCPs and synaptosomes (Katz et al., 1985).

THE REGULATION OF PROTEIN KINASE C ACTIVITY.

A large body of evidence obtained in a variety of systems indicates that protein kinase C activity is stimulated by sn-1,2-diacylglycerol, a cleavage product of phosphorylated forms of phosphatidylinositol (PI). In the case of phosphatidylinositol 4,5-bisphosphate (PIP_2), the second product resulting from this cleavage is inositol 1,4,5-trisphosphate (IP_3), which appears to stimulate the release of calcium from endoplasmic reticulum-like stores (for review see, e.g., Berridge, 1987). Thus, it seems logical to look for the phosphorylation and cleavage of PI in GCPs. Indeed, we find rapid incorporation of ^{32}P from ATP and of ^{3}H-inositol into PIP_2 and its breakdown products, notably inositol phosphates (Hyman and Pfenninger, 1987; Garofalo and Pfenninger, 1986, 1988). In addition, exogenous IP_3 added to intact, permeabilized GCPs stimulates phosphorylation of pp40 and pp80ac, and this stimulation can be blocked by first depleting intracellular calcium stores with the calcium ionophore A23187 (Hyman and Pfenninger, 1987). These results indicate (i) that PI phosphorylation and breakdown are very active in GCPs and, thus, are likely to control protein kinase C activity, and (ii) that IP_3 plays a role in the regulation of calcium within the growth cone.

This raises the further question of the mechanism by which PIP_2 cleavage is activated in nerve growth cones. It is generally believed PIP_2 is cleaved by a receptor-activated phospholipase C (e.g., Berridge, 1987). If this is so, the fetal brain should contain one or more hormone-like factors that activate the PI/protein kinase C cascade. Therefore, a major effort is being made to search for such biological activity in extracts of fetal rat brain. The assay consists of mildly permeabilized GCPs incubated with ^{32}P-ATP, in the presence or absence of fetal brain extract or subfractions thereof. After brief periods an aqueous extract is prepared from the incubation medium, and inositol phosphates are analyzed by high-voltage paper electrophoresis and radioautography (Garofalo and Pfenninger, 1988). Fetal rat brain clearly contains an activity stimulating the release of a compound co-migrating with IP_3, and this factor has a molecular mass below 10,000. In contrast, a variety of known hormones and transmitters such as nerve growth factor, insulin, ACTH, acetylcholine, serotonin, etc., have no influence on inositol phosphate metabolism of GCPs. More recent efforts in this laboratory (K.H. Pfenninger, L.T. Frame, A.J. Vigers and S.M. Helmke, unpublished), using ion exchange chromatography, gel filtration and other methods of peptide purification, have resulted in greater than 10,000-fold purification of an apparently novel factor. The molecular weight of the factor is below 2,000, and it appears to be a small peptide. The factor is now being tested for homogeneity, and amino acid sequence data are expected to be obtained in the near future. Simultaneously, we will pursue studies on the functional effects of the factor on intact growth cones in culture.

CONCLUSIONS.

The observations summarized here indicate that the PI/protein kinase C system is a prominent, and perhaps the major, signal transduction cascade in nerve growth cones isolated from fetal rat brain. This is of particular interest in light of the data suggesting the involvement of this cascade in activation of PC12 cells by nerve growth factor (Traynor, 1984; Hama et al., 1986; cf. Lakshmanan, 1978) and in view of the fact that chemotaxis in leukocytes and thrombin-induced spreading of blood platelets seem to be controlled by the same pathway (e.g., Laskin et al., 1981; Snyderman and Goetzl, 1981; Watson et al., 1984; Berridge, 1987). Furthermore, TPA stimulates neurite outgrowth, at least in some systems (Hsu et al., 1984). These analogies suggest that the PI/protein kinase C pathway may be involved in the regulation of the growth cone's motile activity, perhaps in chemotaxis to an appropriate target area (cf. Pfenninger, 1986). Because of the role of inositol phosphates in calcium regulation, such a hypothesis is consistent with our current knowledge of the influence of calcium on growth cone motility (e.g., Grinvald and Farber, 1981; Anglister et al., 1982; Mattson and Kater, 1987). Yet, the issue of the functional roles of the growth cone's major kinase substrates, especially pp80ac and pp46, is completely unresolved. Protein pp46 is so abundant in GCP membranes that it can be seen easily in Coomassie-blue-stained polyacrylamide gels, and pp80ac is abundant enough to form a large, strikingly intense spot after silver staining. Thus, it does not seem likely that these proteins are part of a signalling mechanism. More probably, these phosphoproteins could be associated with structural proteins, perhaps those involved in the interactions between the plasmalemma and cytoskeletal or extracellular matrix structures.

This last hypothesis cannot be supported by data at the present time and may help only with the definition of future research strategies. However, I hope this report demonstrates that recent progress has made the molecular dissection of the growth cone feasible. In other words, a molecular understanding of the regulation of growth cone function, of neurite outgrowth in general and, perhaps, of neurite regeneration may now be within our reach.

ACKNOWLEDGEMENTS.

I would like to express my gratitude to all those who have contributed to this work, especially my former associates, Drs. Leland Ellis, Robert S. Garofalo, Carolyn Hyman and Flora Katz, and my present associates, Lynn Frame, Dr. Steven Helmke, Alison Vigers and Robert Wheeler. Excellent secretarial assistance by Carmel Montes is also gratefully acknowledged. This work is supported by a Senator Jacob Javits Neuroscience Investigator Award from the NIH (NS24672), and grants from the National Science Foundation (BNS44972) and the American Paralysis Association (RC87-02).

REFERENCES.

Anglister L, Farber I, Shahar A, Grinvald A (1982). Localization of voltage-sensitive calcium channels along developing neurites: Their possible role in regulating neurite elongation. Dev Biol 94: 351-365.

Benowitz LI, Routtenberg A (1987). A membrane phosphoprotein associated with neural development, axonal regeneration, phospholipid metabolism, and synaptic plasticity. Trends Neurosci 10: 527-532.

Berridge, MJ (1987). Inositol trisphosphate and diacylglycerol: two interacting second messengers. Ann Rev Biochem 56: 159-193.

Blackshear PJ, Witters LA, Girard PR, Kuo JF, Quamo, SN (1985). Growth factor-stimulated protein phosphorylation in 3T3-L1 cells. J Biol Chem 260: 13304-13315.

Blackshear PJ, Wen L, Glynn BP, Witters LA (1986). Protein kinase C-stimulated phosphorylation in vitro of a M_r 80,000 protein phosphorylated in response to phorbol esters and growth factors in intact fibroblasts.

J Biol Chem 261: 1459-1469.
Dosemeci A, Rodnight R (1987). Demonstration by phase-partioning in Triton X-114 solutions that phosphoprotein B-50 (F-1) from rat brain is an integral membrane protein. Neurosci Lett 74: 325-330.
Ellis L, Wallis I, Abreu E, Pfenninger KH (1985). Nerve growth cones isolated from fetal rat brain: IV. Preparation of a membrane subfraction and identification of a growth-dependent membrane glycoprotein expressed on sprouting neurons. J Cell Biol 101: 1977-1989.
Garofalo RS, Pfenninger KH (1986). Phosphatidylinositol turnover in nerve growth cones isolated from the CNS. J Cell Biol 103: 454a.
Garofalo RS, Pfenninger KH (1988). Polyphosphoinositide hydrolysis in nerve growth cones from the CNS and its activation by a soluble factor from fetal brain. J Neurosci. In revision.
Gordon-Weeks PR, Lockerbie RO (1984). Isolation and partial characterization of neuronal growth cones from neonatal rat forebrain. Neurosci 13: 119-136.
Greenberger LM, Pfenninger KH (1986). Membrane glycoproteins of the nerve growth cone: diversity and growth-associated oligosaccharides. J Cell Biol 103: 1369-1382.
Grinvald A, Farber I (1981). Optical recording of Ca^{++} action potentials from growth cones of cultured neurons using a laser microbeam. Science 212: 1164-1169.
Gundersen RW, Barrett JN (1980). Characterization of the turning response of dorsal root neurites toward nerve growth factor. J Cell Biol 87: 546-555.
Hama T, Huang KP, Guroff G (1986). Protein kinase C as a component of a nerve growth factor-sensitive phosphorylation system in PC12 cells. Proc Natl Acad Sci USA 83: 2353-2357.
Hsu L, Natyzak D, Laskin JD (1984). Effects of the tumor promoter 12-O-tetradecanoylphorbol-13-acetate on neurite outgrowth from chick embryo sensory ganglia. Cancer Res 44: 4607-4614.
Hughes A (1953). The growth of embryonic neurites. A study on cultures of chick neural tissues. J Anat 87: 150-163.
Hyman C, Pfenninger KH (1985). Intracellular regulators of neuronal sprouting: Calmodulin binding proteins of nerve growth cones. J Cell Biol 101: 1153-1160.
Hyman C, Pfenninger KH (1987). Intracellular regulators

of neuronal sprouting: Protein and lipid phosphorylation in a fraction of nerve growth cones isolated from fetal rat brain. J Neurosci 7: 4076-4083.

Katz F, Ellis L, Pfenninger KH (1985). Nerve growth cones isolated from fetal rat brain: III. Calcium-dependent protein phosphorylation. J Neurosci 5: 1402-1411.

Lakshmanan J (1978). Nerve growth factor induced turnover of phosphatidylinositol in rat superior cervical ganglia. Biochem Biophys Res Comm 82: 767-775.

Laskin DL, Laskin JD, Weinstein IB, Carchman RA (1981). Induction of chemotaxis in mouse peritoneal macrophages by phorbol ester tumor promotors. Cancer Res 41: 1923-1928.

Mattson MP, Kater SB (1987). Calcium regulation of neurite elongation and growth cone motility. J Neurosci 7: 4034-4043.

Meiri KF, Pfenninger KH, Willard MB (1986). Growth-associated protein, GAP-43, a polypeptide that is induced when neurons extend axons, is a component of growth cones and corresponds to pp46, a major polypeptide of a subcellular fraction enriched in growth cones. Proc Nat Acad Sci USA 83: 3537-3541.

Murphy KMM, Gould RJ, Oster-Granite ML, Gearhart JD, Synder SH (1983). Phorbol ester receptors: autoradiographic identification in the developing rat. Science 222: 1036-1038.

Nishizuka Y (1984). The role of protein kinase C in cell-surface signal transduction and tumor promotion. Nature 308: 693-698.

Pfenninger KH, Ellis L, Johnson MP, Friedman LB, Somlo S (1983). Nerve growth cones isolated from fetal rat brain. I. Subcellular fractionation and characterization. Cell 35: 573-584.

Pfenninger KH (1986). Of nerve growth cones, leukocytes and memory: on the growth cone's second messenger systems and growth-regulated proteins. Trends Neurosci 9: 562-565.

Rozengurt E, Rodriguez-Pena M, Smith KA (1983). Phorbol esters, phospholipase C, and growth factors rapidly stimulate the phosphorylation of a M_r 80,000 protein in intact quiescent 3T3 cells. Proc Natl Acad Sci USA 80: 7244-7248.

Simkowitz P, Pfenninger KH (1983). Rapidly transported proteins of nerve growth cones and synaptic endings are markedly different. Neurosci Abst 98: 1422-1433.

Simkowitz P, Ellis L, Pfenninger, KH (1988). Membrane

proteins of the nerve growth cone and their developmental regulation. In submission.

Skene, JHP, Willard M (1981). Axonally transported proteins associated with axon growth in rabbit central and peripheral nervous systems. J Cell Biol 89: 96-103.

Skene JHP, Jacobson RD, Snipes GJ, McGuire CB, Norden JJ, Freeman JA (1986). A protein induced during nerve growth (GAP-43) is a major component of growth-cone membranes. Science 233: 783-786.

Snyderman T, Goetzl EJ (1981). Molecular and cellular mechanisms of leukocyte chemotaxis. Science 213: 830-837.

Traynor AE (1984). The relationship between neurite extension and phospholipid metabolism in PC12 cells. Dev Brain Res 14: 205-210.

Watson SP, McConnell R, Lapetina E (1984). The rapid formation of inositol phosphates in human platelets by thrombin is inhibited by prostacyclin. J Biol Chem 259: 13199-13203.

Wu WC-S, Walaas SI, Nairn AO, Greengard P (1982). Calcium/phospholipid regulates phosphorylation of a M_r "87K" substrate protein in brain synaptosomes. Proc Natl Acad Sci USA 79: 5249-5253.

FAMILIES OF NEURAL ADHESION MOLECULES

Melitta Schachner

Department of Neurobiology, University of Heidelberg, Heidelberg, FRG

To build a complex organ, such as the nervous system, a number of cellular and molecular mechanisms would seem necessary. In terms of cell surface interactions the questions are, how many adhesion molecules are needed for nervous system development, how they may function at the cellular and molecular levels, whether they are dependent on each other in function and whether there are structural and functional similarities among adhesion molecules. One such cue that guided our search came to us in form of a monoclonal antibody designated L2 that recognizes a carbohydrate epitope common to several adhesion molecules (Fig. 1). At the time the L2 monoclonal antibody was discovered, only L1 and N-CAM had been described as bona fide adhesion molecules (Kruse et al., 1984). The myelin associated glycoprotein (MAG), which is one of an unknown number of L2 carbohydrate-positive glycoproteins, had been hypothesized, but experimentally not shown to be involved in axon-myelinating cell interactions (for references, see Poltorak et al., 1987). Based on the observation, that out of two functionally characterized L2 epitope-positive molecules two were indeed adhesion molecules we suggested that other glycoproteins expressing this carbohydrate structure would also be involved in adhesion. To verify this hypothesis we have functionally characterized other, the L2 carbohydrate carrying glycoproteins.

MAG, J1 and other members of the L2 carbohydrate family are adhesion molecules.

That MAG is an adhesion molecule was shown by using antibodies against it to interfere with cell adhesion in vitro (Poltorak et al., 1987). MAG could thus be implicated in oligodendrocyte-neuron and oligodendrocyte-oligodendrocyte, but not oligodendrocyte-astrocyte interactions. MAG could also be incorporated into liposomes and shown to bind to neurites and neurite bundles in cultures of neurons known to engage in myelination, such as spinal cord and dorsal root ganglion neurons. Cerebellar granule cell neurons that are not myelinated in the intact tissue were poor binding partners for these MAG containing liposomes. In situ, MAG could indeed be shown to be localized at the interface between axon and myelinating cell and on opposing surfaces of the turning loops of myelin forming cells, lending support to the notion that MAG is indeed involved in multiple types of cell interactions (Martini and Schachner, 1986). MAG became detectable on myelinating Schwann cells once they had turned approximately 1.5 to 2 loops around the axon signifying a precise timing in the onset of expression. MAG not only acts as a ligand between cell surfaces but also binds to extracellular matrix molecules, such as different types of collagens and heparin (Fahrig et al., 1987). The association of MAG with the extracellular matrix in the peripheral, but not central nervous system is likely to have functional implications (Martini and Schachner, 1986, 1988).

Another adhesion molecule belonging to the L2 family is the J1 complex of glycoproteins (Kruse et al., 1985) that appears to be immunochemically related to tenascin (Faissner et al., 1988), cytotactin (Grumet et al., 1985) and hexabrachion (Erickson and Inglesias, 1984). The J1 glycoproteins are secreted molecules and extracellularly localized, also binding to several types of collagens and heparin (Faissner et al., 1988). During development J1 immunoreactivity shifts from a group of glycoproteins with molecular weights above 200kD to glycoproteins between 190 and 160kD in the adult nervous system. J1 immunoreactive material is found on astrocytes, oligodendrocytes and fibroblast-like cells, but not on neurons. J1 mediates neuron-astrocyte and neuron-Schwann cell, but not astrocyte-astrocyte or neuron-neuron adhesion.

Inferences about functional roles of J1 glycoproteins could be derived from immunohistological observations in the optic nerve and at the neuromuscular junction. In the adult rat optic nerve nodes of Ranvier were preferentially labelled by J1 and L2 antibodies (ffrench-Constant et al., 1986). J1 immunoreactivity appeared concentrated at the site of interdigitation into the nodal region, where the axon is not coverd by myelin and lies free to be contacted by astrocytes. Interestingly, other parts of these astrocytes did not show much J1 immunoreactivity, indicating a high degree of topographically selective deposition of J1. Since J1 is a secreted molecule that is also expressed by oligodendrocytes, conclusions about its mode of synthesis are presently unknown. However, at least its receptor(s) should show this specialized accumulation at the interfaces between oligodendrocyte, astrocyte and axon. The observation that J1 is concentrated at the node of Ranvier has potentially important functional implications in view of the fact that J1 is involved in neuron-glia adhesion in vitro. Taken together, the in vivo and in vitro observations raise the possibility that J1 plays an important part in neuron-glia interactions that are presumably involved in assembly and/or maintenance of the exquisite cytoarchitecture at the node of Ranvier.

J1 also appears to play an important role in neuron-muscle interactions. During development J1 was detectable in small, discrete deposits occupying spaces between myotubes (Sanes et al., 1986). Upon innervation of the muscle these deposits became sparser and disappeared completely after birth. After denervation of adult muscle , however, J1 was re-expressed around the original synaptic site already within two days. Re-expression of J1 was also seen after paralysis of nerve activity by tetrodotoxin. When muscles were re-innervated J1 disappeared again. Thus, muscle activity reverses the denervation-induced accumulation of J1. The accumulation of J1 at original synaptic sites is intriguing in view of the capability of regenerating axons to preferentially re-innervate the muscle at these original synaptic sites. Thus, J1 may be one of the cues that guide the re-growing axon to its target.

Besides MAG and J1, other cell surface glycoproteins have now been recognized to belong to the L2 family. These are the major glycoprotein of peripheral nervous system myelin P_0 (Bollensen and Schachner, 1987), the F11 adhesion molecule involved in fasciculative neurite outgrowth (Chang et al., 1987), the receptor for cytotactin (Hoffman and Edelman, 1987) and two molecules belonging to the integrin family that are cell surface receptors for extracellular matrix constituents, CSAT (Pesheva et al., 1987) and fibronectin receptor (Pesheva et al., submitted for publication). Yet other glycoproteins carry the L2 epitope, but remain to be functionally identified.

The adhesion molecule L1

The observation that one and the same cell can express more than one adhesion molecule at a particular developmental stage and a topographically distinct site on the cell surface (e.g. axon versus dendrite) begs the question why a cell permits itself the luxury of expressing more than one adhesion molecule. One could argue that by varying the steady state levels of a certain adhesion molecule and by its localization at topographically distinct sites, one adhesion molecule would suffice to specify cell surface contacts. Before presenting first hints of evidence that L1 and N-CAM may not act independently of each other within the surface membrane, suggesting cooperativity between the two molecules, a short summary of our present knowledge of L1 appears warranted.

L1 which is immunochemically identical to NILE and Ng-CAM (Bock et al., 1985; Friedlander et al., 1986), is, like N-CAM, involved in Ca^{++}-independent adhesion among neural cells. During central nervous system development L1 appears first and is co-expressed with N-CAM on postmitotic neurons (for previous reviews see Schachner et al., 1985; 1987). L1, in contrast to N-CAM, displays a previously unrecognized restricted expression by particular neurons in that it is found, for instance, in the cerebellum on granule and Purkinje cells, but not on stellate and basket cells (Persohn and Schachner, 1987). Also, L1 is expressed only on axons, but not on dendrites or cell bodies of neurons. L1 is expressed on fasciculating axons in the central and peripheral nervous system. Particularly intriguing is the fact that one and the same axon changes L1 expression along its course. A set of axons in the embryonic spinal cord expresses L1 only when these fasciculate, but not when they are not fasciculated and individually interdispersed among neuroepithelial cells (Schachner et al., 1985, 1987; Holley and Silver, 1987; Holley and Schachner, submitted for publication). Likewise, fasciculating axons in the sciatic and optic nerves express L1, but when they become myelinated more distally they lose L1 expression (Martini and Schachner, 1986, 1988; Bartsch et al., submitted for publication). Thus, one and the same axon is able to express L1 together with N-CAM along its length when fasciculating, and when non-fasciculating or ensheathed by glia L1, but not N-CAM ceases to be detectable. The superposition in expression of L1 onto N-CAM may be responsible for axon-axon interactions.

Two other surface molecules have recently been shown to be also characteristic of fasciculating axons, F11 and neurofascin (Chang et al., 1987; Rathjen et al., 1987a, 1987b), suggesting either redundancy or interdependence in functional mechanisms. Antibodies to these molecules could indeed be shown to interfere with fasciculation and neurite outgrowth on other neurites.

L1 may not only act as key molecule in axon fasciculation, since it has also been observed on single axons in the inner ear and in Vater-Pacini corpuscles in an L1-free territory (Mbiene et al., 1988; Nolte and Martini, unpublished observations), suggesting that L1 may not only interact with other L1-positive structures, such as axons or Schwann cells, but engage also in other interactions. It is pertinent in this respect that L1 is itself a ligand that promotes neurite outgrowth (Lagenaur and Lemmon, 1987; Pohlmann and Schachner, unpublished observations).

The involvement of L1 in cerebellar granule neuron migration (Lindner et al., 1983, 1986) was initially thought to result from an L1 mediated apposition of the migrating neuronal cell body and its leading and trailing processes with Bergmann glia. However, in contrast to Ng-CAM, L1 has so far not been observed to affect neuron-glia, but only neuron-neuron adhesion in vitro (Keilhauer et al., 1985). In fact, in the telencephalic anlage L1 was detectable on neurons only after cessation of neuron migration along radial glial processes (Fushiki and Schachner, 1986). Furthermore, in the developing cerebellum L1 was always found confined to contact sites between apposing neuronal surface membranes and excluded from contacts between L1-positive and L1-negative surface membranes (Persohn and Schachner, 1987). Thus, present evidence suggests that L1 specifies neuron migration in allowing neuronal cell bodies to sort out at the onset and aggregate for the termination of migration.

Interestingly, L1 expression is not confined to nervous tissue, but is expressed on epithelial cells in the intestinal tract, where it is localized on the proliferating epithelial progenitor cell of crypts, but not in the more differentiated epithelial cells of villi (Thor et al., 1987). These epithelial cells constitute another migratory system, in which they are constantly generated in the depth of the crypts, from where they migrate to the villi to be shed from their tips into the intestinal lumen. Since L1 could be shown to engage in crypt cell adhesion, its function may lie in promoting the tight apposition of migratory cells, disappearing from epithelial cells when they prepare for shedding.

L1 and N-CAM interdependence in function

That L1 and N-CAM may not act independently of each other became evident in two functional assay systems in vitro. When aggregation of cell bodies in single cell suspensions was measured, L1 and N-CAM appeared to act synergistically with each other (Faissner et al., 1984). When adhesion between single cell suspensions and substrate attached monolayer cells and migration of cerebellar granule cells was measured, L1 and N-CAM antibodies blocked each other, i.e. in the presence of the two antibodies blocking levels were less than additive (Keilhauer et al., 1985; Lindner et al., 1986). This interdependence in the molecules' action was proposed to result from interactions between the two molecules either between neighbouring partner cells or within the plasma membrane of one cell (Schachner et al., 1985). While up-to-date no evidence could be obtained that L1 and N-CAM interact with each other in a specific manner, association of L1 and N-CAM within the surface membrane of one cell could be demonstrated by antibody-induced re-distribution within the surface membrane of live cells (Thor et al., 1986). These studies showed that L1 was specifically associated with the largest molecular form of N-CAM having a molecular weight of 180kD (N-CAM 180), but not with the lower molecular weight form, N-CAM 140. A close neighbourship between the two molecules may underlie functional cooperativity as it has been seen with the components of the T cell receptor complex in the immune system.

The feature that distinguishes N-CAM 180 from its smaller components is its long cytoplasmic domain, while its extracellular part is supposedly identical to the other two components of N-CAM, N-CAM 140 and N-CAM 120. During development of the cerebellum N-CAM 180 is the latest component to appear, in that it is only detectable in granule cell bodies and axons once migration is finished (Persohn and Schachner, 1987). Thus, N-CAM 180 only becomes apparent when neurons engage to form stable cell contacts. Also, cultured neuroblastoma cells, when promoted into morphological differentiation, shift N-CAM expression towards a predominance of N-CAM 180 (Pollerberg et al., 1985, 1986). Interestingly, L1 and N-CAM 180 were found accumulated together at contact sites between neighbouring cells, whereas N-CAM 140 was more uniformly distributed over the whole cell body (Pollerberg et al., 1985, 1986, 1987). The cytoskeleton membrane linker protein brain spectrin (fodrin) and actin were also accumulated at contact sites, whereas other cytoskeleton-associated proteins, such as neurofilament, alpha-actinin, filamin, vinculin, beta-tubulin, ankyrin, band 4.1 and synapsin I, did not show this accumulation. These observations led to the hypothesis that N-CAM 180 may be involved in stabilization of cell contacts by association with the cytoskeleton. Indeed, brain spectrin could be shown to specifically bind to N-CAM 180, but not to N-CAM 140 or N-CAM 120. Also, N-CAM 180 showed a reduced lateral mobility within the surface membrane, further supporting the notion that it is stabilized within the membrane by its association with the cytoskeleton. It is, therefore, noteworthy that growth cones express N-CAM 180 only, when in contact with the target cell. Conversely, N-CAM 140 is more apparent on growth cones when they are uncontacted and free "searching". Thus, restriction of lateral mobility by association with the cytoskeleton is likely to induce accumulation of N-CAM 180 at contact sites to selectively stabilize cell-cell contacts.

In contrast to N-CAM 180, N-CAM 120, the smallest form of N-CAM, must be at least as mobile within the surface membrane as N-CAM 120, since it lacks a transmembrane domain and is anchored to the surface membrane via phosphatidylinositol (He et al., 1986; Sadoul et al., 1986). The functional role of N-CAM 120 in the context of its particular membrane anchor remains, however, to be established.

Regeneration

In the mammalian nervous system neurons of both peripheral and central nervous system origin show the capacity for functional re-growth, but it is the unique feature of Schwann cells that allows re-growth and regeneration (Aguayo, 1985; Ramon y Cajal, 1928a, 1928b). In contrast to the peripheral glia, central nervous system glial cells beyond a certain developmental stage do not support re-growth (Smith et al., 1986). In lower vertebrates, however, axon re-growth in the central nervous system takes place even in adulthood. These observations have led us to search for the cellular and molecular signals that regulate adhesion molecule expression on Schwann cells during development and regeneration.

Our immunohistological observations showed that L1 and N-CAM are expressed on Schwann cells already before the establishment of a 1:1 relationship with axons (Martini and Schachner, 1986) and remain expressed in the non-myelinating state into adulthood (Bollensen and Schachner, 1987; Martini and Schachner, 1986; Mirsky et al., 1986). P_0 then becomes expressed on Schwann cells when these establish a 1:1 ratio with axons (Martini et al., submitted for publication). When Schwann cell processes have turned 1.5 to 2 loops around the axons, L1 and N-CAM are reduced in their expression on both axons and Schwann cells. Thereafter, neither axons nor Schwann cells can be detected to express L1, whereas N-CAM is found periaxonally and, more weakly, in compact myelin, thus exemplifying again the principle of a broader range of expression. With the disappearance of L1 MAG becomes detectable periaxonally and on the turning loops of Schwann cells to disappear again once compaction occurs. P_0, on the contrary, remains detectable in compact myelin. These studies show that axon-Schwann cells interactions are characterized by a very precisely timed appearance of adhesion molecules in various compartments of Schwann cell and axon. From this sequence it may be deduced that L1 and

N-CAM are involved in the initial interaction between axon and Schwann cell and P_0 in the segregation of axon fascicles for ensheathment by Schwann cells on a 1:1 basis, apposition of turning loops of Schwann cells and the maintenance of compact myelin, while MAG in conjunction with P_0 may be involved in the spiralling of Schwann cell processes.

After lesioning peripheral nerves by cut or crush re-expression of adhesion molecules is reminiscent of development. Within several days after transection, L1 and N-CAM appear again on all Schwann cells, even if they are still in association with degenerating myelin (Martini and Schachner, 1988). The temporal sequence and spatial distribution of adhesion molecule expression on axons and Schwann cells is then the same as during development.

The re-expression of L1 and N-CAM on Schwann cells at the time of axon re-growth requires validation of its functional significance. It is likely that expression of L1 and N-CAM is a prerequisite for successful re-growth of axons and that the capacity for regeneration in the peripheral nervous system may be attributed to the plasticity in re-expression of these adhesion molecules. It is, therefore, interesting that both, L1 and N-CAM are involved in adhesion of dorsal root ganglion neurons and Schwann cells (Seilheimer and Schachner, 1988). Only L1, however, appears to be involved in promoting neurite outgrowth, reminiscent of the involvement of L1 in axon growth on other L1-positive axons.

Elucidation of cellular and molecular signals that underlie re-expression of adhesion molecules on Schwann cells is a prerequisite for understanding the remarkable plasticity of these cells to re-juvenate after incurrence of a lesion. As a first step in this direction we have studied the influence of nerve growth factor (NGF) on adhesion molecule expression by Schwann cells in culture. These experiments were instigated by the observation that upon denervation NGF is synthesized by Schwann cells (Rush, 1984) and that Schwann cells may express NGF receptors at early developmental stages (Rohrer, 1985). Furthermore, we knew that PC12 pheochromocytoma cells are induced by NGF to synthesize increased levels of NILE/L1 (Lee et al., 1981). It was, therefore, gratifying to find that NGF also leads to an increased expression of L1 in pure cultures of

Schwann cells (Seilheimer and Schachner, 1987). Since antibodies to NGF reduce L1 expression in these cultures, NGF is likely to act by an autocrine mechanism. These experiments show for the first time that a neuronotrophic factor directly influences a functionally meaningful parameter, namely adhesion molecule expression, in a non-neuronal cell, the Schwann cell. Thus, NGF may play a dual role in regeneration: Increase in L1 expression by both axons and Schwann cells to enhance successful neurite outgrowth.

Family traits

Of the three functionally characterized Ca^{++}-independent adhesion molecules, N-CAM, MAG and L1, all three carry five or six immunoglobulin homologous domains (Fig. 1) (Arquint et al., 1987; Lai et al., 1987; Salzer et al., 1987; Tacke et al., 1987; Moos et al., submitted for publication). The functional role of these domains characteristic of all members of the immunoglobulin superfamily (Williams, 1987) remains obscure, however. That members of the immunoglobulin superfamily in the immune system have been reported to interact with each other (not themselves) is an incentive to look at similar types of interactions in the nervous system. Among the Ca^{++}-dependent adhesion molecules, E- and P-cadherin, considerable degrees of homology have also been found (Takeichi, 1987).

The L2 carbohydrate epitope is another family trait that is found in common among several Ca^{++}-independent adhesion molecules (Fig. 1). One could argue that since this carbohydrate is shared by functionally important molecules, it itself may be functionally important. The carbohydrate epitope is not confined to the nervous system, but is also present on subpopulations of lymphoid cells, among them natural killer cells, giving it the name HNK-1 (Abo and Balch, 1981). On neural adhesion molecules, the carbohydrate is regulated during develoment independently of the protein backbone (Martini and Schachner, 1986, Wernecke et al., 1985; Martini et al., submitted for publication). Also, in the adult state, N-CAM, L1 and MAG are heterogenous with respect to the expression of the L2/HNK-1 epitope in that only subpopulations of each adhesion molecule express the carbohydrate (Faissne, 1987;

Kruse et al., 1984; Poltorak et al., 1986). The carbohydrate is carried by the 65kD amino-terminal fragment of N-CAM, but is not present in the amino-terminal 24kD region that contains the heparin binding domain (Cole and Schachner, 1987). Sera from patients with gammopathy and peripheral polyneuropathy also react with the carbohydrate (for references see Bollensen et al., 1988; Wernecke et al., 1985). On glycolipids, the L2/HNK-1 carbohydrate epitope contains a 3'-sulphated glucuronic acid (Ariga et al., 1987; Chou et al., 1986).

Indications that the L2/HNK-1 domain is involved in cell interactions came from studies that investigated the effect of L2 antibodies on neural cell adhesion (Faissner, 1987; Keilhauer et al., 1985) or HNK-1 antibodies on neurite outgrowth (Riopelle et al., 1986). However, since antibodies do not only cover the epitope that they are directed against, but may sterically block neighbouring molecular domains from function, a more direct demonstration of the importance of the L2/HNK-1 carbohydrate for cell interactions appeared necessary. We, therefore, took advantage of the possibility to assay the effects of the L2 glycolipid and tetrasaccharide derived from this glycolipid on cell-cell interactions in culture. The isolated carbohydrate structures could, indeed, be shown to interfere not only with cell to cell, but, more strikingly even, cell to substrate interactions (Künemund et al., 1988). Since the inhibitory effects in adhesion assays observed with the glycolipid or tetrasaccharide were qualitatively and quantitatively amazingly similar to those observed with the L2 antibodies, the most straightforward interpretation of our findings is that the L2/HNK-1 carbohydrate is itself involved as a ligand in cell interactions. However, the involvement of carbohydrate structures in adhesion and recognition may be more complex and subtle (for review, see Rademacher and Dwek, 1988), so that direct inferences about the molecular mechanisms of the carbohydrate's function may be premature. At the moment, the possibility that the L2/HNK-1 carbohydrate structure may share certain structural and functional properties with glycosaminoglycans would make it a likely candidate for binding to extracellular matrix molecules (Bronner-Fraser, 1987; Künemund et al., 1988). Furthermore, it likely also modulates protein-protein interactions, possibly by fine tuning the extent and quality of affinities between adhesion molecules. Indeed, subsets of axons in the sciatic nerve express different carbohydrate epitopes that may correlate with distinct modalities conveyed by these axons (Martini and Schachner, 1986, 1988; Martini et al., submitted for publication).

The adhesion molecule on glia (AMOG) and the L3 carbohydrate family

AMOG is a neural cell adhesion molecule that mediates neuron-astrocyte interaction in vitro (Antonicek et al., 1987; Antonicek and Schachner, 1988). It is expressed by astrocytes in the cerebellum at critical developmental stages of granule cell neuron migration. AMOG is not expressed on Bergmann glial cells before the onset of migration and disappears from these cells after migration has ceased. At the end of the migratory period AMOG becomes detectable on astrocytic processes in the internal granular layer and remains there in adulthood. Granule neuron migration is strongly inhibited by monoclonal AMOG antibody, probably by disturbing neuron-glia adhesion. Thus, AMOG is yet another cell adhesion molecule involved in granule cell migration.

AMOG does not express the L2/HNK-1 carbohydrate epitope, but expresses another carbohydrate structure recognized by the monoclonal antibody L3. The L3 carbohydrate is expressed by several adhesion molecules from mouse brain, including L1 and MAG, but, interestingly, not by J1 and N-CAM (Kücherer et al., 1987) at the levels of detectability. The occurrence of this epitope thus makes AMOG the founding member of another family of cell adhesion molecules based on a carbohydrate structure that is common to members within this family, but also shared by some, but not all members of the other, the L2 family. The number of members in the L3 family is yet unknown, but appears to consist of at least nine glycoproteins in the adult mouse brain.

Several other features of the L3 carbohydrate epitope are reminiscent of those of the L2/HNK-1 epitope. Like L2/HNK-1, the L3 carbohydrate domain appears to be involved in cell interactions, since L3 antibodies have been found to inhibit cell adhesion and cellular outgrowth patterns in explant cultures (Weber and Schachner, unpublished observations). Consistent with its functional importance is its phylogenetic conservation and occurrence in invertebrates (Dennis et al., 1988; Dennis et al., unpublished observations). It is N-glycosidically linked and its expression is regulated independently of the protein backbone. Thus, not all molecules of each member in this family express the epitope. Consistent with these findings is the observation that only 10 to 20% of all MAG-positive oligodendrocytes express the L3 epitope. Similarly, in cultures of early postnatal mouse cerebellum, AMOG-positive astrocytes do not express the L3 epitope. Since the L3 carbohydrate epitope is expressed on both the L2-negative and -positive L1 molecules, a simple relationship between the L2 and L3 carbohydrate epitope carrying variants of adhesion molecules appears unlikely.

These observations point to questions that need to be answered in the future: Is the next, functionally characterized member of the L3 family also an adhesion molecule? What is the structure and function of the L3 carbohydrate? How many families of adhesion molecules exist that are combined by a common family feature in form of a distinct carbohydrate structure? Is it possible that adhesion molecules are "presenters" of functionally important carbohydrate structures with immense combinatorial possibilities? And, how do protein backbones and carbohydrates interact with each other? Elucidation of the functional and structural complexities in the rapidly expanding list of adhesion molecules will yield important insights into the morphogenetic mechanisms that underlie formation, maintenance and plasticity of the nervous system.

REFERENCES

Abo T, Balch CM (1981). A differentiation antigen of human NK and K cells identified by a monoclonal antibody (HNK-1). J Immunol 127:1024-1029.
Aguayo AJ (1985). Axonal regeneration from injured neurons in the adult mammalian central nervous system. In Cotman CW (ed): Synaptic Plasticity, The Guilford Press, pp.457-483.
Antonicek H, Persohn E, Schachner M (1987).

Biochemical and functional characterization of a novel neuron-glia adhesion molecule that is involved in neuronal migration. J Cell Biol 104: 1587-1595.

Antonicek H, Schachner M (1988). The adhesion molecule on glia (AMOG) incorporated into lipid vesicles binds to subpopulations of neurons. J Neurosci (in press).

Ariga T, Kohriyama T, Freddo L, Latov N, Saito M, Kon K, Ando S, Suzuki M, Hemling ME, Rinehart KL, Kusunoki S, Yu RK (1987). Characterization of sulfated glucuronic acid containing glycolipids reacting with IgM M proteins in patients with neuropathy. J Biol Chem 262:848-853.

Arquint M, Roder J, Chia LS, Down J, Wilkinson D, Bayley H, Braun P, Dunn R (1987). Molecular cloning and primary structure of myelin-associated glycoprotein. Proc Natl Acad Sci USA 84:600-604.

Bock E, Richter-Landsberg C, Faissner A, Schachner M (1985). Demonstration of immunochemical identity between the nerve growth factor-inducible large external (NILE) glycoprotein and the cell adhesion molecule L1. EMBO J 4:2765-2768.

Bollensen E, Schachner M (1987). The peripheral myelin glycoprotein P0 expresses the L2/HNK-1 and L3 carbohydrate structures shared by neural adhesion molecules. Neurosci Lett 82:77-82.

Bollensen E, Steck A, Schachner M (1988). Reactivity with the peripheral myelin glycoprotein P0 in sera from patients with monoclonal IgM gammopathy and polyneuropathy. Neurology (in press).

Bronner-Fraser M (1987). Perturbation of cranial neural crest migration by the HNK-1 antibody. Dev Biol 123:321-331.

Chang S, Rathjen FG, Raper JA (1987). Extension of neurites on axons is impaired by antibodies against specific neural cell surface glycoproteins. J Cell Biol 104:355-362.

Chou DKH, Ilyas AA, Evans JE, Costello C, Quarles RH, Jungalwala FB (1986). Structure of sulfated glucuronyl glycolipids in the nervous system reacting with HNK-1 antibody and some IgM paraproteins in neuropathy. J Biol Chem

261:383-388.
Cole GJ, Schachner M (1987). Localization of the L2 monoclonal antibody binding site on N-CAM and evidence for its role in N-CAM-mediated cell adhesion. Neurosci Lett 78:227-323.
Dennis RD, Antonicek H, Yu RK, Wiegandt H, Schachner M (1988). Detection of the L2/HNK-1 carbohydrate epitope on glycoproteins and acidic glycolipids of the insect, Calliphora vicina. J Neurochem (in press).
Erickson HP, Inglesias JL (1984). A six-armed oligomer isolated from cell surface fibronectin preparations. Nature 311: 267-269.
Fahrig T, Landa C, Pesheva P, Kühn K, Schachner M (1987). Characterization of binding properties of the myelin-associated glycoprotein to extracellular matrix constitutents. EMBO J 6:2875-2883.
Faissner A (1987). Monoclonal antibody detects carbohydrate microheterogeneity on the murine neural cell adhesion molecule L1. Neurosci Lett 83:327-332.
Faissner A, Kruse J, Chiquet-Ehrismann R, Mackie E (1988). The high molecular weight J1 glycoproteins are immunochemically related to tenascin. Differentiation (in press).
Faissner A, Kruse J, Goridis C, Bock E, Schachner M (1984). The neural cell adhesion molecule L1 is distinct from the N-CAM related group of surface antigens BSP-2 and D2. EMBO J 3:733-737.
ffrench-Constant C, Miller RH, Kruse J, Schachner M, Raff MC (1986). Molecular specialization of astrocyte processes at nodes of Ranvier in rat optic nerve. J Cell Biol 102:844-852.
Friedlander DR, Grumet M, Edelman GM (1986). Nerve growth factor enhances expression of neuron-glia cell adhesion molecule in PC12 cells. J Cell Biol 102:413-419.
Fushiki S, Schachner M (1986). Immunocytological localization of cell adhesion molecules L1 and N-CAM and the shared carbohydrate epitope L2 during development of the mouse neocortex. Devel Brain Res 289:153-167.
Grumet M, Hoffman S, Crossin KL, Edelman GM (1985). Cytotactin, an extracellular matrix

protein of neural and non-neural tissues that mediates glia-neuron interaction. Proc Natl Acad Sci USA 82:8075-8079.

He, H-T, Barbet J, Chaix J-C, Goridis C (1986). Phosphatidylinositol is involved in the membrane-attachment of NCAM-120, the smallest component of the neural cell adhesion molecule. EMBO J 5:2489-2494.

Hoffman S, Edelman GM (1987). A proteoglycan with HNK-1 antigenic determinants is a neuron-associated ligand for cytotactin. Proc Natl Acad Sci USA 84:2523-2527.

Holley JA, Silver J (1987). Growth pattern of pioneering chick spinal cord axons. Dev Biol 123:375-388.

Keilhauer G, Faissner A, Schachner M (1985). Differential inhibition of neurone-neurone, neurone-astrocyte and astrocyte-astrocyte adhesion by L1, L2 and N-CAM antibodies. Nature 316:728-730.

Kruse J, Keilhauer G, Faissner A, Timpl R, Schachner M (1985). The J1 glycoprotein - a novel nervous system cell adhesion molecule of the L2/HNK-1 family. Nature 316:146-148.

Kruse J, Mailhammer R, Wernecke H, Faissner A, Sommer I, Goridis C, Schachner M (1984). Neural cell adhesion molecules and myelin-associated glycoprotein share a common carbohydrate moiety recognized by monoclonal antibodies L2 and HNK-1. Nature 311:153-155.

Kücherer A, Faissner A, Schachner M (1987). The novel carbohydrate epitope L3 is shared by some neural cell adhesion molecules. J Cell Bio 104: 1597-1602

Künemund V, Jungalwala FB, Fischer G, Chou DKH, Keilhauer G, Schachner M (1988). The L2/HNK-1 carbohydrate of neural cell adhesion molecules is involved in cell interactions. J Cell Biol (in press).

Lagenaur C, Lemmon V (1987). An L1-like molecule, the 8D9 antigen, is a potent substrate for neurite extension. Proc Natl Acad Sci USA 84: 7747-7753.

Lai C, Brown MA, Nave K-A, Noronha AB, Quarles RH, Bloom FE, Milner RJ, Sutcliffe JG (1987). Two forms of 1B 236H/myelin-associated glycoprotein cell adhesion molecule for postnatal neural development are produced by alternative splicing. Proc Natl Acad Sci USA 84:4337-4341.

Lee, VM, Greene LA, Shelanski ML (1981). Identification of neural and adrenal medullary surface membrane glycoproteins recognized by antisera to cultured rat sympathetic neurons and PC12 pheochromocytoma cells. Neurosci 6:2773-2786.

Lindner J, Rathjen FG, Schachner M (1983). L1 mono- and polyclonal antibodies modify cell migration in early postnatal mouse cerebellum. Nature 305:427-430.

Lindner J, Zinser G, Werz W, Goridis C, Bizzini B, Schachner M (1986). Experimental modification of postnatal cerebellar granule cell migration in vitro. Brain Res 377:298-304.

Martini R, Schachner M (1986). Immunoelectron microscopic localization of neural cell adhesion molecules (L1, N-CAM, MAG) and their shared carbohydrate epitope and myelin basic protein (MBP) in developing sciatic nerve. J Cell Biol 103:2439-2448.

Martini R, Schachner M (1988). Immunoelectron microscopic localization of neural cell adhesion molecules (L1, N-CAM and myelin associated glycoprotein) in regenerating adult mouse sciatic nerve. J Cell Biol (in press).

Mbiene JP, Dechesne CJ, Schachner M, Sans A (1988). Immunocytological characterization of cell adhesion molecule L1 expression during early innervation of mouse otocysts. J Neurocytol (in press).

Mirsky R, Jessen KR, Schachner M, Goridis C (1986). Distribution of the adhesion molecules N-CAM and L1 on peripheral neurons and glia in adult rats. J Neurocytol 15:799-815.

Persohn E, Schachner M (1987). Immunoelectronmicroscopic localization of the neural cell adhesion molecules L1 and N-CAM during postnatal development of the mouse cerebellum. J Cell Biol 105:569-576.

Pesheva P, Horwitz AF, Schachner M (1987). Integrin, the cell surface receptor for fibronectin and laminin, expresses the L2/HNK-1 and

L3 carbohydrate structures shared by neural adhesion molecules. Neurosci Lett 83:303-306.

Pollerberg E, Burridge K, Krebs K, Goodman S, Schachner M (1987). The 180 kD component of the neural cell adhesion molecule N-CAM is involved in cell-cell contacts and cytoskeleton-membrane interactions. Cell Tiss Research 250:227-236.

Pollerberg E, Sadoul R, Goridis C, Schachner M (1985). Selective expression of the 180-kD component of the neural cell adhesion molecule N-CAM during development. J Cell Biol 101:1921-1929.

Pollerberg E, Schachner M, Davoust J (1986). Differentiation-state dependent surface mobilities of two forms of the neural cell adhesion molecule. Nature 324:462-465.

Poltorak M, Sadoul R, Keilhauer G, Landa C, Fahrig T, Schachner M (1987). The myelin-associated glycoprotein (MAG), a member of the L2/HNK-1 family of neural cell adhesion molecules, is involved in neuron-oligodendrocyte and oligodendrocyte-oligodendrocyte interaction. J Cell Biol 105:1893-1899.

Poltorak M, Steck AJ, Schachner M (1986). Reactivity with neural cell adhesion molecules of the L2/HNK-1 family in sera from patients with demyelinating diseases. Neurosci Lett 65: 199-203.

Rademacher T, Dwek R (1988). Glycobiology. Annu Rev Biochem (in press).

Ramon y Cajal S (1928a). Degeneration and regeneration of the nervous system Vol.I, 1-396, Oxford University Press

Ramon y Cajal S (1928b). Degeneration and regeneration of the nervous system Vol. II, 397-769, Oxford University Press

Rathjen FG, Wolff JM, Chang S, Bonhoeffer F, Raper JA (1987a). Neurofascin: A novel chick cell-surface glycoprotein involved in neurite-neurite interactions. Cell 51:841-849.

Rathjen FG, Wolff JM, Frank R, Bonhoeffer F, Rutishauser U (1987b). Membrane glycoproteins involved in neurite fasciculation. J Cell Biol 104:343-353.

Riopelle RJ, McGarry RC, Roder JC (1986). Adhesion properties of a neuronal epitope recog-

nized by the monoclonal antibody HNK-1. Brain Res 367: 20-25.
Rohrer H (1985). Nonneuronal cells from chick sympathetic and dorsal root sensory ganglia express catecholamine uptake and receptors for nerve growth factor during development. Dev Biol 111:95-107.
Rush, RA (1984) Immunohistochemical localization of endogenous nerve growth factor. Nature 312: 364-367
Sadoul K, Meyer A, Low MG, Schachner M (1986). Release of the 120 kD component of the neural cell adhesion molecule N-CAM from cell surfaces by phosphatidylinositol-specific phospholipase C. Neurosci Lett 72:341-346.
Salzer JL, Holmes WP, Colman DR (1987). The amino acid sequence of the myelin-associated glycoproteins: homology to the immunoglobulin gene superfamily. J Cell Biol 104:957-965.
Sanes JR, Schachner M, Covault J (1986). Distribution of several adhesive macromolecules in embryonic, adult, and denervated adult skeletal muscles. J Cell Biol 102:420-431.
Schachner M, Antonicek H, Fahrig T, Faissner A, Fischer G, Künemund V, Martini R, Meyer A, Persohn E, Pollerberg E, Probstmeier R, Sadoul K, Sadoul R, Seilheimer B, Thor G (1987). Families of neural cell adhesion molecules. In Edelman GM, Thiery J-P (eds): The Cell in Contact II, John Wiley & Sons, Ltd., (in press).
Schachner M, Faissner A, Fischer G, Keilhauer G, Kruse J, Künemund V, Lindner J, Wernecke H (1985). Functional and structural aspects of the cell surface in mammalian nervous system development. In Edelman GM, Thiery J-P (eds): The Cell in Contact, John Wiley & Sons, Ltd., pp. 257-275.
Seilheimer B, Schachner M (1987). Regulation of neural cell adhesion molecule expression on cultured mouse Schwann cells by nerve growth factor. EMBO J 6:1611-1616.
Seilheimer B, Schachner M (1988). Studies of adhesion molecules mediating interactions between cells of peripheral nervous system indicate a major role for L1 in mediating

sensory neuron growth on Schwann cells. J Cell Biol (in press).

Smith GM, Miller RH, Silver J (1986). Changing role of forebrain astrocytes during development, regenerative failure, and induced regeneration upon transplantation. J Comp Neurol 251:23-43.

Tacke R, Moos M, Früh K, Scherer H, Bach A, Schachner M (1987). Isolation of cDNA clones of the mouse neural cell adhesion molecule L1. Neurosci Lett 82:89-94.

Takeichi MC (1987). Cadherins: A molecular family essential for selective cell-cell adhesion and animal morphogenesis. Trends in Genetics 3:213-217.

Thor G, Pollerberg E, Schachner M (1986). Molecular association of two neural cell adhesion molecules, L1 antigen and the 180 kD component of N-CAM, within the surface membrane of cultured neuroblastoma cells. Neurosci Lett 66:121-126.

Thor G, Probstmeier R, Schachner.M (1987). Characterization of the cell adhesion molecules L1, N-CAM and J1 in the mouse intestine. EMBO J 6:2581-2586.

Wernecke H, Lindner J, Schachner M (1985). Cell type specificity and developmental expression of the L2/HNK-1 epitopes in mouse cerebellum. J Neuroimmunol 9:115-130.

Williams AF (1987). A year in the life of the immunoglobulin superfamily. Immunology Today 8:298-303.

NCAM AS A GENERAL REGULATOR OF CELL CONTACT

Urs Rutishauser, Ann Acheson, Alison K. Hall,
Dennis M. Mann and Jeffrey Sunshine
Neuroscience Program
Department of Developmental Genetics and Anatomy
Case Western Reserve University School of Medicine
Cleveland, Ohio 44106

Cell adhesion molecules (CAMs) are ligands that can participate in cell-cell recognition during the formation of tissue structures. In the nervous system, a number of membrane glycoproteins have been identified as CAMs. Most of these molecules are associated with specific aspects of development, such as axon fasciculation or target recognition. In contrast, the function of NCAM, one of the most abundant adhesion molecules, appears to affect a wide variety of different cellular events. To understand the biological role of NCAM, it is necessary to explain how and why so many different types of interactions appear to be influenced by its function.

The interpretation of NCAM-associated phenomena previously has emphasized adhesive preferences that directly reflect variations in NCAM's binding (Rutishauser, 1986). However, as illustrated below, both NCAM expression and its polysialic acid (PSA) content may in addition serve as indirect and permissive regulatory elements in other cell interactions. Experimental evidence and a model are presented suggesting that this situation reflects changes in the overall state of membrane-membrane contact, as well as direct alteration of a specific ligation event.

NCAM BINDING CAN AFFECT THE FUNCTION OF ANOTHER CELL-CELL ADHESION MECHANISM.

While adhesion mediated by NCAM is calcium-independent, a different class of CAM that requires calcium often exists on the same cell surface (Takeichi, 1987;

Brackenbury et al 1981). To investigate a possible
functional interdependence between these two adhesion
mechanisms, cells were prepared such that one or both of
these CAMs was present. Cells with only NCAM showed
calcium-independent aggregation which was blocked by anti-
NCAM Fab, and cells without NCAM on their surfaces displayed
a purely calcium-dependent aggregation which was not
affected by anti-NCAM. As expected, when both classes of
molecule were present, aggregation was enhanced and included
both a calcium-dependent and a calcium-independent
component. However, in this case, *both* types of adhesion
were blocked by anti-NCAM Fab, whereas NCAM-mediated binding
was not affected by removal of calcium.

BOTH NCAM BINDING AND PSA CONTENT INFLUENCE CELL CONTACT-DEPENDENT BIOCHEMICAL CHANGES.

Membrane-membrane contact regulates the levels of
neurotransmitter biosynthetic enzymes *in vitro* for a variety
of neural crest-derived cells (Acheson and Thoenen, 1983;
Sadaat and Thoenen, 1986; Adler and Black, 1986). We have
found that membrane contact-mediated increases in choline
acetyltransferase requires both NCAM binding function and
the presence of the molecule in its adhesion-promoting, low
PSA form. Moreover, the ability of anti-NCAM Fab to block
increased ChAT levels can be reversed by addition of a plant
lectin, but again only when the PSA content of the
endogenous NCAM is low (Acheson and Rutishauser, in press).
Thus, NCAM appears to serve as a permissive regulatory
factor in this system in two different ways: its binding
function holds membranes together, and its PSA content
independently regulates the ability of cells to transmit the
relevant biochemical signal.

NCAM PSA CONTENT ALONE CAN REGULATE THE FUNCTION OF OTHER CELL SURFACE LIGANDS.

Additional evidence for an influence of NCAM PSA on
cell-cell interactions involving molecules other than NCAM
has been obtained in studies of the bundling patterns of
neurites on a laminin substrate. The size of these bundles
reflects two opposing adhesive forces, neurite-neurite
binding mediated by several adhesion molecules including
NCAM (Rutishauser et al., 1985; Stallcup and Beasley, 1985;
Fischer et al, 1986; Rathjen et al., 1987), versus the pull
exerted by the individual growth cones as they adhere to and

migrate along the substrate (Rutishauser et al., 1978). With embryonic chick spinal cord neurites, whose NCAM is heavily sialylated, large fascicles are obtained. This observation is surprising since a high PSA content would be expected to decrease NCAM-mediated adhesion (Hoffman and Edelman, 1983; Rutishauser et al., 1985). Moreover, removal of PSA from these axons by endo N actually reduces fasciculation. The most consistent explanation of the neurite patterns obtained is that removal of NCAM PSA indirectly augments a second cell interaction, in this case an increase in growth cone-substrate adhesion.

A second illustration of this phenomenon is the effect of PSA on an artificial cell-cell interaction, wheat germ lectin (WGA)-mediated agglutination of embryonic chick brain membrane vesicles. In these experiments, the ability of WGA to agglutinate membranes in the absence of NCAM binding function was examined as a function of NCAM PSA content. Removal of NCAM PSA greatly facilitated the ability of WGA to promote aggregation. This effect did not reflect a change in the number of lectin receptors on membranes but rather an enhanced ability of the lectin to function when PSA was removed from the endogenous NCAM.

MEMBRANE AND MOLECULAR PARAMETERS IN NCAM-MEDIATED ADHESION.

It is known that NCAM mediates cell-cell binding, and that the rate of adhesion is enhanced by the removal of PSA from the molecule (Hoffman and Edelman, 1983; Rutishauser et al., 1985), but how are these effects manifested in terms of membrane-membrane contacts? Electron microscopic examination of aggregates formed by embryonic chick brain cells, which express NCAM with a high PSA content, showed intermittent regions of close membrane-membrane apposition between neighboring cells. Specific removal of the NCAM PSA by endo N resulted in a large increase in the area of these closely apposed regions. In contrast, addition of anti-NCAM Fab fragments completely prevented the formation of such areas of close contact. Therefore, as might be expected for an abundant adhesion ligand with a uniform distribution on the cell surface (van den Pol et al., 1986), there is a gross physical change in the overall degree of membrane apposition as a result of either enhanced or decreased NCAM function.

The observation that alterations in PSA content affect other cell-cell interactions even when NCAM's binding function is blocked is a striking phenomenon. This carbohydrate comprises up to one third of the molecule's mass (Hoffman et al., 1982), and causes a very large decrease in the molecule's electrophoretic mobility in SDS-PAGE (Hoffman and Edelman, 1983; Hoffman et al., 1982; Rothbard et al., 1982) and an increase in its apparent excluded volume in gel filtration chromatography. On this basis it would appear that the steric properties of the PSA moiety are not only likely to affect NCAM-NCAM binding, but in view of the abundance of NCAM in the membrane, could produce a thin screen of carbohydrate around the cell.

PROPOSED MECHANISM FOR NCAM-MEDIATED REGULATION.

On the basis of these observations, we have proposed that the presence of NCAM on the cell surface can have either a positive or negative effect on its overall interaction with other cells or substrates, depending on the molecule's PSA content. To account for these phenomena, two mechanisms are proposed (Figure 1).

For NCAM with relatively low PSA content, as found predominantly in early development and adult tissues (Rothbard et al.; 1982, Sunshine et al., 1987), the molecule's presence would increase the extent or duration of membrane contact and thereby promote other interactions (Figure 1a). This mechanism is consistent with the present findings on the relationship between NCAM and calcium-dependent adhesion, which has been linked to the formation of adherens-type junctions (Boller et al., 1985; Volk and Geiger, 1986; Gumbiner and Simons, 1986). We have also reported two other examples of the ability of NCAM expression to regulate the formation of specialized cell-cell contacts. Antibody perturbation studies suggest that NCAM-mediated adhesion is required for the onset of extensive junctional communication among neuroepithelial cells (Keane et al., in press). A role for NCAM has also been proposed in the initial innervation of limb muscles by motoneurons (Tosney et al.; 1986, Grumet et al.; 1982, Covault and Sanes, 1985).

For molecules with high PSA content, the large volume occupied by the carbohydrate would impede membrane-membrane contact so that the function of some ligands, and probably even that of NCAM itself, is hindered (Figure 1b). In this case, interactions could be initiated by a reduction in the amount of PSA. At present it is not possible to distinguish whether the effects of PSA involve changes in the extent, intimacy or duration of cell-cell contact. Each could, in principle, enhance the efficiency of a particular cell interaction.

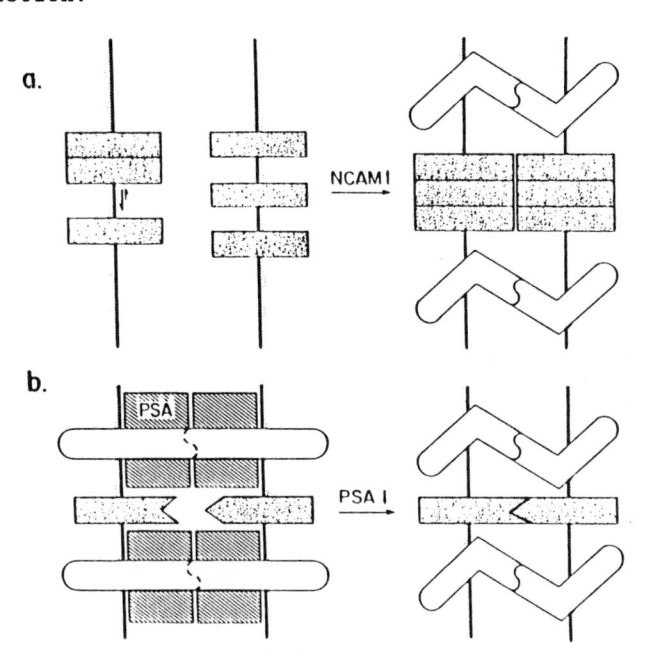

Figure 1. Two mechanisms for the regulation of cell-cell interactions by NCAM. A. Expression of NCAM on cell surfaces and the resultant formation of NCAM-NCAM bonds enhances the probability of junction formation from interacting subunits (*shaded rectangles*) by increasing the extent or duration of membrane-membrane contact. B. Initiation of cell interactions via specific ligands by a reduction in NCAM PSA content (*hatched areas*). The ability of the ligands to engage is enhanced by reducing the excluded volume of carbohydrate between membranes, which impedes close cell-cell contact. The presence and absence of a bend in NCAM is based on electron micrographs of the molecule and the proposal that such a flexible hinge could allow for changes in membrane-membrane distances (Hall and Rutishauser, 1987).

DISCUSSION.

Our findings provide evidence for the importance of *permissive hierarchies* of cell-cell interaction, in which the degree of cell-cell contact required to initiate one interaction is provided by a second molecule. NCAM can function in such a hierarchy in two ways. First, its expression can enhance cell interactions by increasing membrane-membrane adhesion. A useful feature of this type of permissive regulation is that if a particular cell interaction requires several components, they can be synthesized independently and then functionally activated by expression of a single polypeptide.

Second, NCAM PSA can mediate global regulation of membrane events via its steric or repulsive properties, by producing an oligosaccharide coating around the cell. Such alterations of the overall degree of close membrane apposition could allow differential use of several ligand-receptor systems according to their properties. For example, a receptor that is small, relatively immobile, or present in low amounts may require a low NCAM PSA content in order to function, while an abundant and mobile extracellular protein receptor, or a soluble ligand, would be independent of this type of control. Embryonic axons, which have a particularly high PSA content during the formation of tracts and connections (Sunshine et al., 1987), may illustrate this type of selection. As an axon grows through a complex environment, it must be able to avoid inappropriate interactions, such as formation of stable junctions, yet remain responsive to guidance and target cues. The fact that mammalian adult axons lack large amounts of PSA may therefore represent an important impediment to their ability to regenerate after injury. (supported by grants HD18369 and EY06107 from the USPHS)

REFERENCES

Acheson A and Thoenen H (1983). Cell contact-mediated regulation of tyrosine hydroxylase synthesis in cultured bovine adrenal chromaffin cells. J Cell Biol 97:925-928.
Acheson A and Rutishauser U (in press). NCAM regulates cell contact-mediated changes in choline aceytltransferase activity of embryonic chick sympathetic neurons. J Cell Biol.
Adler JE and Black IB (1986). Membrane contact regulates transmitter phenotypic expression. Dev Brain Res 30:237-

241.
Boller K, Vestweber D, Kemler, R (1985). Cell-adhesion molecule uvomorulin is localized at the intermediate junctions of adult intestinal epithelial cells. J Cell Biol 100:327.
Brackenbury R, Rutishauser U, Edelman, GM (1981). Distinct calcium-independent and calcium-dependent adhesion systems of chick embryo cells. Proc Nat Acad Sci USA 78:387.
Covault J, Sanes JR (1985). Neural cell adhesion molecule (NCAM) accumulates in denervated and paralyzed skeletal muscles. Proc Natl Acad Sci USA 82:4544.
Fischer G, Kunemund V, Schachner M (1986). Neurite outgrowth patterns in cerebellar microexplant cultures are affected by the antibodies to the cell surface glycoprotein L1. J Neurosci 6:605-612.
Grumet M, Rutishauser U, Edelman GM (1982). N-CAM mediates adhesion between embryonic nerve and muscle cell in vitro. Nature(Lond) 295:693-695.
Gumbiner B, Simons K (1986). A functional assay for proteins involved in establishing an epithelial occluding barrier: Identification of a uvomorulin-like peptide. J Cell Biol 102:457-468.
Hall A, Rutishauser U (1987). Visulaization of neural cell adhesion molecule by electron microscopy. J Cell Biol 104:1579-1586.
Hoffman S, Sorkin BC, White PC, Brackenbury R, Mailhammer R, Rutishauser U, Cunningham BA, Edelman GM (1982). Chemical characterization of a neural cell adhesion molecule (N-CAM) purified from embryonic brain membranes. J Biol Chem 257:7720-7729.
Hoffman S, Edelman GM (1983). Kinetics of homophilic binding by embryonic and adult forms of the neural cell adhesion molecule. Proc Natl Acad Sci USA 80:5762-5766.
Keane RW, Mehta PP, Rose B, Honig LS, Lowenstein WR, Rutishauser U (in press). Neural differentiation, NCAM-mediated adhesion and gap junctional communication in neuroectoderm. A study in vitro. J Cell Biol.
Rathjen FG, Wolff JM, Frank R, Bonhoeffer F, Rutishauser U (1987). Membrane glycoproteins involved in neurite fasciculation. J Cell Biol 104:343-353.
Rothbard JB, Brackenbury R, Cunningham BA, Edelman GM (1982). Differences in the carbohydrate structures of neural cell-adhesion molecules from adult and embryonic chicken brains. J Biol Chem 257:11064-11069.
Rutishauser U (1986). Differential cell adhesion through spatial and temporal variations of NCAM. Trends in Neurosci 9:374-378.
Rutishauser U, Gall WE, Edelman GM (1978). Adhesion among

neural cells of the chick embryo. IV. Role of the cell surface molecules CAM in the formation of neurite bundles in cultures of spinal ganglia. J Cell Biol 79:382-393.

Rutishauser U, Watanabe M, Silver J, Troy FA, Vimr ER (1985). Morpholgy, motility and surface behavior of lymphocytes bound to nylon fibers. J Cell Biol 101:1842-1849.

Saadat S, Thoenen H (1986). Selective induction of tyrosine hydroxylase by cell-cell contact in bovine adrenal chromaffin cells is mimicked by plasma membranes. J Cell Biol 103:1991-1997.

Stallcup WB, Beasley L (1985). Involvement of the nerve growth factor-inducible large external glycoprotein (NILE) in neurite fasciculation in primary culture of rat brain. Proc Natl Acad Sci USA 82:1276.

Sunshine J, Balak K, Rutishauser U, Jacobson M (1987). Changes in neural cell adhesion molecule (NCAM) structure during vertebrate neural development. Proc Natl Acad Sci USA 84:5986-5990.

Takeichi M (1987). Cadherins: a molecular family essential for selective cell-cell adhesion and animal morphogenesis. Trends in Genetics 3:213-217

Tosney KW, Watanabe M, Landmesser L, Rutishauser U (1986). The distribution of NCAM in the chick hindlimb during axon outgrowth and synaptogenesis. Dev Biol 114:437.

van den Pol AN, DiPorzio U, Rutishauser U (1986). Growth cone localization of neural cell adhesion molecule on central nervous system neurons in vitro. J Cell Biol 102:2281-2294.

Volk T, Geiger B (1986). A-CAM: A 135-KD receptor of intercellular adherens junctions. II. Antibody-mediated modulation of junction formation. J Cell Biol 103:1451-1464.

DEVELOPMENTAL REGULATION OF EXPRESSION OF THE NEURAL CELL
ADHESION MOLECULES NCAM AND L1

E. Bock, O. Nybroe and D. Linnemann

The Protein Laboratory, University of Copenhagen, Copenhagen, Denmark

INTRODUCTION

   The cell adhesion molecules NCAM and L1 have been implicated in cell surface interactions during development of the nervous system (Edelman, 1986). NCAM is expressed already at early developmental stages and on all major neural cell types in the central and peripheral nervous system. It mediates aggregation of single cells and histotypic deployment in neural tissue culture. NCAM is identical to the BSP-2 antigen and the D2-protein (Noble et al., 1985). L1 appears later during development and has a more restricted set of roles. In the central nervous system, L1 expression is restricted to post-mitotic neurons (Rathjen and Schachner, 1984). It is involved in migration of granular neurons in the early postnatal mouse cerebellar cortex (Lindner et al., 1983) and in fasciculation of neurites (Linnemann et al., 1987). L1 is immunochemically identical to the nerve growth factor-inducible large external (NILE) glycoprotein (Bock et al., 1985).

MOLECULAR GENETICS

   By radio-iodination of whole brain homogenates with subsequent immunoisolation, NCAM appears as three polypeptides of 190 kd (Polypeptide A), 140 kd (Polypeptide B) and 115 kd (Polypeptide C) in SDS-polyacrylamide gel electrophoresis. Occasionally, small amounts of one to three polypeptides of 250-300 kd can be observed. L1 appears by the same procedure as three polypeptides of 200, 140 and

80 kd.

In vitro translation of membrane bound polysomes has shown that NCAM A, B, and C chains are synthesized from three individual mRNA species (Hansen et al., 1985). This has been confirmed by isolation of NCAM cDNA clones (Murray et al., 1984; Goridis et al., 1985). In contrast there is only one copy of the NCAM gene in the chicken and mouse genome. The mechanism behind the occurrence of NCAM A, B, and C is differential splicing of one primary transcript. The amino acid sequence of NCAM (Cunningham et al., 1987) indicates that NCAM is a member of the immunoglobulin gene superfamily. Members of this superfamily all share a common structure called the immunoglobulin homology unit. NCAM has five homology unit sequences and it has been suggested (Hunkapiller and Hood, 1986) that the homophilic and polyvalent nature of NCAM binding may result from receptor-ligand binding analogous to the paired homology unit associations observed for other molecules of the superfamily.

Less is known so far about L1. However, by metabolic labelling in cell culture the molecule is seen as one single polypeptide of 200 kd indicating that the lower molecular weight polypeptides of 140 and 80 kd probably are the result of posttranslational modulations or artefacts (Faissner et al., 1985).

POST-TRANSLATIONAL MODULATIONS

Both NCAM and L1 undergo several post-translational modifications, see Table 1. All polypeptides of both proteins are glycosylated. Co-translational N-linked glycosylation has been shown to take place for NCAM A, B, and C and for the 200 kd polypeptide of L1 (Lyles et al., 1984; Faissner et al., 1985). An interesting feature of NCAM and L1 is the presence of a carbohydrate epitope recognized by two monoclonal antibodies: HNK1 and L2. This epitope has been shown to include a terminal 3-sulphoglucoronyl residue. The epitope has been demonstrated on other adhesion molecules including myelin associated glycoprotein and the J1 cell adhesion molecule (Kruse et al., 1985).

TABLE 1. Co- and Post-Translational Modulations of NCAM and L1.

	NCAM			L1		
	190 kd	140 kd	115 kd	200 kd	140 kd	80 kd
N-linked glycosylation	+	+	+	+	+	+
Polysialation	+	+	n.d.	–	–	–
Sulphation	+	+	+	+	n.d.	n.d.
Phosphorylation	+	+	–	+	–	+
Membrane insertion	+	+	–	+	–	+

n.d. = not determined

Furthermore, NCAM in rat brain contains several sialosyl residues in a polysialic alpha-2,8 ketosidic linkage (Lyles et al., 1984). Polysialation cannot be demonstrated on L1 (Linnemann et al., 1987). Both NCAM and L1 are sulphated and phosphorylated (Linnemann et al., 1987 and 1988; Lyles et al., 1984). Two of the three NCAM polypeptides are integral membrane proteins, whereas the NCAM polypeptide C lacks a membrane spanning domain (Nybroe et al., 1985). It has been demonstrated that at least a fraction of polypeptide C is held in the membrane by a covalently bound phosphatidyl-inositol anchor (He et al., 1986; Sadoul et al., 1986; Hemperly et al., 1986). Phosphatidylinositol-specific phospholipase C releases a substantial proportion of NCAM-C from brain membranes (He et al., 1986). The release of polypeptide C may interfere with already established NCAM mediated cell-cell bonds.

The 200 kd and 80 kd L1-polypeptides are integral membrane proteins, whereas the membrane association of 140 kd L1 still remains to be determined (Faissner et al., 1985).

DEVELOPMENTAL CHANGES IN BIOSYNTHESIS OF NCAM AND L1

Both cell adhesion molecules are submitted to developmental changes in concentration, glycosylation and phosphorylation (Linnemann et al., 1985, 1987, 1988; Linnemann and Bock, 1986; Lyles et al., 1984). Furthermore, NCAM changes during development in polypeptide composition, polysialation, sulphation and in solubility of polypeptide C. The changes are summarized in Tables 2 and 3.

TABLE 2. Developmental Changes in NCAM Expression in Rat Brain

	Embryonic day 17	Postnatal day 4-5	Postnatal day 15-25	Postnatal day 40
mg NCAM per g protein	8	16	12	10
NCAM Polypeptides	A,B,(C)*	A,B,C	A,B,C	A,B,C
NCAM-C Solubility				
in buffer pH 7.2	n.d.	+	(+)	−
in buffer pH 8.6	n.d.	+	+	−
in detergent	n.d.	+	+	(+)
Polysialation	+	+	−	−
Sulphation	+	(+)	−	n.d.
Phosphorylation	++	+	+	n.d.

n.d. = not determined.

*C is not detectable in mouse or chicken brain at this stage. In chicken retina embryonic day 6 only polypeptide B is expressed (Friedlander et al., 1985).

Polysialation of NCAM is temporally regulated. A functional importance has been demonstrated for this modification. During development NCAM sialylation decreases at least three fold (Linnemann et al., 1985). This decrease is accompanied by an increased NCAM adhesivity (Sadoul et al., 1983).

TABLE 3. Developmental Changes in L1 Expression in Rat Brain

	Embryonic day 17	Postnatal day 4	Postnatal day 15	Postnatal day 40
A.u.L1 per g protein*	190	325	170	100
Sulphation	+	+	+	n.d.
Phosphorylation	++	+	+	n.d.

n.d. = not determined

*The amount of L1 per g protein at postnatal day 40 was set to 100 arbitrary units (a.u.).

In contrast to NCAM, it has been found that biosynthesis of L1 decreases relatively more than total protein biosynthesis indicating that the decrease in L1 biosynthesis not merely reflects a general decrease in metabolism during development (Linnemann et al., 1988).

The amount of L1 in rat brain changes during development in a manner comparable to NCAM. Expressed relative to total protein the amount of both proteins increases to a peak value at postnatal day 4 and then decreases. However, while NCAM concentration stabilizes at a level close to the level at embryonic day 17 (Linnemann and Bock, 1986) L1 decreases to 50% of this level (Linnemann et al., 1988). L1 expression is restricted to certain postmitotic neurons (Faissner et al., 1984) and some of the changes in L1 concentration may be explained by developmentally changing ratios between cell populations in the brain. Consequently, the postnatally decreasing amount of L1 as well as NCAM may reflect an increasing glial contribution to total brain protein as CNS glial cells contain no L1 (Rathjen and Schachner, 1984) and only minor amounts of NCAM compared to neurons (Noble et al., 1985). The more pronounced decrease in L1 amount compared to NCAM may partly be explained by the glial contribution to NCAM amount.

Both NCAM and L1 are sulphated and phosphorylated. However, sulphation of NCAM decreases during development, whereas L1 sulphation does not seem to decrease more than

L1 biosynthesis. Thus, while the degree of sulphation may be of importance for regulation of NCAM function, L1 function may not be developmentally regulated by this modification. Phosphorylation of both adhesion molecules, on the other hand, decreases during development and may, thus, be assumed to be of importance for temporal modulation of their function.

In conclusion, it appears that the many cell interactions involved in early development do not require an extensive repertoire of ligand binding specificities. In the nervous system f.ex., NCAM and L1 contribute to the morphogenetic events through a complex regulation of both the expression and the structure of the molecules.

REFERENCES

Bock E, Richter-Landsberg C, Faissner A, Schachner M (1985). Demonstration of immunochemical identity between the nerve growth factor-inducible large external (NILE) glycoprotein and the cell adhesion molecule L1. EMBO J 4: 2765-2768.

Cunningham BA, Hemperly JJ, Murray BA, Prediger EA, Brackenbury R, Edelman GM (1987). Neural cell adhesion molecule: Structure, immunoglobulin-like domains, cell surface modulation, and alternative RNA splicing. Science 236: 799-806.

Edelman GM (1986). Cell adhesion molecules in neural histogenesis. Ann Rev Physiol 48: 417-430.

Faissner A, Kruse J, Nieke J, Schachner M (1984). Expression of neural cell adhesion molecule L1 during development, in neurological mutants and in the peripheral nervous system. Devl Brain Res 15: 69-82.

Faissner A, Teplow DB, Kubler D, Keilhauer G, Kinzel V, Schachner M (1985). Biosynthesis and membrane topography of the neural cell adhesion molecule L1. EMBO J 4: 3105-3113.

Goridis C, Hirn M, Santoni M-J, Gennarini G, Deagostini-Bazin H, Jordan BR, Kiefer M, Steinmetz M (1985). Isolation of mouse N-CAM related cDNA. Detection and cloning using monoclonal antibodies. EMBO J 4: 631-635.

Hansen OC, Nybroe O, Bock E (1985). Cell-free synthesis of the D2-cell adhesion molecule: evidence for three primary translation products. J Neurochem 44: 712-717.

He HT, Barbet J, Chaix JC, Goridis C (1986). Phosphatidylinositol is involved in the membrane attachment of NCAM-

120, the smallest component of the neural cell adhesion molecule. EMBO J 5: 2489-2494.
Hemperly JJ, Edelman GM, Cunningham BA (1986). cDNA clones of the neural cell adhesion molecule (N-CAM) lacking a membrane-spanning region consistent with evidence for membrane attachment via a phosphatidylinositol intermediate. Proc Natl Acad Sci 83: 9822-9826.
Hunkapiller T, Hood L (1986). The growing immunoglobulin gene superfamily. Nature (London) 323: 15-16.
Lindner J, Rathjen FG, Schachner M (1983). L1 mono- and polyclonal antibodies modify cell migration in early postnatal mouse cerebellum. Nature (London) 305: 427-430.
Linnemann D, Bock E (1986). Developmental study of the solubility and polypeptide composition of the neural cell adhesion molecule. Dev Neurosci 8: 24-30.
Linnemann D, Edvardsen K, Bock E (1988). Developmental study of the cell adhesion molecule L1. Dev Neurosci, in press.
Linnemann D, Lyles JM, Bock E (1985). A developmental study of the biosynthesis of the neural cell adhesion molecule. Dev Neurosci 7: 230-238.
Linnemann D, Nybroe O, Gibson A, Rohde H, Jørgensen OS, Bock E (1987). Characterization of the biosynthesis, membrane association and function of the cell adhesion molecule L1. Neurochem Int 10: 113-120.
Lyles JM, Linnemann D, Bock E (1984). Biosynthesis of the D2-cell adhesion molecule. Posttranslational modifications, intracellular transport and developmental changes. J Cell Biol 99: 2082-2091.
Murray BA, Hemperly JJ, Gallin WJ, MacGregor JS, Edelman GM, Cunningham BA (1984). Isolation of cDNA clones for the chicken neural cell adhesion molecule (N-CAM). Proc Natl Acad Sci 81: 5584-5588.
Noble M, Albrechtsen M, Møller C, Lyles J, Bock E, Goridis C, Watanabe M, Rutishauser U (1985). Glial cells express N-CAM/D2-CAM-like polypeptides in vitro. Nature (London) 316: 725-728.
Nybroe O, Albrechtsen M, Dahlin J, Linnemann D, Lyles JM, Møller CJ, Bock E (1985). Biosynthesis of the neural cell adhesion molecule: characterization of polypeptide C. J Cell Biol 101: 2310-2315.
Rathjen FG, Schachner M (1984). Immunocytological and biochemical characterization of a new neuronal cell surface component (L1 antigen) which is involved in cell adhesion. EMBO J 3: 1-10.

Sadoul R, Hirn M, Deagostini-Bazin H, Rougon G, Goridis C (1983). Adult and embryonic mouse neural cell adhesion molecules have different binding properties. Nature (London) 304: 347-349.

Sadoul K, Meyer A, Low MG, Schachner M (1986). Release of the 120 kDa component of the mouse neural cell adhesion molecule N-CAM from cell surfaces by phosphatidylinositol-specific phospholipase C. Neurosci Lett 72: 341-346.

Friedlander DR, Brackenbury R, Edelman GM (1985). Conversion of embryonic form to adult forms of N-CAM in vitro: results from de novo synthesis of adult forms. J Cell Biol 101(2): 412-419.

Kruse J, Keilhauer G, Faissner A, Timpl R, Schachner M (1985). The J1 glycoprotein - a novel nervous system cell adhesion molecule of the L2-HNK-1 family. Nature (London) 316: 146-148.

ASTROCYTIC RESPONSE TO INJURY

ASTROCYTIC RESPONSE TO INJURY

Lawrence F. Eng

Department of Pathology, Stanford University
School of Medicine, Stanford, CA 94305 and
Veterans Administration Medical Center,
Palo Alto, CA 94304

INTRODUCTION

Astrocytes comprise as much as 25% of the cells and 35% of the total mass of the central nervous system (CNS). Astrocytes form barriers around blood vessels and connections between nerve cells. Based on classical morphological critera, astrocytes can be classified into three types: the protoplasmic astrocyte present in gray matter, the fibrous astrocyte present in white matter, and the reactive astrocyte which can derive from the protoplasmic or fibrous astrocyte in response to injury or disease. Numerous functions have been assigned to the astrocyte depending on its stage of maturation, location in the CNS, and response to CNS insult. These functions for the most part attempt to maintain and support the normal function of the CNS. In some instances, however, these beneficial responses may compete and inhibit the regeneration response of the oligodendrocytes and neurons. Current investigations are directed toward characterization of the normal functions and properties of the astrocyte and the specific factors which induce its reactive response to injury.

Astrocytic functions suggested from early anatomical observations include (1) a cytoskeletal role in structural support for neurons and isolation of neurons, (2) a physiological role of channeling nutrients from the vascular to neuronal elements, (3) inactivation of substances used in neuronal communication, and (4) detoxification of substances entering the brain. Experimentally observed functions include: (1) proliferation and space filling during repair, (2) guidance of the migrating neurons and the growth of their processes during ontogenesis, (3) release of interleukin-1 following stimulation by various antigens, and (4) presentation of antigens (specific, major-histocompatibility-complex-restricted, antigens). Putative functions include: (1) maintenance of the proper ionic environment for neuronal communication, (2) provision of trophic and nutrient factors required for neuronal function, (3) synthesis, accumulation, metabolism and release of neurotransmitters, (4) modulation of the extracellular distribution of neuronally released neurotransmitters by changing in cell shape and volume, and (5) direction or guide for differentiating neurons in developing tissue.

REACTIVE ASTROGLIOSIS

Reactive astrogliosis is a stereotypic reaction of astrocytes within and adjacent to the site of injury. It also occurs in CNS demyelination such as multiple sclerosis and the degenerative diseases -- Alzheimer's disease, Creutzfeldt-Jakob disease (CJD), and Huntington's disease. Astrogliosis is characterized by astrocyte proliferation and extensive hypertrophy of the cell body and cytoplasmic processes (Hortega and Penfield, 1927; Latov et al., 1979; Oehmichen, 1980; Barrett et al., 1981; Nathaniel and Nathaniel, 1981; Polak et al., 1982). Activated, reactive astrocytes exhibit cytological, histochemical, and biochemical transformations which include the following: 1) increases in nuclear diameter (Hortega and Penfield, 1927; Cavanagh, 1970), 2) elevated DNA levels (Lapham and Johnstone, 1964), 3) accumulation of intermediate filaments (Nathaniel and Nathaniel, 1977), 4) heightened oxidoreductive enzyme activity (Oehmichen, 1980), 5) increased immunostaining (Bignami and Dahl, 1976; Amaducci et al., 1981) and transcription of glial fibrillary acidic protein (GFAP) (Kretzschmar et al., 1986; Manuelidis et al., 1987), (6) increased content of vimentin (Dahl et al., 1981, 1982), glutamine synthetase (Norenberg, 1983), and glycogen (Nathaniel and Nathaniel, 1981).

Astrogliosis may participate in the healing phase following CNS injury by actively monitoring and controlling the molecular and ionic contents of the extracellular space of the CNS. Important extracellular constituents which may be regulated by reactive astrocytes include potassium ions, neurotransmitters, trophic factors, nutrients and metabolic waste products. (For reviews, see Kimelberg and Ransom, 1986; Manthorpe et al., 1986; Nathaniel and Nathaniel, 1981; Reier, 1986). Astrocytes are also thought to participate in the removal of myelin and neuronal debris from injured areas (Gray and Guillery, 1966; Anderson and Westrum, 1972; Cook and Wisniewski, 1973; Nathaniel and Nathaniel, 1977). They can wall off areas of the CNS that are exposed to non-CNS tissue environments following trauma (i.e., Schultz and Pease, 1959; Matthews et al., 1979; Reier et al., 1983, Berry et al., 1983; Mathewson and Berry, 1985). On the other hand, astrogliosis may have pathological effects by interfering with the function of residual neuronal circuits, by preventing remyelination, or by inhibiting axonal regeneration (Reier et al., 1983; Reier, 1986).

Astrogliosis is characterized by extensive synthesis of GFAP intermediate filaments and by hypertrophy of the astrocytic cytoplasmic processes. The functional significance for this increase in intermediate filaments (IFs) is not known. Evidence from studies with rat optic nerve astrocyte cultures suggests that the content and subcellular distribution of IFs are important for cytoplasmic process formation and for structural stability of astrocytes. The relatively slow metabolic turnover rate for GFAP is consistent with such a structural role (DeArmond et al., 1983,1986; Smith et al., 1984). Ultrastructural and immunocytochemical studies of astrocytic differentiation *in vitro* show that the flat, polygonal astroblast contains abundant microtubules and actin stress fibers; however, these elements progressively decrease while GFAP increases during the change in shape of this astroblast to a stellate cell having slender, unbranched processes (Trimmer et al, 1982; Ciesielski-Treska et al., 1982a; Ciesielski-Treska et al., 1982b; Fedoroff, 1985).

GFAP is the intermediate filament in differentiated astrocytes. Extensive use of mono- and polyclonal antibodies to GFAP in neurobiology has established GFAP as a prototype brain antigen in CNS immunocytochemistry and as a standard astrocyte marker for neuroscience research. Comprehensive treatment of this subject can be found in the following reviews and books: Bignami et al. (1980); Bock (1978); Dahl and Bignami (1983, 1985); Dahl et al (1986); DeArmond and Eng (1984); Duffy (1983); Eng and Bigbee (1978); Eng (1979a and b, 1980, 1985); Eng and DeArmond (1982, 1983); Traub (1985); and Schliwa (1986).

Our working hypothesis is that control of astrocyte proliferation, differentiation, and astrogliosis may be linked to GFAP synthesis. One might be able to modulate astrogliosis to promote healing and functional recovery of neuronal pathways. For example, inhibition of GFAP synthesis immediately following injury might delay astrogliosis, thereby allowing the neurons the opportunity to regenerate and oligodendrocytes to proliferate and remyelinate. The ability to induce GFAP synthesis and differentiation in anaplastic astrocyte tumors might cause terminal differentiation and mitotic arrest.

ASTROGLIOSIS FOLLOWING CNS INJURY

Any type of insult to the CNS can induce astrogliosis whether it results from physical trauma such as a liquid nitrogen lesion (Amaducci et al., 1981), light-induced photoreceptor degeneration in the rat retina (Eisenfeld et al., 1984) or spinal cord transsection (Reier, 1986), immunologic cellular insult such as experimental allergic encephalomyelitis (EAE) (Smith et al., 1983) or experimental allergic uveitis (EAU) (Wacker et al., 1977; Chan et al., 1985), CJD infection (Manuelidis et al, 1987), or biochemical alteration due to a genetic defect (Eisenfeld et al., 1984). Once the blood-brain barrier is broken, numerous factors can activate the astrocytes: (1) anoxia may occur due to the disruption of the blood supply, (2) dilution of inhibitory "chalones" around the site of edema may occur, (3) blood-born substances can enter the CNS, (4) cell-derived substances from infiltrating cells can be released, (5) mitogenic and non-mitogenic substances from degenerating neurons and fibers can be released, and (6) astrocytes can be released from contact inhibition due to increase in space. A flow chart illustrating the possible factors which could activate the astrocyte and cause astrogliosis is shown in Figure 1.

CNS INJURY RESULTING FROM:

TRAUMA —— Physical, Chemical
CELLULAR —— Immunologic: EAE, EAU
INFECTION —— Viral, Bacteria
BIOCHEMICAL — Metabolic Defect

Disruption of the BBB

Activated or Injured Endothelial Cells
Factors Lymphokines

Anoxia
Edema *
Blood Borne Agents
Change in Ionic Composition

Death of Neurons and Glia

Toxic Agents
Stimulation
Microglia and Macrophage Responses
Factors Lymphokines

ASTROCYTES ACTIVATED

Hyperplasia
Vimentin
GFAP

Hypertrophy
GFAP

ASTROGLIOSIS

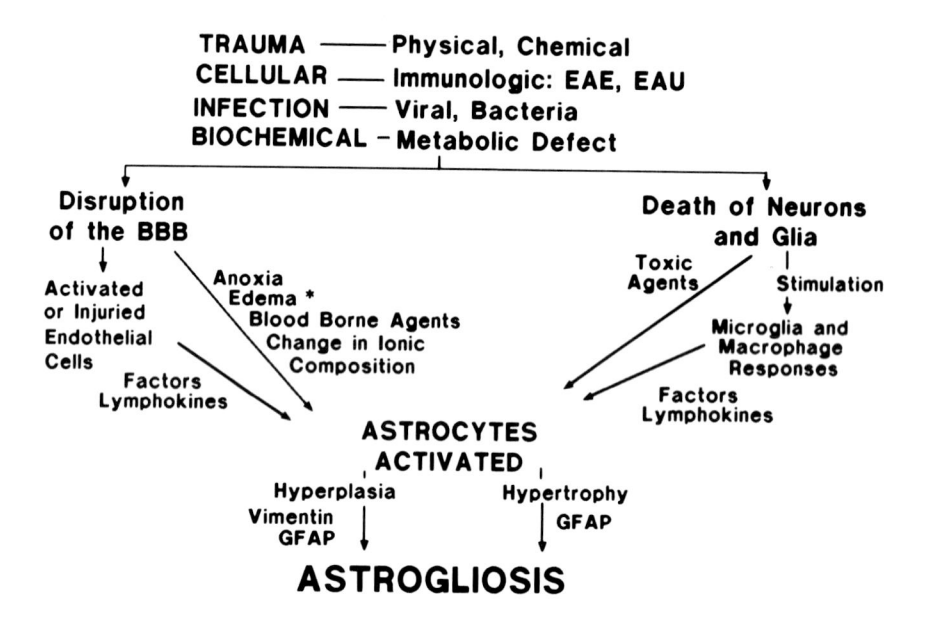

Figure 1. Flow chart for astrogliosis.

The next six chapters expand on some of these issues related to the activation of astroglia following trauma or disease, as well as the ability of young astrocytes to foster axonal outgrowth. Dr. de Vellis reviews the various hormones and growth factors which activate astrocytes with special emphasis on the early molecular events. Dr. Silver reports that immature astrocytes exhibit mobility, plasticity, and the ability to serve as a bridge or guide for migrating neuronal processes. Dr. Kalderon shows that immature astrocytes express high levels of plasminogen activator and that this protease is involved in the process of axon migration. Dr. Giulian provides good evidence that mononuclear phagocytes and ameboid microglia release Interleukin-1 which stimulates astrogliosis. Dr. Smith demonstrates that in the chronic-relapsing model of EAE, astrocyte division and growth of the fibrous processes extends over a long period of time (months) resulting in the formation of gliotic plaques similar to those seen in multiple sclerosis. Finally, Dr. Nieto-Sampedro proposes that the activity of protein factors which cause astrocyte proliferation and morphological changes at the site of injury may be due in part to a decrease in the concentration of inhibitory protein molecules.

Acknowledgements: Thanks are due to Donna Buckley for typing the manuscript. Supported in part by the VA and NINCDS Grant NS-11632.

REFERENCES

Amaducci, L, Forno KI, Eng LF (1981). Glial fibrillary acidic protein in cyrogenic lesions of the rat brain. Neurosci Letts 21:27-32.
Anderson CA, Westrum LE (1972). An elecron microscopic study of the normal synaptic relationships and early degenerative changes in the rat olfactory tubercle. Z Zellforsch 127:462-482.
Barrett CP, Guth L, Donati EJ, Krikorian JG (1981). Astroglial reaction in the gray matter lumbar segments after midthoracic transection of the adult rat spinal cord. Exp Neurol 73:365-377.
Berry M, Maxwell WL, Logan A, Mathewson A, McConnell P, Ashhurst DE, Thomas GH (1983). Deposition of scar tissue in the cenral nervous system. Acta Neurochirurgica Suppl 32:31-53.
Bignami A, Dahl, D (1976). The astroglial response to stabbing. Immunofluorescence studies with antibodies to asrocyte- specific protein (GFA) in mammalian and submammalian vertebrates. Neuropathol Appl Neurobiol 2:99-111.
Bignami A, Dahl D, Rueger DG (1980). Glial fibrillary acidic (GFA) protein in normal neural cells and in pathological conditions. Adv Cell Neurobiol 1:285-310.
Bock E (1978). Nervous system specific proteins. J Neurochem 30:7-14.

Cavanagh JB (1970). The proliferation of astrocytes around a needle wound in the rat brain. J Anat 106:471-487.

Chan C-C, Mochizuki M, Nussenblatt RB, Palestine AG, McAllister C, Gery I, Benezra D (1985). T-lymphocyte subsets in experimental autoimmune uveitis. Clin Immunol Immunopathol 35:103-110.

Ciesielski-Treska J, Bader M-F, Aunis D (1982a). Microtubular organization in flat epitheloid and stellate process-bearing astrocytes in culture. Neurochem Res 7:275-286.

Ciesielski-Treska J, Guerold B, Aunis (1982b). Immunofluorescence study on the organization of actin in astroglial cells in primary cultures. Neuroscience 7:509-522.

Cook RD, Wisniewski HM 1973). The role of oligodendroglia and astroglia in Wallerian degeneration of the optic nerve. Brain Res 61:191-206.

Dahl D, Bignami A (1983). The glial fibrillary acidic protein and astrocytic 10 nanometer filaments. In Lajtha A (ed): "Handbook of Neruochemistry," 2nd Ed, Vol 5, New York: Plenum Press, pp. 127-151.

Dahl D, Bignami A (1985). Intermediate filaments in nervous tissue. In Shay JW (ed): "Cell and Muscle Motility," Vol 6, New York: Plenum, pp. 75-96.

Dahl D, Bjorklund H, Bignami A (1986). Immunological markers in astrocytes. In Fedoroff S, Vernadakis A (eds): "Astrcoytes, Cell Biology and Pathology of Astrcoytes," Vol 3, Orlando, Florida: Academic Press, pp 1-25.

Dahl D, Cosby CJ, Bignami A (1981). Filament proteins in rat optic nerves undergoing Wallerian degeneration. Exp Neurol 71:421-430.

Dahl D, Strocchi P, Bignami A (1982). Vimentin in the central nervous system. A study of the mesenchymal-type intermediate filament-protein in Wallerian degeneration and in postnatal rat development by two-dimensional gel electrophoresis. Differentiation 22:185-190.

DeArmond SJ, Eng LF (1984). Immunohistochemistry: Techniques and application to neurooncology. Prog Exp Tumor Res 27:92-117.

DeArmond SJ, Lee Y-L, Eng LF(1983). Turnover of glial fibrillary acidic protein in the mouse. J Neurochem 41 (Suppl) S3.

DeArmond SJ, Lee Y-L, Kretzschmar HA, Eng LF (1986). Turnover of glial filaments in mouse spinal cord. J Neurochem 47:1749-1753.

Duffy PE (1983). "Astrocytes: Normal, Reactive, and Neoplastic." New York: Raven Press.

Eisenfeld AJ, Bunt-Milam AH, Sarthy PV (1984). Muller cell expression of glial fibrillary acidic protein after genetic and experimental photoreceptor degeneration in the rat retina. Invest Ophthalmol Vis Sci 25:1321-1328.

Eng LF (1979a). A reply to the comments of Bignami and Dahl ("Isolation of GFA protein from normal brain -- A comment"). J Histochem Cytochem 27:694-696.

Eng LF (1979b). Brain related antigens. In Thomas D, Graham D (eds): "Brain Tumors: Scientific Basis, Clinical Investigation, and Current Therapy," London: Butterworth, pp 109-120.

Eng LF (1980). The glial fibrillary acidic protein (GFA) protein. In Bradshaw RA, Schneider DM (eds): "Proteins of the Nervous System," 2nd Ed, New York: Raven Press, pp 85-117.

Eng LF (1985). Glial fibrillary acidic protein: The major protein of glial intermediate filaments in differentiated astrocytes. J Neuroimmunol 8:203-214.

Eng LF, Bigbee JW (1978). Immunohistochemistry of nervous system-specific antigens. Adv Neurochem 3:43-98.

Eng LF, DeArmond SJ (1982). Immunocytochemical studies of astrocytes in normal development and disease. Adv Cell Neurobiol 3:145-171.

Eng LF, DeArmond SJ (1983). Immunochemistry of the glial fibrillary acidic protein. Prog Neuropathol 5:19-39.

Fedoroff S (1985). Macroglial cell lineages. In: G.M. Edelman, W.E. Gall, W.M. Cowan, eds., Molecular Bases of Neural Development, Neurosciences Research Foundation, Inc., Raven Press, New York, pp. 91-117.

Gray EG, Guillery RW (1966). Synaptic morphology in the normal and degenerating nervous system. Int Rev Cytol 19:111-182.

Hortega P del Rio, Penfield W (1927). Cerebral cicatrix. The reaction of neuroglia and microglia to brain wounds. Bull Johns Hopkins Hosp 31:278-303.

Kimelberg HK, Ransom BR (1986). Physiological and pathology aspects of astrocytic swelling. In Fedoroff S, Vernadakis A (eds): "Astrocytes. Cell Biology and Pathology of Astrocytes," Vol 3, Orlando, Florida: Academic Press, pp. 129-166.

Kretzschmar HA, Prusiner SB, Stowring LE, DeArmond SJ (1986). Scrapie prion proteins are synthesized in neurons. Am J Pathol 122:1-5.

Lapham LW, Johnstone MA (1964). Cytologic and cytochemical studies of neuroglia. III. The DNA content of fibrous astrocytes with implication concerning the nature of these cells. J Neuropathol Exp Neurol 23:419-430.

Latov N, Nilaver G, Zimmerman A (1979). Fibrillary astrocytes proliferate in response to brain injury. Dev Biol 72:381-384.

Manthorpe M, Rudge JS, Varon S (1986). Astroglial cell contributions to neuronal survival and neuritic growth. In Fedoroff S, Vernadakis A (eds): "Astrocytes, Biochemistry, Physiology, and Pharmacology of Astrocytes,", Orlando, Florida: Academic Press, pp 315-376.

Manuelidis L, Tesin DM, Sklaviadis T, Manuelidis EE (1987). Astrocyte gene expression in Creutzfeldt-Jakob disease. Proc Natl Acad Sci USA 84:5937-5941.

Mathewson AJ, Berry M (1985). Observations on the astrocyte response to a cerebral stab wound in adult rats. Brain Res 327:61-69.

Matthews MA, St Onge MF, Faciane CL, Geldred JB (1979). Axon sprouting into segments of rat spinal cord adjacent to the site of a previous transection. Neuropathol Appl Neurobiol 5:181-196.

Nathaniel EJH, Nathaniel DR (1977). Astroglial response to degeneration of dorsal root fibers in adult rat spinal cord. Exp Neurol 54:60-76.

Nathaniel EJH, Nathaniel DR (1981). The reactive astrocyte. In: S. Fedoroff, L. Hertz, eds., Advances in Cellular Neurobiology,Vol. 2, Academic Press, New York, pp. 249-301.

Norenberg MD (1983). Immunohistochemistry of glutamine synthetase. In: L. Hertz, E. Kvamme, E.G. McGeer, A. Schousboe, eds., Glutamine, Glutamate, and GABA in the Central Nervous System, Alan R. Liss, N.Y.,pp. 95-111.

Ochmichen M (1980). Enzyme-histochemical differentiation of neuroglia and microglia: A contribution to the cytogenesis of microglia and globoid cells. Pathol Res Pract 168:344-373.

Polak M, Haymaker W, Johnson JE, D'Amilio F (1982). Neuroglia and their reactions. In: W. Haymaker, R. Adams, eds., Histology and histopathology of the nervous system, Charles Thomas Publ., Springfield, IL.

Reier PJ (1986). Gliosis following CNS injury: The anatomy of astrocytic scars and their influences on axonal elongation. In Fedoroff S, Vernadakis A (eds): "Astrocytes. Cell Biology and Pathology of Astrocytes," Vol 3, Orlando, Florida: Academic Press, pp. 263-324.

Reier PJ, Stensaas LJ, Guth L (1983). The astrocytic scar as an impediment to regeneration in the central nervous system. In Kao CC, Bunge RP, Reier PJ (eds): "Spinal Cord Reconstruction," New York: Raven Press, pp. 163-196.

Schliwa M (1986). "The Cytoskeleton: An Introductory Survey," Cell Biology Monographs, Vol 13. Berlin and New York: Springer-Verlag.

Schultz RL, Pease DC (1959). Cicatrix formation in rat cerebral cortex as revealed by electron microscopy. Am J Pathol 35:1017-1041.

Smith ME, Somera FP, Eng LF (1983). Immunocytochemical staining for glial fibrillary acidic protein and the metabolism of cytoskeletal proteins in experimental allergic encephalomyelitis. Brain Res 264:241-253.

Smith ME, Perret V, Eng LF (1984). Metabolic studies in vitro of the CNS cytoskeletal proteins: Synthesis and degradation. Neurochem Res 9:1493-1507.

Traub P (1985). "Intermediate Filaments: A Review." Berlin and New York: Springer-Verlag.
Trimmer PA, Reier PJ, Oh TH, Eng LF (1982). An ultrastructural and immunocytochemical study of astrocytic differentiation in vitro. Changes in the composition and distribution of the cellular cytoskeleton. J Neuroimmunol 2:235-260.
Wacker WB, Donoso LA, Kalsow CM, Yankeelov JA, Jr, Organisciak DT (1977). Experimental allergic uveitis. Isolation, characterization, and localization of a soluble uveitopathogenic antigen from bovine retina. J Immunol 119:1949.

ASTROCYTE RESPONSE TO GROWTH FACTORS AND HORMONES: EARLY MOLECULAR EVENTS

Alaric T. Arenander, Robert Lim, Brian Varnum, Ruth Cole, Harvey R. Herschman and Jean de Vellis

Departments of Biological Chemistry (A.T.A., R.L., B.V, H.R.H), Anatomy and Psychiatry (A.T.A., J.deV.), Laboratory of Biomedical and Environmental Sciences, Mental Retardation Research Center (A.T.A., R.C. J.deV.) and Brain Research Institute (A.T.A., H.R.H., J.deV.), UCLA School of Medicine, University of California, Los Angeles, CA 90024

INTRODUCTION

Astrocytes are called upon to perform a wide range of functions on demand (For review see Arenander and de Vellis, 1983). For instance, astrocytes are known to proliferate and hypertrophy as a response to perturbation of the adult central nervous system (CNS). This reaction can involve astrocytes far away from the site of injury, suggesting that diffusible factors trigger the response (Pixley and de Vellis, 1984; Nieto-Sampedro et al., 1985). The cellular complexity of the CNS, the blood-brain-barrier and the difficulty in controlling the chemical composition of the CNS extracellular fluid have hampered the characterization of hormones and growth factors potentially involved in regulating astrocyte functions.

The availability of pure cultures of astrocytes, oligodendrocytes and neurons (Saneto and de Vellis, 1987) has allowed us to dissect hormonally regulated phenomena and determine the cellular specificity of hormones and growth factors. In serum-free chemically defined media, cultured astrocytes are responsive to a wide spectrum of mitogenic factors, including: epidermal growth factor (EGF), basic and acidic fibroblast growth factors (b and aFGF) insulin, insulin-like growth factor I(IGF-I), platelet-derived growth factor, glial growth factor (GGF) and interleukin-1 (IL-1)(Saneto and de Vellis, 1985). Serum, brain and pituitary extracts, and injury-induced factors are mitogenic and may add other candidates to the list of astroglial mitogens. In contrast, oligodendrocytes display a much more restricted repertoire. They are unresponsive to serum, IL-1, GGF and EGF (Saneto and de Vellis, 1985; Saneto et al., 1986).

Previous studies by several laboratories on the regulation of phenotypic expression in astrocytes have been focused on glutamine synthetase (GS), the intermediate filaments, glial fibrillary acidic protein (GFAP) and vimentin, and to a lesser extent S-100 protein (de Vellis et al., 1986). In addition to molecular changes, the shape of astrocytes in culture can be dramatically altered by a wide range of substances. For instance, the addition of insulin and bFGF to a serum-free medium transforms the flat polygonal shaped astrocytes (Fig. 1A) into stellate process-bearing cells (Fig. 1B). This stellation process is associated with de novo synthesis of GFAP (Morrison et al., 1985). Similarly, thyroid hormone, T3, by itself induces stellation. But this effect is accentuated by insulin (Aizenman and de Vellis, 1987). GFAP content and stellation are increased by dibutyryl cAMP (de Vellis et al., 1986). The level of cAMP in astrocytes is increased by ß-adrenergic agonists, adenosine (A2 receptor), prostaglandin E, substance P, somatostatin, VIP, secretin and numerous other peptides while α-adrenergic agonists, adenosine (A1 receptor) and melatonin decrease cAMP levels (Hamprecht, 1986). In addition to its effect on GFAP content, cAMP increases the phosphorylation of GFAP and vimentin which may alter the function of the cytoskeleton.

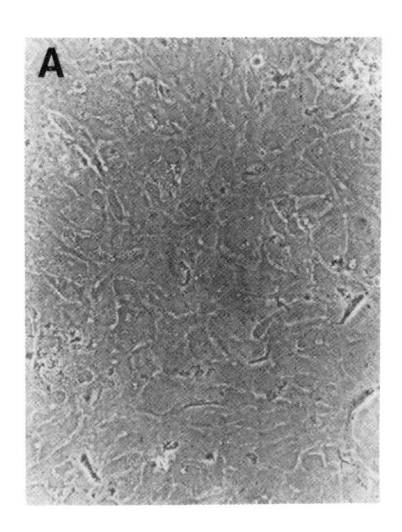

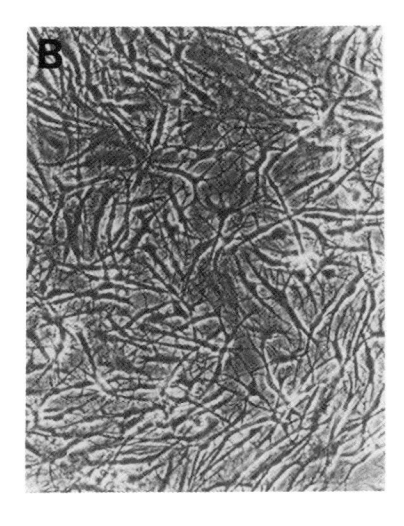

Figure 1. Cultures of purified astrocytes grown for one week in either: A, serum-free medium or B, insulin (5 µg/ml) and bFGF (50 ng/ml) supplemented serum-free medium. Note hormone-induced stellation.

The regulation of GS has been more thoroughly investigated than GFAP (For review see de Vellis et al., 1986). The pioneering work on GS was done in the retina by Moscona and his collaborators. GS in the retina is developmentally induced by glucocorticoids and reaches a level higher than in any other organ. The activity is localized in Müller cells. In the rest of the CNS, GS is also a marker for astrocytes and is inducible by hydrocortisone (HC). The effect is receptor mediated and involves a primary gene response (Yamamoto and Alberts, 1976). Other factors influence GS expression, but they have not been well characterized yet. Interestingly, insulin induces GS and acts synergistically with HC.

Furthermore, cAMP (de Vellis et al., 1986) and neuronal astroglial cell surface interactions (Wu et al., 1988) can independently induce GS. The above examples suggest that astrocyte differentiation and function are influenced by numerous hormones and growth factors, often acting in concert.

The molecular mechanisms underlying these changes in astrocyte physiology can be better understood if viewed in a temporal framework. The immediate events of cellular activation following ligand-receptor interaction are coupled to various cytoplasmic pathways of signal transduction. These pathways can then lead to intermediate and late events which are represented by increases in the production and turnover of GS and GFAP mRNA and protein content and the changes in morphology (stellation), respectively. In this presentation, we will focus on a set of cellular processes which represent some of the earliest changes in RNA transcription following the interaction of agents with astrocytes. These early events are of interest because they may play an important role in coordinating the changes in the state of astrocyte physiology following treatment with various neuro-active agents and hormones.

EARLY MOLECULAR EVENTS

In an attempt to characterize the early nuclear events which may be important in controlling developmental decisions that are induced by various growth factors, a family of Transiently (T) Induced (I) Sequences (S) were examined in rat astrocytes treated with various factors and hormones. The TIS genes were isolated from a cDNA library constructed from mRNAs induced in density arrested Swiss mouse 3T3 cells following a 3 hour exposure to the mitogen and tumor-promoting agent tetradecanoyl phorbol acetate (TPA) and cycloheximide (Lim et al, 1987). These primary response genes (Yamamoto and Alberts, 1976) represent distinct mRNAs whose levels of expression are rapidly and transiently increased following exposure of cells to TPA or other mitogens. Seven clones of the TIS genes have been isolated and characterized (see table 1). One of the TIS genes (TIS 28) was identified as the cellular c-fos proto-oncogene.

TABLE 1. CHARACTERIZATION OF TIS CLONES

CLONE	MESSAGE SIZE	IDENTITY
TIS 1	3.3kb	unique
TIS 7	2.2kb	unique
TIS 8	4.0kb	unique
TIS 10	5.8kb	unique
TIS 11	2.2kb	unique
TIS 21	3.6kb	unique
TIS 28	2.2kb	c-fos

Since proto-oncogenes are postulated to play important regulatory roles in normal growth patterns (Weinberg, 1985) as well as in a variety of differentiated functions of the nervous system such as information signalling (Morgan et al.,1987; Hunt et al., 1987) and storage (Berridge, 1986; Goelet et al., 1986), the study of the TIS family in developing astrocytes may well provide further insight into the sequence of early molecular events that underlie the processes of proliferation and differentiation.

In addition, it has recently been reported that the TIS genes are rapidly induced in the rat pheochromocytoma cell line PC12 by TPA as well as by various neuro-active agents (Kujubu et al., 1987). Differentiation of PC12 cells into sympathetic-like neurons with neurite processes induced by nerve growth factor is preceded by rapid and transient expression of six of the TIS genes, including c-fos. Also, depolarizing PC12 cells with elevated K+ levels, which is linked to activation of voltage-dependent Ca++ channels and c-fos transcription (Greenberg, et al., 1985; Morgan and Currant et al., 1986) induces the same six TIS genes. These data suggest that induction of the TIS family of genes may represent a set of early molecular events that may be involved in transducing the immediate and rapid factor-induced effects into later occurring and longer lasting biological responses in nerve cells.

We have examined time course of induction of the TIS genes in pure cultures of rat astrocytes derived from neonatal cerebral cortices (McCarthy and de Vellis, 1980). Total cell RNA isolated from astrocyte cultures following the technique of Chomczynski and Sacchi (1987) is analyzed using formaldehyde agarose gels followed by northern blotting and hybridization against nick-translated probes for the various TIS clones using standard methods (Lim et al., 1987).

We first studied the response of astrocytes to treatment with TPA. Northern blots demonstrate that the pattern of TPA-induction of TIS genes is similar to previously described results in 3T3 and PC12 cells (fig. 2). The induction of the mRNA in astrocytes represents a primary response (they occur in the presence of cycloheximide). It is evident that the expression is both rapid, occurring within 10 to 20 minutes and transient, the message disappearing within 3 hours. More importantly, the TIS genes exhibit differential patterns of response. For example, as illustrated in figure 2 and graphically in figure 3, the pattern of TPA-induction of the TIS genes is different when comparing the culture conditions of serum-free (SFM) vs. 10% fetal calf serum (FCS) supplemented media. While the onset of mRNA during TPA induction is similar for the two TIS genes under differing conditions of serum support, the levels and duration of induction appear to be different. Whereas, the pattern of induction of TIS 8 (fig. 3A) does not appear to be sensitive to serum conditions, c-fos mRNA reach higher levels and are detected for longer periods in SFM than in FCS.

TPA (100ng/ml)   SFM   10% FCS

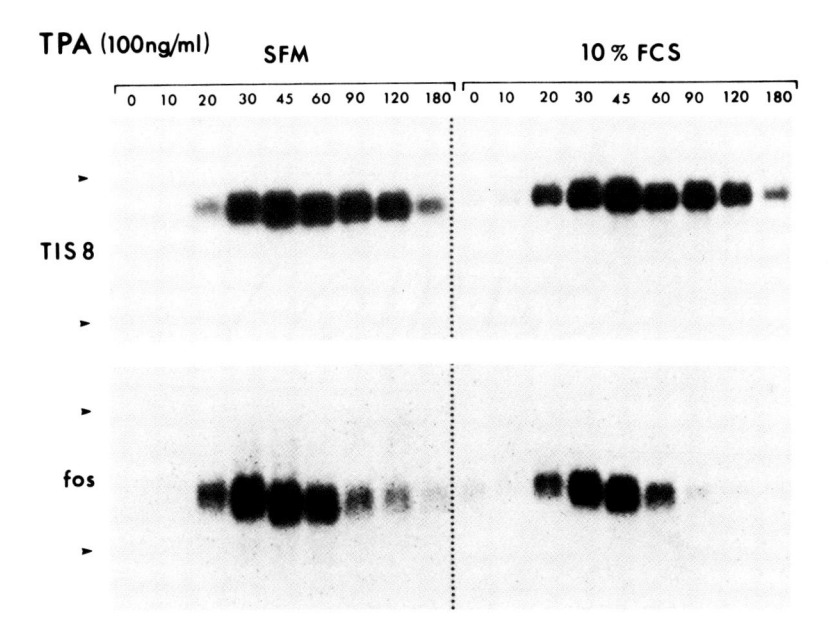

         0 10 20 30 45 60 90 120 180   0 10 20 30 45 60 90 120 180

TIS 8

fos

Figure 2. Time-course of induction of TIS 8 and TIS 28 (c-fos) in response to TPA. Total RNA was isolated from secondary astrocytes at various times (10 to 180 minutes) after addition of TPA (100 ng/ml), run on agarose gels, blotted on nitrocellulose and probed with nick-translated cDNA TIS gene or v-fos plasmid probe. The autoradiograph is shown. Each lane contains 11 ug of RNA. Cells were grown in 10% fetal calf serum (FCS) and then incubated in either FCS or serum-free medium (SFM) for 2 days before the treatment.

The value of such time-course experiments is also evident in that a comparison of c-fos and TIS 8 using a single time point could support different, possibly erroneous, conclusions regarding TPA inducibility of the two genes and their differential sensitivity to culture conditions: at 30 minutes little difference would be evident, while at 60 minutes possibly significant differences are observed.

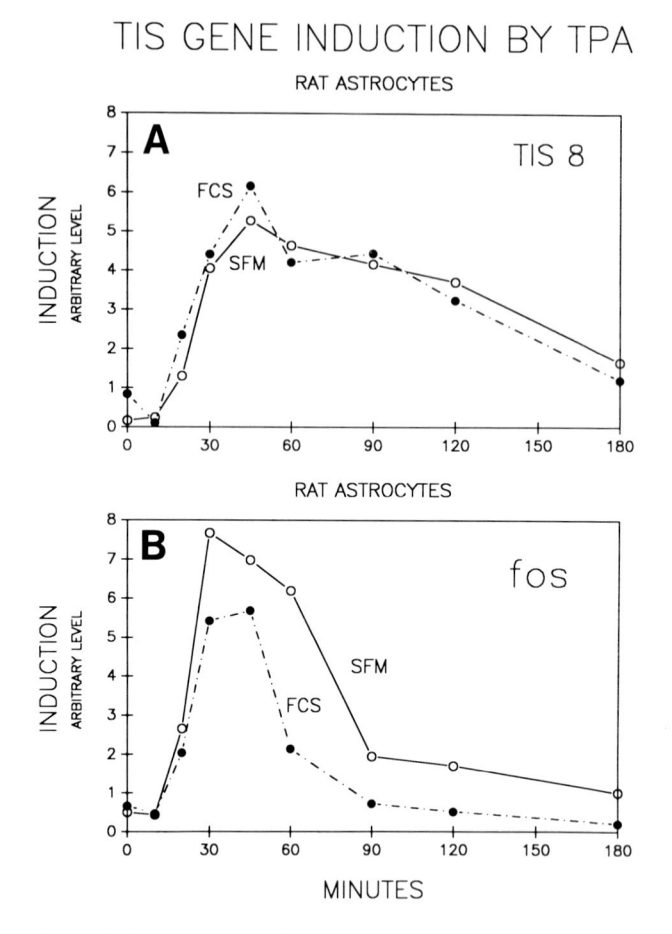

Figure 3. Kinetics of induction of TIS 8 (A) and TIS 28 (c-fos, B) in response to TPA. The autoradiograph shown in figure 2 was analyzed by laser densitometric scanning. The level of induction corresponds to the area under the curve for each band plotted against the duration of TPA treatment. Examination of RNA loading indicate no significant differences between levels of mRNA of the different samples on the northern blot.

Astrocytes in culture can rapidly alter their morphology when treated with a variety of factors. In particular, dibutyryl cyclic AMP (dbcAMP) and forskolin, which activates cAMP generating systems, induce morphological conversion of astrocytes from flat, epitheloid to star-shaped cells (see Skaper et al., 1986). This in vitro transformation may be related to rapid alterations that can occur during the onset of pathologies in vivo, for example, in reactive gliosis. To determine whether TIS gene expression can be induced in astrocytes by agents which modulate cell morphology, we examined the response of the TIS genes to dbcAMP and forskolin. Analysis of northern blots from time-course studies showed that the TIS genes are rapidly and transiently induced by these agents. Surprisingly, treatment of astrocytes with GM1 ganglioside, reported to block or reverse dbcAMP-induced morphological transformation, also resulted in a very rapid and short-lived induction of the TIS genes.

As discussed earlier, T3 and insulin are also capable of modulating astrocyte differentiation. T3 transform the flat, polygonal astrocytes into stellate cells associated with changes in GFAP immunostaining pattern (Aizenman and de Vellis, 1987). However, in contrast to the rapid dbcAMP-induced morphological changes noted above, the T3-induced effects were slower, occurring over a period of 3-8 days. Insulin alone was observed to have no influence on astrocyte morphology but was able to accentuate the effects of T3. It was also noted that hydrocortisone (HC), which had no effect on astrocyte morphology, increased glutamine synthetase (GS) levels in both control and in insulin-treated cultures of astrocytes. In the later condition, HC acted synergistically with insulin in its action on GS.

We asked whether the TIS genes could be induced by these hormones in astrocytes and if the pattern of induction revealed any inter-actions among the hormones in their ability to induce changes. Preliminary findings suggest that some of the TIS genes can be induced by T3, insulin and HC. Furthermore, the pattern of induction of the TIS genes show that some of the genes respond in a manner suggestive of synergistic interaction among these hormones. Experiments in progress are designed to further document the nature of these hormonal interactions for all the TIS genes

SUMMARY

We feel that studying the pattern of expression of the TIS genes in astrocytes will provide valuable information regarding the early nuclear events in the overall sequence of molecular events regulating cellular proliferation and differentiation (Fig. 4).

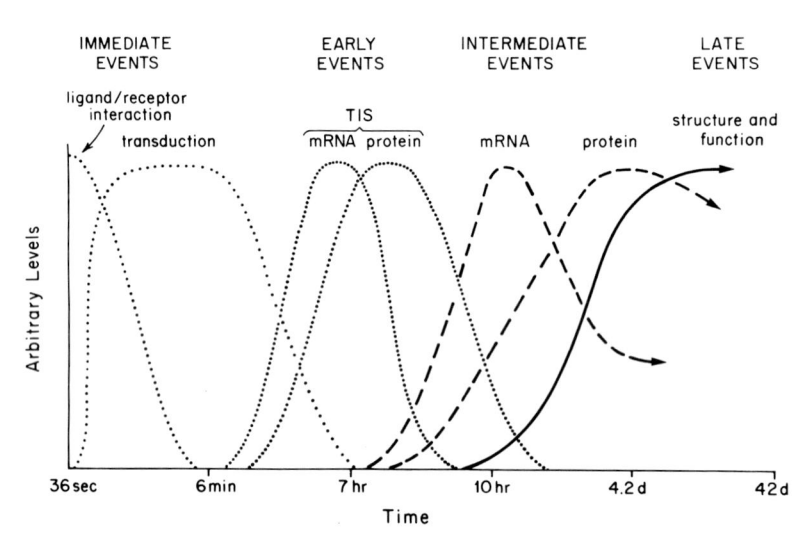

Figure 4. Sequence of Molecular Events in Cellular Differentiation. This figure illustrates four major stages in the sequence of responses of an astrocyte following exposure to an active agent during development. The pattern of physiological changes is graphed using a log time scale in order to cover the entire range of events

stemming from immediate receptor-ligand interaction to long-term changes in cell structure and function. A similar sequence of events can be envisioned to occur in the adult brain during normal or regenerative states.

It is clear from our initial exploration of TIS gene inducibility in astrocytes that this family of transiently induced sequences are sensitive to a wide range of growth factors known to play important roles in brain development. Future studies are aimed at investigating the various possible pathways of signal transduction which link receptor-ligand binding and genomic induction. We will be comparing the activity of agents which modulate monovalent and divalent cation flux and the inducing activities of peptide growth factors. In addition, the possible causal relationship of the TIS genes in the induced proliferation and/or differentiation of transformed astrocytes or PC12 cells will be examined using inducible antisense vectors to interfere with TIS gene expression.

It is probable that the TIS genes represent a subset of a larger family of early nuclear mechanisms by which growth factors control not only normal growth and differentiation of astrocytes in vivo, but also the mechanisms by which astrocytes contribute to the processes of neural regeneration.

ACKNOWLEDGEMENTS: The authors research was supported by the Department of Energy contract DE-AC03-76-00012 (HRH and JdeV) and NIH grant HD 06576 (JdeV) and MIU Research Support Fund 011-705 (ATA).

REFERENCES

Aizenman Y, de Vellis J (1987). Synergistic action of thyroid hormone, insulin and hydrocortisone on astrocyte differentiation. Brain Res 414:301.
Arenander AT, de Vellis J (1983). Frontiers of

glial physiology. In Rosenberg R (ed.): The Clinical Neurosciences., Section V., "Neurobiology" (WD Willis, Assoc. ed.) Chapter IV, New York: Churchill Livingstone, p 53.

Berridge M (1986). Second messenger dualism in neuromodulation and memory. Nature 323:294.

Chomczynski P, Sacchi N (1987). Single-step method of RNA isolation by acid quanidinium thiocyanate-phenol-chloroform extraction. Anal Biochem 162:156.

de Vellis J, Wu DK, Kumar S (1986). Enzyme induction and regulation of protein synthesis. In Federoff S, Vernadakis A (eds.): "Astrocytes," Vol. 2, New York: Academic Press, p 209.

Goelet P, Castellucci F, Schacher S, Kandel ER (1986). The long and the short of long-term memory--a molecular framework. Nature 322:419.

Greenberg M, Green L, Ziff E (1985). Nerve growth factor and epidermal growth factor induce rapid transient changes in proto-oncogene transcription in PC-12 cells. J Biol Chem 260:14101.

Hamprecht B (1986). Astroglial cells in culture: Receptors and cyclic nucleotides in astrocytes In Federoff S, Vernadakis A (eds.): "Astrocytes," Vol. 2. New York: Academic Press, p77.

Hunt SP, Pini A, Evan G (1987). Induction of c-fos-like protein in spinal cord neurons following sensory stimulation. Nature 328:632.

Kujubu DA, Lim RW, Varnum BC, Herschman HR (1987). Induction of transiently expressed genes in PC-12 pheochromocytoma cells. Oncogene 1:257.

Lim R, Varnum BC, Herschman HR (1987). Cloning of sequences induced as a primary response following mitogen treatment of density arrested Swiss 3T3 cells. Oncogene 1:263.

McCarthy KD, de Vellis J (1980). Preparation of separate astroglial and oligodendroglial cell cultures from rat cerebral tissue. J Cell Biol 85: 890.

Morgan J, Curran T (1986). Role of ion flux in the control of c-fos expression. Nature 322:552.

Morgan J, Cohem DR, Hempstead JL, Curran T (1987). Mapping patterns of c-fos expression

in the central nervous system after seizure. Science 237:192.
Morrison RS, de Vellis J, Lee YL, Bradshaw RA, Eng LF (1985). Hormones and growth factors induce the synthesis of glial fibrillary acidic protein in rat brain astrocytes. J Neurosci Res 14:167.
Nieto-Sampedro M, Saneto RP, de Vellis J, Cotman CW (1985). The control of glial populations in brain: Changes in astrocyte mitogenic and morphogenic factors in response to injury. Brain Res 343:320.
Pixley SKR, de Vellis J (1984). Transition between immature radial glia and mature astrocytes studied with a monoclonal antibody to vimentin. Develop Brain Res 15:201.
Saneto RP, de Vellis J (1985). Hormonal regulation of the proliferation and differentiation of astrocytes and oligodendrocytes in primary culture. In Bottenstein J, Sato G (eds.): "Cell Culture in the Neurosciences." New York: Plenum Press, p 125.
Saneto, RP, de Vellis, J (1987). Neuronal and glial cells: Cell culture of the central nervous system. In Turner AJ, Bachelard HS (eds.): "Neurochemistry - A Practical Approach." Washington, D.C.: IRL Press, p 27.
Saneto RP, Altman A, Knobler RL, Johnson HM, de Vellis J (1986). Interleukin 2 mediates the inhibition of oligodendrocyte progenitor cell proliferation in vitro. Proc Natl Acad Sci USA 83: 9221.
Skaper SD, Facci L, Rudge J, Katoh-Semba R, Manthorpe M, Varon S (1986). Morphological modulation of cultured rat brain astroglial cells: Antagonism by ganglioside GM1. Dev Brain Res 25:21.
Weinberg RA (1985). The action of oncogenes in the cytoplasm and nucleus. Science 230:770.
Wu DK, Scully S, de Vellis J (1988). Induction of glutamine synthetase in rat astrocytes by co-cultivation with embryonic chick neurons. J Neurochem In Press.
Yamamoto K, Alberts B (1976). Steroid receptors: Elements for modulation of eukaryotic transcription. Ann Rev Biochem 45:721.

ASTROGLIA AND PLASMINOGEN ACTIVATOR ACTIVITY: DIFFERENTIAL ACTIVITY LEVEL IN THE IMMATURE, MATURE AND "REACTIVE" ASTROCYTES.

Nurit Kalderon, Kenneth Ahonen, Anna Juhasz, Joseph P. Kirk, and Sergey Fedoroff

The Rockefeller University, New York, New York 10021, and University of Saskatchewan (S.F.), Saskatoon, Saskatchewan, Canada S7N 0W0

The control of nervous system histogenesis, on the molecular level, is accomplished by common extracellular biochemical machineries, by: cell adhesion molecules which provide the glue (e.g., fibronectin), proteases which enable the breakdown of bonds (e.g., plasmin), and modulators which serve as growth and mitogenic factors (e.g, insulin). Regeneration of a nervous system is attained presumably by a recapitulation of the histogenic process. On the molecular level, a failure of a nervous tissue to regenerate, is due to a deficiency in one or more of the biochemical machineries which participate in and regulate histogenesis. In contrast with the peripheral nervous system (PNS), the mammalian central nervous system (CNS) lacks the capacity to regenerate. Hence, upon maturation, adult CNS, but not adult PNS, has lost one or more of the biochemical machineries that were instrumental in the process of development of the immature tissue. Further, transplantation experiments provide indirect evidence that this deficiency of the adult CNS can be partially supplemented by grafts of peripheral nerve (e.g., Aguayo et al., 1987), embryonic CNS tissue (e.g., Reier et al., 1986), and immature astrocytes (Smith et al., 1987). That is, embryonic CNS tissue, Schwann cells and immature astrocytes express the biochemical machineries that are necessary and sufficient to support axonal regrowth.

Our research is concerned with the extracellular proteolytic system, which regulates cell migration processes. One of the most common physiological mechanisms for generating localized extracellular proteolytic activity is the production and secretion by the cells of the protease, plasminogen activator (PA). PA activates plasminogen to generate the protease, plasmin; plasmin in turn can degrade a wide range of extracellular matrix proteins and/or activate other latent proteases such as latent collagenase (Mullins and Rohrlich, 1983). The temporary increase in PA activity levels in several biological systems, together with plasmin activity have been proven to be the driving force for cell migration/invasion processes (e.g., Mignatti et al., 1986).

Tissue remodelling events such as cell migration/invasion are essential in the process of nervous tissue formation. Indeed, it was established in recent years that developing nervous tissues produce PA. Kalderon (1979) observed that dissociated chick embryonic spinal cord cells produce extracellular PA, and that the expression of plasmin activity in the growth medium of these neural cells leads to some significant changes in their organization on the substratum. Developing rodent brain tissue (Soreq and Miskin, 1981), and embryonic chick spinal cord (Kalderon and Williams, 1986) express PA activity. It was found in those studies that PA-activity levels of the tissues are developmentally regulated, that is, the tissue-specific activity is enhanced and reduced at certain developmental stages, and upon maturation is decreased to a low plateau level.

Schwann cells produce and secrete PA; they do so during development and regeneration of peripheral nerves. It was demonstrated that the proliferating Schwann cell populations (e.g., the differentiating cells) express increased PA activity levels, 3 to 4-fold higher than those measured in the nondividing populations (Kalderon, 1984). No PA activity was found in adult sciatic or optic nerve (Bignami et al., 1982). In that study, with histological PA assay, it was found that in response to injury, a tightly ligated sciatic nerve (for prevention of neural regeneration) expresses PA activity. This proteolysis was attributed to the proliferating Schwann cells. However, no PA activity was found in the injured, degenerating, optic nerve.

In the studies described in the present article, the role of the astrocyte (immature and mature) in tissue remodelling processes in developing and regenerating CNS will be examined. Biochemical data which demonstrate the capacity of the astroglia to express and modulate their PA activity and its protease inhibitory activity levels at different developmental and physiological stages will be presented.

These will include results showing that among immature, mature and "reactive" astrocytes, the immature astrocyte is the sole source of high levels of PA activity. Furthermore, studies on mature and "reactive" astrocytes in culture suggest that in the adult injured CNS, the reactive astrocyte expresses low levels of PA activity with protease inhibitory activity. In all, data will be submitted to support the idea that the inability of the adult CNS to regenerate is due, in part, to the deficiency in the extracellular proteolytic machinery. A machinery which is provided during histogenesis by the immature astrocyte but is not expressed by the mature cell.

The following experiments focus on the characterization of the expression of PA activity by the CNS glia during the differentiation period of these cells in culture. The study was done in a cell culture assuming that as according to Abney et al., (1981) glial cells differentiate and mature in culture on schedule in a sequence similar to the one observed in situ. The studies were performed on cell preparations of both rat glia and mouse astroglia. Studies described in this article were performed on the cellular PA activity. PA activity which is associated with the cells and obtained by cell extraction or solubilization is referred to as the cellular activity; whereas PA activity which is released by the cells into the growth medium is referred to as the extracellular activity. Detailed experimental procedures are summarized in Kalderon et al., (1987a).

Differentiating purified rat glia were obtained from the developing cerebrum of 1-3 day old rat pups (McCarthy and de Vellis, 1980). The glioblasts were plated in flasks and after 7-10 days in culture the flasks were shaken to remove the loosely attached cells, e.g., oligodendrocytes, microglia, dividing cells. The detached cells were collected and replated. The purified astroglial cells in the flasks were either maintained in these flasks or subcultured onto new dishes. Temporal PA specific activities were determined at different ages on the following cell populations: I. heterogeneous glial cell populations at ages corresponding to postnatal (P) 5-31 days; II. enriched population of oligodendroglial cells at P11-18 days; III. purified astroglial cells at P10-45 days; IV. subcultured astroglial cells at P10-38 days which were passaged once at three different stages at P10, P11 and P15; and V. subcultured astroglial cells at P21-32 days which were passaged twice, first at P11 and then at P18.

The results from these experiments can be summarized as follows: Purified astroglia express PA activity, while no PA activity was found in the oligodendroglial cell populations. The cellular PA activity levels of the differentiating rat astroglia are developmentally regulated. PA specific activity of the astroglia reached its highest level at a cell age of P24-31 days (Table 1). Then, upon cell maturation, the specific activity declined (4-fold decrease) to a low plateau value. PA activity levels in the purified astroglia was slightly higher than those observed in the heterogeneous cell populations (Table 1).

TABLE 1. PA specific activities of the glial and of the purified astroglial preparations as function of their age.

Postnatal age (days)	PA specific activity (arbitrary units/mg protein) *	
	Astroglia (N)	Glia (N)
10	—	41.2 ± 5.8 (3)
17	33.2 ± 4.2 (5)	30.0 (2)
24	42.1 ± 4.2 (6)	33.5 (2)
31	36.4 ± 9.3 (6)	43.1 (2)
38	27.2 ± 3.8 (6)	—
45	10.8 ± 2.5 (6)	—

* Mean ± S.D.; N number of samples.

In many cell types, e.g., Schwann cell, stimulation of cell division is accompanied by an increase in the cells' PA specific activity. Subculturing of the astroglia and stimulation of cell proliferation, however, did not lead to an increase in PA activity; rather, beyond a certain developmental stage it resulted in a 3-fold irreversible decline in the PA specific activity of the daughter cells (Fig. 1). It seems that the subcultured astroglia, those which were passaged after age P 15, may represent a "reactive" astrocytic population. Rat cerebral glia in situ were found to proliferate mainly during the first and second postnatal weeks

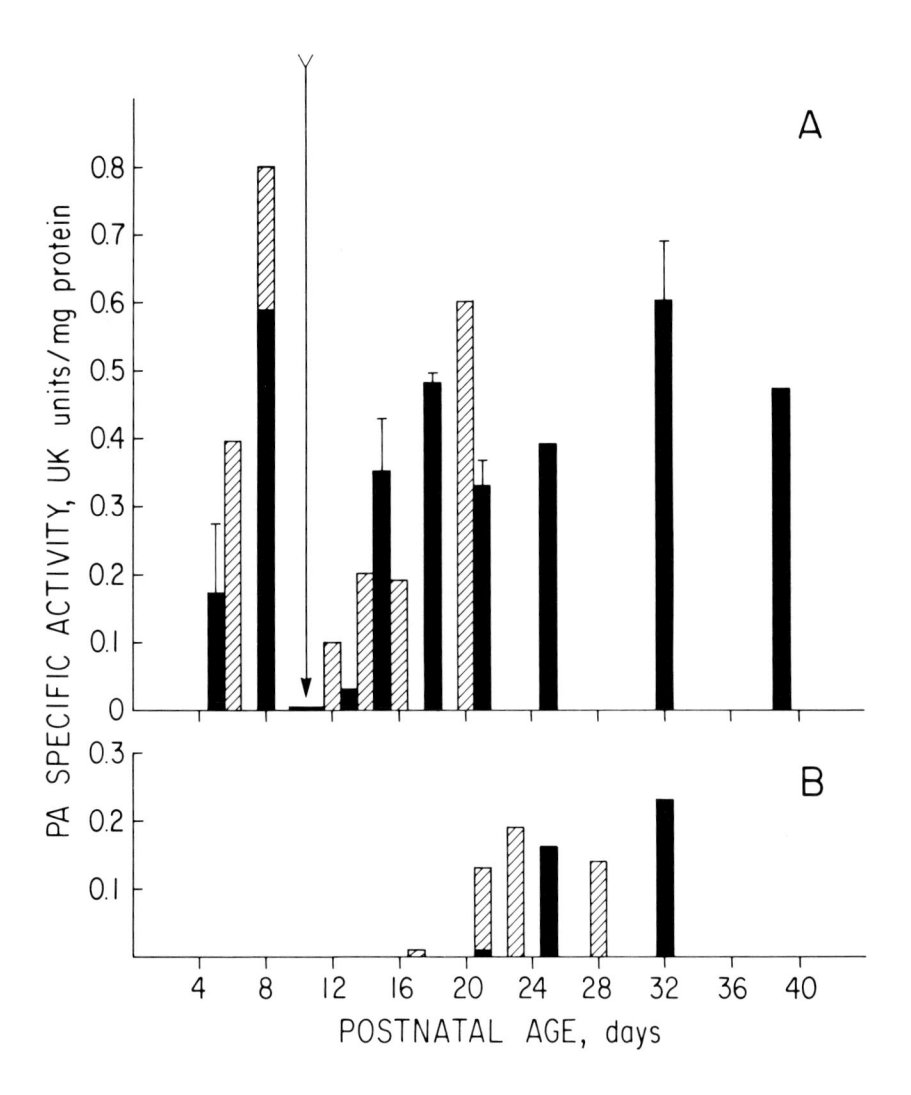

Figure 1. Summary of the temporal PA activity levels which were monitored in the heterogeneous glial cells, and after the cell separation stage (arrow) in the various astroglial cultures. The astroglial cells were subcultured at different ages: early (A) -- at P10 and P11 , and late (B) -- at P15 and P18. The solid and hatched bars represent two different cell culture preparations. Error bars are S.D.s from the mean values.

(Ichikawa and Hirata, 1982). Based on these findings we can assume that the majority of the astroglia in our study quit the mitotic cycle by day 15, and any stimulation of cell division after this stage will result in abnormal cells.

PA specific activities of the developing rat cerebrum, the tissue from which the astroglia were purified, were determined at ages P0-35 days. Several peaks of activity were detected. These were at the range of 0.45-0.5 Ploug units/mg protein, and were similar in size to the maximum values obtained in the differentiating astroglia (Fig. 1). Upon maturation, at age P31, PA activity levels declined and reached a plateau of 0.26 Ploug units/mg protein.

The temporal PA cellular content of the differentiating mouse astroglia in culture (Fedoroff, 1977), was determined. The study was performed on two different types of astrocytic cultures, cell cultures which were obtained from 16 day old embryos and from newborn pups. The two temporal patterns of PA specific activity of the different astroglial cell preparations revealed two distinct peaks, corresponding to 8 and 12-14 postnatal days. These peaks appeared at the same age in both cell preparations. Thus, in mouse astroglia, as in rat astroglia, PA activity levels are developmentally regulated, they reach a maximum value and then, at day 16 they start to decline to a low plateau level. A 2-fold decrease in the specific activity was observed.

It has been established that cells which normally express PA activity, for example, fibroblast cells also produce several types of PA inhibitors (Pollanen et al., 1987). Astroglia produce protease inhibitors. So far, two of these inhibitors have been identified -- protease nexin (Rosenblatt et al., 1987) and α_2-macroglobulin (Gebick-Haerter et al., 1987). We have examined whether PA inhibitory (PAI) activity can be detected in various astroglial populations. The method employed to monitor PAI activity in our studies was to measure PA activity of a sample at different protein concentrations of the sample. The measured value of an enzyme specific activity should not be affected by the sample concentration unless this sample contains inhibitory activity. Few of these data are summarized in Fig. 2. PAI activity was found in mouse astroglia (in the newborn cell culture), this activity seems to be developmentally regulated. No activity was found at age P12; however, PAI activity was found at later ages at P14-20. PAI activity was found in astroglial cell samples which can be regarded as reactive "astrocytes", that is, in mature subcultured rat astrocytes (P80), and in mouse astrocytes which were treated with dibutyrylcAMP (Fedoroff et al., 1984). PAI activity was also detected in glial scar tissue, in degenerating rat optic nerve. This glial scar was obtained by eye enucleation.

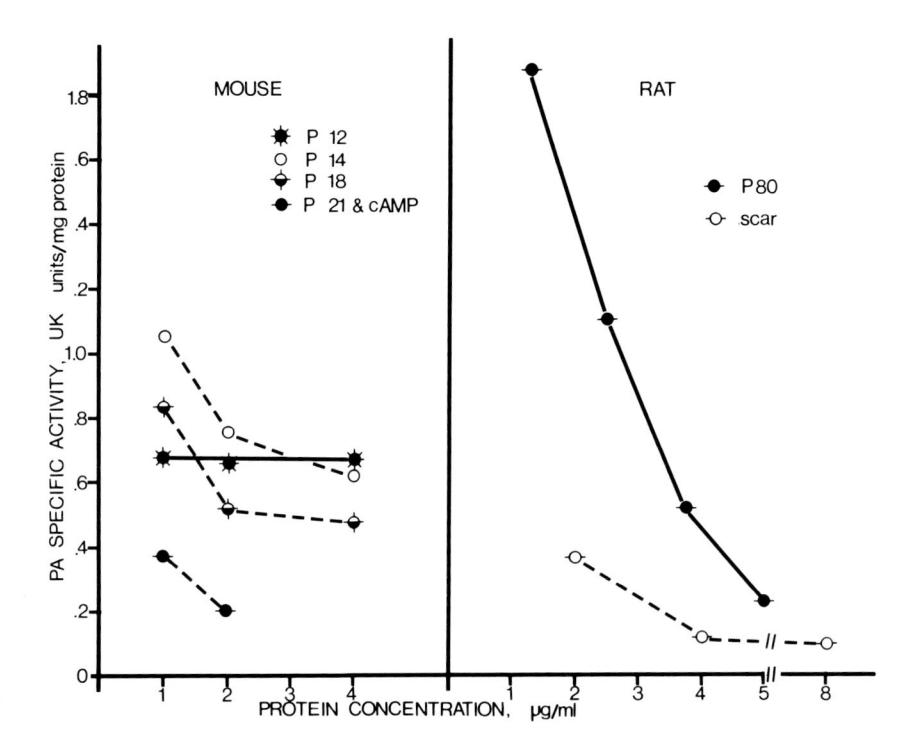

Figure 2. PA inhibitory activity in mouse and rat astroglial cell preparations, and in rat glial scar.

The idea that the Schwann cells and the immature astrocytes employ PA/plasmin activities for cell migration purposes as a crucial step leading to a successful regeneration, is being examined. This is performed in a model system, sciatic nerve regenerating through a silicone chamber. The Schwann cell plays a crucial role in the fate of neuronal regeneration. It has been demonstrated in numerous studies of transplantation, into both the peripheral and the central nervous systems, that this cell provides and supports axonal growth (ibid.). In the regenerating sciatic nerve, the Schwann cell precedes and seems to be "going" in front of the growing axons (Williams et al., 1983).

To examine the role of extracellular proteolysis in regeneration we are studying the effects of protease inhibitors on rat sciatic nerve regeneration through a 10mm silicone chamber (Kalderon et al, 1987b). The inhibitors were injected into the chamber at 7 days postsurgery, at which time a massive cell migration was about to occur, and their effect on nerve regeneration was examined a week later. None of the tested inhibitors showed any adverse effect on Schwann cells in culture. The plasmin inhibitors D-Lys(Bz)-Lys(Bz)-LysCH$_2$Cl (Ganu and Shaw, 1987) (1µM) and ε-aminocaproic acid (7.6mM) inhibited cell migration at 58% and 31% correspondingly, as compared with control samples; accordingly, axonal regrowth was impaired. These results indicate that plasmin activity is elaborated by the Schwann cells for migration/invasion and is essential for successful nerve regeneration.

In a separate set of experiments the effect of different astroglial cell populations on sciatic nerve regeneration was examined. Immature and mature astrocytes were inoculated within the silicone chamber between the sciatic nerve stumps at the time of surgery and a few weeks later neural regeneration within the chamber was analyzed (Kalderon, 1987). Nerve regeneration was significantly inhibited by the mature astrocytes whereas it did take place in the presence of the immature cells. In the cases where neural regrowth was blocked, the mature astrocytes encapsulatd the nerve stumps forming glial scar tissue.

In conclusion, it seems that PA activity is differentially expressed in the astroglia. Namely, among differentiating, mature and "reactive" astroglial cells the immature astrocyte appears to be the sole source of high levels of PA activity. The astroglia express this enhanced activity level in a limited developmental period only, and upon maturation or in "reactivation" lose this capacity. We would like to propose, by deduction from the data of our studies in the PNS regenerating model system, that immature astrocytes which support neural regeneration (Silver et al., ibid.) may function like the Schwann cells as "bulldozers" which pave the way in front of the regrowing axons. Furthemore, that PA activity levels of the astroglia are determinative in the fate of neural regeneration.

REFERENCES

Abney ER, Bartlett PP, Raff MC (1981). Astrocytes, ependymal cells, and oligodendrocytes develop on schedule in dissociated cell cultures of embryonic rat brain. Dev Biol 83:301.
Aguayo AJ, Vidal-Sanz M, Villegas-Perez MP, Bray GM (1987). Growth and connectivity of axotomized retinal neurons in adult rats with optic nerves substituted by PNS grafts linking the eye and the midbrain. Ann NY Acad Sci 495:1.
Bignami A, Cella G, Chi NH (1982). Plasminogen activators in rat neural tissues during development and in Wallerian degeneration. Acta Neuropathol (Berl) 58:224.
Fedoroff S, McAuley WAJ, Houle JD, Devon RM (1984). Astrocyte cell lineage. V. Similarity of astrocytes that form in the presence of dBcAMP in cultures to reactive astrocytes in vivo. J Neurosci Res 12:15.
Fedoroff S (1977). Tracing glial cell lineages by colony formation in primary cultures. In Fedoroff S, Hertz L(eds): "Cell Tissue and Organ Cultures in Neurobiology," New York: Academic Press, p.215.
Ganu VS, Shaw E (1987). Improved synthetic inactivators of plasmin. Thromb Res 45:1.
Gebick-Haerter PJ, Bauer J, Brenner A, Gerok W (1987). α_2-Macroglobulin synthesis in an astrocyte subpopulation.
Ichikawa M, Hirata Y (1982). Morphology and distribution of postnatally generated glial cells in the somatosensory cortex of the rat: an autoradiographic and electron microscopic study. Dev Brain Res 4:369.
Kalderon N (1979). Migration of Schwann cells and wrapping of neurites *in vitro*: a function of protease activity (plasmin) in the growth medium. Proc Natl Acad Sci USA 76:5992.
Kalderon N (1984). Schwann cell proliferation and localized proleolysis: expression of plasminogen-activator activity predominates in the proliferating cell populations. Proc Natl Acad Sci USA 81:7216.
Kalderon N (1987). The astrocyte and the failure of CNS neural regeneration. A study of inoculated astrocytes in a PNS regenerating model system. Ann NY Acad Sci 495:722.
Kalderon N, Williams CA (1986). Extracellular proteolysis: developmentally regulated activity during chick spinal cord histogenesis. Dev Brain Res 25:1.

Kalderon N, Ahonen K, Fedoroff S (1987a). The immature astrocyte as the predominant source of plasminogen-activator activity: studies in differentiating rodent cell culture systems. Submitted for publication.

Kalderon N, Kirk JP, Juhasz A (1987b). Impairment of sciatic nerve regeneration by protease inhibitor treatment: inhibition of Schwann cell migration. Soc Neurosci Abstr 13:1208.

Mignatti P, Robbins E, Rifkin DB (1986). Tumor invasion through the human amniotic membrane: requirement for a proteinase cascade. Cell 47:487.

McCarthy KD, de Vellis J (1980). Preparation of separate astroglial and oligodendroglial cell cultures from rat cerebral tissue. J Cell Biol 85:890.

Mullins DE, Rohrlich ST (1983). Role of protinases in cellular invasiveness. Biochim Biophys Acta 695:177.

Pollanen J, Saksela O, Salonen E-M, Andereasen P, Nielsen L, Dano K, Vaheri A (1987). Distinct localization of urokinase-type plasminogen activator and its type 1 inhibitor under cultured human fibroblasts and sarcoma cells. J Cell Biol 104:1085.

Reier PJ, Bregman BS, Wujek JR (1986). Intraspinal transplantation of embryonic spinal cord tissue in neonatal and adult rats. J Comp Neurol 247:275.

Rosenblatt DE, Cotman CW, Nieto-Sampedro M, Rowe JW, Knauer DJ (1987). Identification of a protease inhibitor produced by astrocytes that is structurally and functionally homologous to human protease nexin-I. Brain Res 415:40.

Smith GS, Miller RH, Silver J (1987). Astrocyte transplantation induces callosal regeneration in postnatal acallosal mice. Ann NY Acad Sci 495:185.

Soreq H, Miskin R (1981). Plasminogen activator in the rodent brain. Brain Res 216:361.

Williams LR, Longo FM, Powell HC, Lundborg G, Varon S (1983). Spatial-temporal progress of peripheral nerve regeneration within a silicone chamber: Parameters for a bioassay. J Comp Neurol 218:460.

The research reported herein was supported by the National Institutes of Health, grants NS 23064 (N.K.) and in part BRSG SO7 RR07065 (N.K.), by The Spinal Cord Research Foundation (N.K.), and by M.R.C. Canada grant MT-4235 (S.F.). N.K. is the recipient of Career Scientist Award from the Irma T. Hirschl Trust.

IMMUNOSUPPRESSION AS A TREATMENT FOR ACUTE INJURY
OF THE CENTRAL NERVOUS SYSTEM

Dana Giulian

Department of Neurology and
Program of Neuroscience
Baylor College of Medicine

Houston, Texas 77030

Trauma and stroke often lead to permanent loss of function in the central nervous system (CNS). The tissue reaction to these types of injuries involves an acute inflammatory response followed by astrogliosis (Rio Hortega, 1932; Bignami and Dahl, 1976; Oehmichen, 1983). Recent studies suggest that inflammatory cells play an important role in mediating the acute phase of CNS injury (Giulian and Baker, 1985; Giulian and Baker, 1986; Giulian, 1987; Giulian et al; 1988b). As described in this chapter, the suppression of inflammatory cell activity may limit the degree of tissue destruction and thus, preserve function of the nervous system.

The Response of Mononuclear Phagocytes to CNS Injury

Normal brain of adult mammal contains very few mononuclear phagocytes which are identified as active cells by such criteria as the ability to present antigens, appearance of cell surface markers, phagocytic capability, or presence of hydrolytic enzymes (Ling, 1981; Oehmichen, 1983; Giulian, 1987). After injury the CNS contains two major classes of active mononuclear phagocytes, the ameboid microglia which are **intrinsic** to the nervous system and the blood borne macrophage which are **extrinsic** to the nervous system (Giulian, 1987). The type of inflammatory response appears to depend upon the type of injury. For example, a wound penetrating the blood-brain barrier is dominated by an invasion of macrophage (Konigsmark and Sidman, 1963) while axonal degeneration stimulates a microglial response (Kreutzberg and Barron, 1976).

Microglia first appear within the CNS during the embryonic stage of development as ameboid cells (Rio-Hortega, 1932; Matsumoto and Ikuta, 1985; Giulian et al, 1988a). Later ameboid microglia undergo differentiation with the formation of multiple thin processes (Murabe and Sano, 1982; Giulian and Baker, 1986); such ramified microglia are found throughout the CNS of adult mammals and are considered to be quiescent cells. Rio-Hortega (1932) first proposed that the ramified cells revert to active ameboid forms as part of the glial reaction to brain injury. It is likely that signals produced within the CNS attract extrinsic mononuclear phagocytes as well as reactivate the intrinsic cell population to attack damaged tissue (North, 1978).

Our laboratory has been keenly interested in deciphering the cellular and biochemical events associated with acute CNS injury. We have developed techniques to isolate ameboid microglia from newborn brain of rat (Giulian and Baker, 1986). Characterization of these isolated cells has led to insights concerning the role of microglia in brain function (Giulian and Baker, 1985; Giulian et al, 1986b; Giulian et al, 1988a). Cell surface morphology, mitogenic responses, and histochemistry indicate that ameboid microglia are a class of mononuclear phagocytes which can be distinguished from tissue macrophage and blood monocytes (Giulian and Baker, 1986).

Many of the tissue responses which occur during acute brain injury may be mediated by the intrinsic and extrinsic mononuclear phagocytes (Giulian, 1987). For example, we found that microglia when activated release several astroglia-stimulating growth factors (Giulian and Young, 1986) including the immunomodulator Interleukin-1 (IL-1) (Dinarello, 1984; Giulian and Lachman, 1985; Giulian et al, 1986b). Cell cultures studies (Giulian et al, 1986a) and in vivo infusion of IL-1 (Giulian et al, 1988b) show that microglial secretion products help to regulate astrogliosis at wound sites.

In addition to secretion of growth factors, macrophage release a number of cytopathic agents including proteases, arachidonic acid metabolites and superoxide anion (Nathan et al, 1980; Davis, 1981). We have made similar observations on isolated ameboid microglia (Giulian and Baker, 1986). It is quite likely that such secretion products help mediate cell killing and remodeling of damaged brain (Giulian, 1987).

Clinically, the acute phase of injury is the most difficult to manage for it is during this period that patients develop tissue edema, vascular compromise, and deteriorating neurologic function (Raichle, 1983). We suggest that the control of brain mononuclear phagocytes will check this neuropathic state and reduce the likelihood of disability and death.

Drug Suppression of Mononuclear Phagocytes In Vitro

Mononuclear phagocytes attack the CNS through a variety of mechanisms such as phagocytosis of injured neurons and the release of cytotoxins. We believe that the complexity of this cellular attack upon the CNS limits the usefulness of drugs that block only a single cellular event. For example, agents that selectively reduce the production of superoxide anion would not alter the potentially harmful effects of secreted proteases or arachidonic acid metabolites. It is for this reason we searched for therapeutic agents that would block activating or chemotaxic signals, retard cell engulfment, and inhibit the release of cytotoxins. The suppression of endocytosis, phagocytosis, and secretion (Figure 1) should reduce tissue destruction associated with CNS inflammation.

In order to develop suitable therapeutic regimens, we screened a variety of drugs for their ability to inhibit activity of cultured ameboid microglia and peritoneal macrophage. In agreement with numerous reports, dexamethasone and chloroquine, but not colchicine, stop secretion of IL-1 (Norris, 1977; Dinarello, 1984; Bochner et al, 1987).

ENDOCYTOSIS

PHAGOCYTOSIS

SECRETION

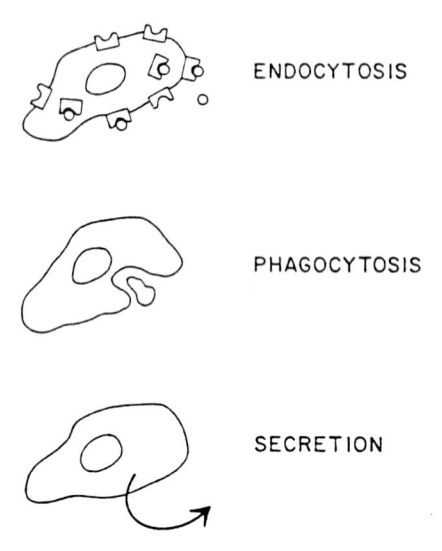

Figure 1) Drug strategies to inhibit mononuclear phagocytes. Three cellular functions are necessary for the mononuclear phagocytic attack upon damaged CNS. We have selected drugs to inhibit one or more of these functions. Blockage of endoctyosis inhibits such receptor-mediated events such as activation by immunomodulators, mitogens, or chemotaxic factors. Blockage of phagocytosis limits the ability of mononuclear phagocytes to engulf and destroy injured neurons. It also reduces the ability of phagocytic signals to stimulate release of cytotoxins. Blockage of secretory function decreases the release of interleukin-1, proteases, leukotrienes, superoxide anion and a variety of other substances that mediate the inflammatory response. In vitro studies show that chloroquine and colchicine block endocytosis, chloroquine and colchicine block phagocytosis, and chloroquine and dexamethasone block secretion. In vivo studies suggest that chloroquine or chloroquine plus colchicine is more effective in inhibiting the activity of CNS mononuclear phagocytes than dexamethasone.

In contrast to the glucocorticoid dexamethasone, colchicine and chloroquine effectively blocked phagocytosis and endocytosis in vitro (Table 1).

Table 1. Drug Effects Upon Mononuclear Phagocytes

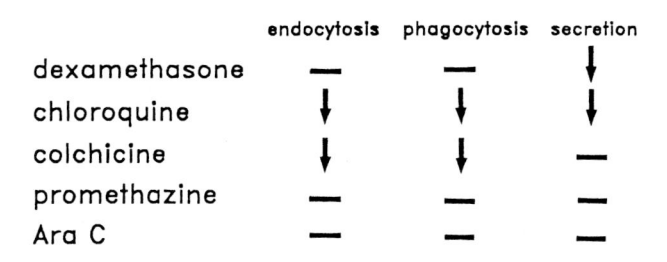

	endocytosis	phagocytosis	secretion
dexamethasone	—	—	↓
chloroquine	↓	↓	↓
colchicine	↓	↓	—
promethazine	—	—	—
Ara C	—	—	—

Although the precise mechanisms of action of dexamethasone and chloroquine upon cell membranes and lysosomal enzymes are complex and controversial (Lie and Schofield, 1973; Norris, 1977; Wildfeur, 1983; Schleimer, 1985), colchicine is thought to retard phagocytosis and chemotaxis by binding to cytoskeleton proteins (Malawista, 1971). Colchicine had a synergistic effect when combined with chloroquine in blocking phagocytic, endocytotic, and secretory functions of brain mononuclear phagocytes.

Effects of Immunosuppression Upon Penetrating Brain Injury

We extended the in vitro observations by testing the effects of mononuclear phagocyte-inhibiting drugs upon penetrating brain injury. A flammed, 26 gauge needle was placed stereotaxically at a depth of 1.0 mm into the cerebral cortex of adult albino rats (Giulian, 1987). Biopsies taken from injury sites of drug treated and untreated control groups were examined for inflammation.

We observed that colchicine, chloroquine, or colchicine-chloroquine significantly reduced the number of mononuclear phagocytes at injury sites when compared to controls (Table 2). Importantly, the number of mononuclear phagocytes found at wound sites were often greater in animals treated with dexamethasone than the number of cells found in biopsy sites of controls. That is to say, more inflammatory cells attack the brain when animals were treated with dexamethasone; far less cells appeared in brains treated with colchicine or chloroquine. In agreement with our in vitro observations, chloroquine or dexamethasone decreased the amount of IL-1 produced at the site of brain injury with chloroquine as the more effective agent (Table 2).

Clearance of debris is an important function of brain mononuclear phagocytes (Rio-Hortega, 1932; Oehmichen, 1983) and involves a series of cellular behaviors including chemotaxis to the site of injury, debris recognition, phagocytosis, and movement of debris-laden cells. We examined phagocytic cell function in vivo by monitoring the clearance of microspheres injected into the site of penetrating brain injury. Colchicine or chloroquine blocked the engulfment and clearance of microspheres from brain by about 80% whereas dexamethasone had no significant effect (Table 2).

Table 2. Drug Effects Upon Brain Injury

	cell number	Il-1 release	clearance
dexamethasone	—	↓	—
chloroquine	↓	↓	↓
colchicine	↓	—	↓

CONCLUSIONS

Glucocorticoids are the drugs most commonly used to reduce inflammation of the CNS. The in vitro and in vivo observations described here show that although dexamethasone decreases secretory function, it neither reduces the number of inflammatory cells nor inhibits phagocytic activity. The limited effectiveness of dexamethasone as a mononuclear phagocyte-inhibitor may explain in part the limited benefit dexamethasone (or other classes of glucocorticoids) offers to patients with traumatic or ischemic injury of the CNS (Norris and Hachinski, 1985). We propose that chloroquine alone or in combination with colchicine is more effective than dexamethasone in suppressing the attack of mononuclear phagocytes upon the CNS.

In summary, damage to the CNS involves an early appearance of mononuclear phagocytes. Microglia and macrophage are thought to regulate neural tissue reaction to injury by controlling scar formation, immune responses, protein degradation, cell death, capillary permeability and vascular flow. Drug regimens which suppress such functions of mononuclear phagocytes as the clearance of tissue debris, the secretion of growth factors, and the release of cytotoxic agents may help patients with acute injury of the nervous system.

REFERENCES

Bignami A, Dahl D (1976). The astroglial response to stab injury. Immunofluorescence studies with antibodies to astrocyte-specific protein (GFA) in mammalian and submammalian vertebrates. Neuropath Apllied Neurobiol 2:99.

Bochner BS, Rutledge BK, Schleimer RP (1987). Interleukin-1 production by human lung tissue. II. Inhibition by anti-inflammatory steroids. J Immunol 139:2303.

Davis P. Secretory functions of mononuclear phagocytes: overview and methods for preparing conditioned supernatants. In: Methods for Studying Mononuclear Phagocytes, edited by Adams, D.O., Edelson, P.J. and Koren, H. New York: Academic Press, 1981, p. 549-559.

Dinarello CA (1984). Interleukin-1. Rev Inf Dis 6:51.

Giulian D (1987). Ameboid microglia as effectors of inflammation in the central nervous system. J Neurosci Res 18:155.

Giulian D, Baker TJ (1985). Peptides released by ameboid microglia regulate astroglial proliferation. J Cell Biol 101:2411.

Giulian D, Baker TJ (1986). Characterization of ameboid microglia isolated from the developing mammalian brain. J Neurosci 6:2163.

Giulian D, Allen RJ, Baker TJ, Tomozawa Y (1986a). Brain peptides and glial growth. 1) Glia-promoting factors as regulators of gliogenesis in the developing and injured central nervous system. J Cell Biol 102:803.

Giulian D, Baker TJ, Shih LN, Lachman LB (1986b). Interleukin-1 of the central nervous system is produced by ameboid microglia. J Exp Med 164:594.

Giulian D, Lachman LB (1985). Interleukin-1 stimulates astroglial proliferation after brain injury. Sci 228:497.

Giulian D, Young D (1986). Brain peptides and glial growth. 2) Identification of cells that secrete glia-promoting factors. J Cell Biol 102:812.

Giulian D, Young DG, Woodward J, Brown D, Lachman LB (1988a). Interleukin-1 is an astroglial growth factor in developing brain. J Neurosci, in press.

Giulian D, Woodward J, Young DG, Krebs JF, Lachman LB (1988b). Interleukin-1 injected into mammalian brain stimulates astrogliosis and neovascularization. J Neurosci, in press.

Konigsmark, B.W. and R.L. Sidman (1963) Origin of brain macrophage in the mouse. J Neuropath. 22:643-676.

Kreutzberg GW, Barron ICD (1976). 5' nucleotidase of microglial cells in the facial nucleus during axonal reaction. J Neurocytol 7:601.

Lie SO, Schofield B (1973). Inactivation of lysosomal function in normal cultured human fibroblasts by chloroquine. Biochem Pharm 22:3109.

Ling EA. The origin and nature of microglia. In: Advances in Cellular Neurobiology, Edited by Fedoroff, S. and Hertz, L. New York: Academic Press, 1981, p. 33-82.

Malawista SE (1971). Vinblastine and colchicine effects on human blood leukocytes during phagocytosis. Blood 37:519.

Matsumoto Y, Ikuta F (1985). Appearance and distribution of fetal brain macrophages in mice. Cell Tis Res 239:271.

Murabe Y, Sano Y (1982). Morphological studies on neuroglia: Postnatal development of microglial cells. Cell Tis Res 225:464.

Nathan C, Murray H, Cohn Z (1980). The macrophage as an effector cell. N Eng J Med 303:622.

Norris DA (1977). The effect of immunosuppression and anti-inflammatory drugs upon monocyte function in vitro. J Lab Clin Med 90:569.

Norris JW, Hachinski VC (1985). Megadose steroid therapy in ischemic stroke. Stroke 16:150.

North RJ (1978). Concept of activated macrophage. J Immunol 121:806.

Oehmichen M (1983). Inflammatory cells in the central nervous system. Prog Neuropath 5:277.

Raichle ME (1983). The pathophysiology of brain ischemia. Ann Neurol 13:2.

Rio-Hortega P. Microglia. In: Cytology and Cellular Pathology of The Nervous System, edited by Penfield, W. New York: Paul P. Hocker, Inc., 1932, p. 481-584.

Schleimer RP (1985). The mechanisms of anti-inflammatory steroid action in allergic diseases. Ann Rev Pharm Toxicol 25:381.

Wildfeur A (1983). Action of anti-rheumatic drugs on the function of the human leukocytes. Drug Res 33:780.

THE DEVELOPMENT OF THE GLIOTIC PLAQUE IN EXPERIMENTAL ALLERGIC ENCEPHALOMYELITIS

Marion E. Smith* and Lawrence F. Eng**

Departments of Neurology* and Pathology**
Veterans Administration Medical Center
Palo Alto, CA 94304

HISTORICAL INTRODUCTION

The astrocytic response in multiple sclerosis was first described by Charcot. In his lecture delivered in 1868 at La Salpetriere on disseminated sclerosis he said: "The central region of the sclerosed patch, you are aware, is that in which the most marked alterations are observed. Here all vestige of fibroid reticulum has disappeared; we no longer meet with distinct trabeculae or cell-forms; the nuclei are less numerous and less voluminous than in the external zones; they are shrunken in every direction, appear shriveled and do not take so deep a tint as usual under the action of carmine. They may be observed forming little groups here and there in the interspaces between the bundles of fibrillae. The latter, however, have invaded every part. They now fill up the aveolar spaces from which the medullary matter has completely disappeared." (Charcot, 1877). In the ensuing discussion he described the fibers as extremely thin, opaque and smooth, and "are frequently interwoven and entangled so as to form a kind of felted tissue." He also raised the question whether the fibers are derived from "pre-existing amorphous matter or from a newly formed blasteme. In other words, is there metamorphosis or substitution?" He noticed that the fibers have sometimes appeared to take root in the substance of nuclei or cells.

About a hundred years later Lumsden wrote a chapter in the Handbook of Clinical Neurology on "The Neuropathology of Multiple Sclerosis." By then it was known that the fibrillary processes emanate from the astrocytes. The author remarked that swollen astrocytes and the production of gliofibrillae are found very early in the disease, and can even precede the stage of sudanophilia, the time when macrophages have ingested the myelin and have synthesized neutral lipids. Thus the gliofibrillogenesis is already vigorous when the fragmentation of the myelin lamellae is still only partial. He raised the question as to whether these astrocytes multiply, and showed two pictures of nuclear duplication (Lumsden, 1970).

ASTROCYTE ACTIVATION IN EAE

Several years ago we began the study of the astrocytic response in experimental allergic encephalomyelitis (EAE) which has in common many of the features of multiple sclerosis. We now have the invaluable tool for the selective visualization of astrocytes, the antibody to the glial fibrillary acidic protein (GFAP), and can easily see the source and the extent of hypertrophy of the gliotic fibers. When the astrocytes were visualized in the spinal cord of the rat with acute EAE we were surprised at the extent of astrocyte hypertrophy, even early when rats were first showing clinical signs of the disease. This gliotic reaction was quite vigorous for about a week, then gradually faded. At the time of acute EAE, about 12-14 days after immunization with purified myelin, and up to 18 days when recovery was progressing, no increase in the amounts of GFAP could be measured by radioimmune assay (Smith et al., 1983).

The chronic relapsing models of EAE more closely resemble the human disease, therefore we turned to the SJL/J mouse which develops a chronic relapsing disease after a series of immunizations with whole spinal cord administered shortly after weaning (Brown and McFarlin, 1981). Although some spontaneous relapses occur, these episodes can be scheduled and the disease exacerbated by periodic injections of mouse spinal cord. The chronic disease results in such clinical symptoms as limp tails, hind leg stiffness or paralysis, and loss of the righting ability. In the first episode of EAE which occurs shortly after the initial series of immunizations, small inflammatory lesions were seen in CNS tissues, especially in the spinal cord and the periventricular areas of the brain. Astrocytes in these areas as well as in the hippocampus and cerebellum became prominently stained with antibody to the GFAP. These cells became hypertrophied and developed convoluted processes. As the disease progressed dense gliotic plaques formed in the spinal cord, periventricular areas and cerebellum. Although much of the forebrain was not involved, measurement of total GFAP in the whole CNS of the mouse with chronic relapsing EAE six months post injection showed an increase by a factor of more than two (Smith and Eng, 1987; Smith et al., in press).

RADIOAUTOGRAPHY OF EAE TISSUES

<u>Acute disease</u>. The density of the areas overgrown with GFAP fibrous material again provoked the question raised earlier by Lumsden: is the overgrowth of astrocytic processes a result of hypertrophy of existing astrocytes or does astrocyte multiplication also occur? To gain insight into this problem we turned to radioautography. Lewis rats in early and late stages of acute EAE were injected intraperitoneally with 2.5 mCi ^{3}H-thymidine, then autopsied two days later. Spinal cord tissues were embedded in paraffin, immunostained for GFAP, dipped in photographic emulsion, and allowed to expose for three weeks.

Upon examination of these tissues it was apparent that very few cells in the central nervous system of control rats injected with Freund's adjuvant alone were labeled with ^{3}H-thymidine. Only a few endothelial cells and some small dark cells, possibly microglia, showed label. Large numbers of mononuclear cells in the EAE spinal cords showed intense uptake of ^{3}H-thymidine. Many of these were associated with the perivascular lesions of EAE, but others were found in regions far removed from any lesion sites. These mononuclear cells appeared to be inflammatory cells invading the CNS, which are known to include monocytes, macrophages, and lymphocytes. Small numbers of GFAP-stained cells were also labeled. Both small and large hypertrophied astrocytes were included among the labeled cells. These were seen throughout the time course of the acute disease, and as many labeled astrocytes were seen at eleven days early in the disease as at 17 days when the animal was recovering (Smith et al., 1987).

We concluded that since spinal cord tissues of rats injected one time only with ^{3}H-thymidine contained rather small numbers of labeled astrocytes compared to the much more extensive label in the mononuclear cells, it is likely that only occasional astrocytes undergo cell division. More recently, however, several animals eleven days after immunization were injected three times within thirty hours with one mCi/injection ^{3}H-thymidine, and the tissues were processed as described above. Again, very few cells and no astrocytes in the control tissue showed radioactive label. In the EAE tissue, however, large numbers of labeled cells in areas of intense gliosis could be seen (Fig. 1). In most microscopic fields where astrocytes were prominent a number of GFAP-stained cells showing radioactive label could be identified (Figs. 2 and 3), indicating cell division was taking place.

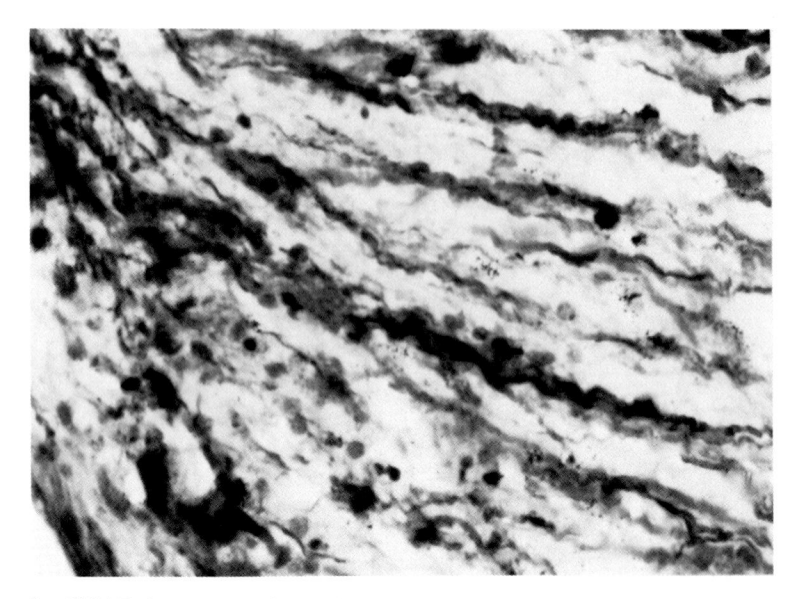

Fig. 1. GFAP-immunostained fibers in spinal cord Lewis rat 12 days after immunization with purified myelin. Cell bodies associated with the fibers have incorporated ^{3}H-thymidine.

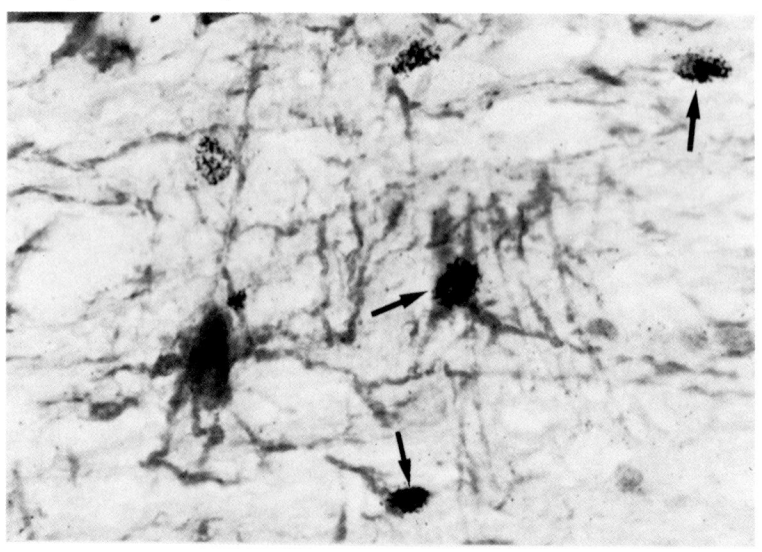

Fig. 2. Cells in spinal cord of Lewis rat with acute EAE showing ^{3}H-thymidine label. Arrows indicate GFAP-stained cells.

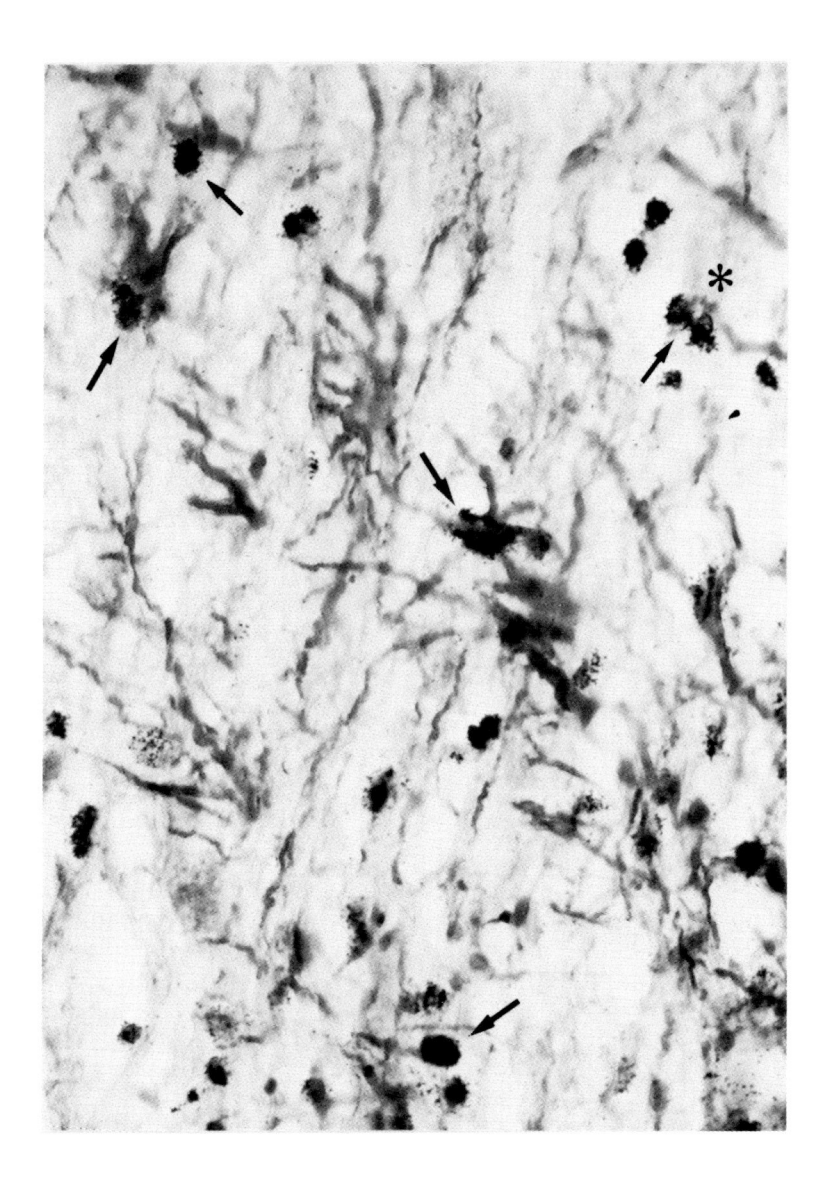

Fig. 3. ^{3}H-thymidine-labeled cells in spinal cord of Lewis rat with acute EAE. Arrows show GFAP-immunostained cells. Asterisk indicates astrocyte in possible mitosis.

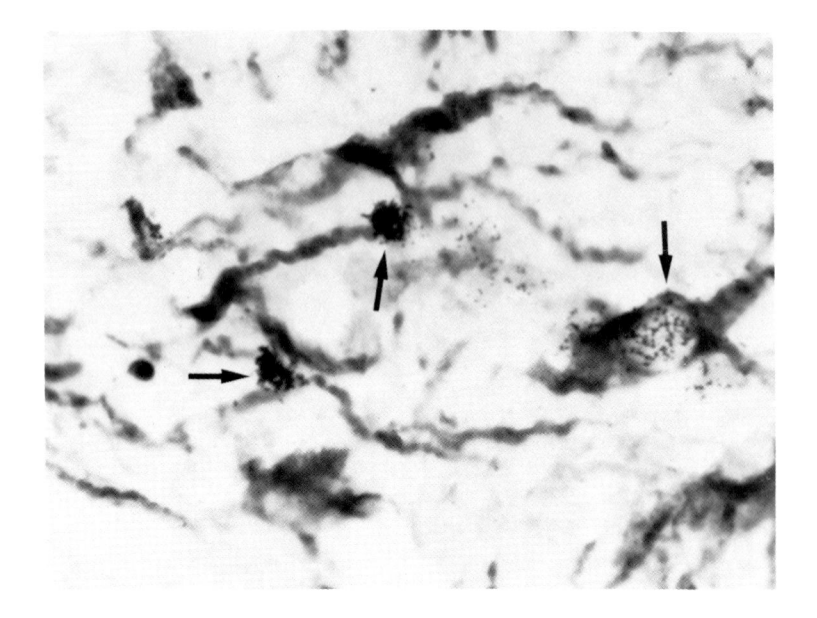

Fig. 4. GFAP-immunostained cells in brain of SJL/J mouse with chronic relapsing EAE of eight months duration. Three astrocytes have incorporated ^{3}H-thymidine.

Chronic EAE. In previous studies of mice with chronic relapsing EAE autoradiographs have revealed very few labeled astrocytes (Smith et al., in press), even though dense gliotic plaques were present within three months after immunization. When these mice were injected with ^{3}H-thymidine more frequently over a longer period, labeled astrocytes could be found in small numbers distributed throughout the plaque areas in the brains and spinal cords. Generally, only one to three labeled cells were seen in any one area, and these active areas were far removed from each other. It appeared that astrocytes in different areas became active at different times. In most mice studied the tissues were prepared for radioautography only during a relapse after reimmunization, but the CNS of one mouse with chronic EAE of eight months duration was examined without reimmunization. Labeled astrocytes were visible in several areas of the brain and spinal cord, indicating that an immunological boost was not necessary and that astrocyte division may occur occasionally, but continuously over a long period of time (Fig. 4).

ELECTRON MICROSCOPY OF ASTROCYTES IN EAE

Electron microscopic examination of the early EAE lesion revealed a typical reactive astrocytic response expressed by an enlarged watery cytoplasm, particularly at the level of the processes surrounding neurons and blood vessels. The astroglial processes contained numerous glycogen particles (aggregates and single particles). Glial filaments were also conspicuous and were arranged in small bundles or loose thin filaments adjacent to the bundles, as if dissociated by the pressure exercised by the intracellular fluid. The glial filaments which normally appear as tight bundles have expanded and appear less dense (Figs. 5 and 6) (Eng et al., 1988).

DISCUSSION

Astrocyte hypertrophy and proliferation of cell processes appears very early in EAE, coincidently with the first inflammatory foci. In the rat the activation of astrocyte staining for the GFAP is general and not limited to the site of the lesion. In the chronic relapsing EAE mouse, on the other hand, astrocyte activation appears only in certain areas which are generally in the vicinity of the inflammatory lesion. These lesions are much milder than the acute inflammatory lesions of the rat.

The cause of the early astrocyte hypertrophy is unknown, but one likely factor is the onset of edema due to breakdown of the blood-brain barrier and leakage of blood-borne substances into the central nervous sytem. It was shown twenty years ago that leakage of gamma globulin and leukocytes occurs very early in EAE (Cutler et al., 1967). Brain edema may be reflected by the swollen astrocyte fibers clearly seen by electron microscopy. These may expose additional antigenic sites, resulting in increased immunostaining at the initial stages of the disease.. It is difficult, however, to link this process with the vigorous hypertrophy and cell division demonstrated here in the reactive astrocytes.

It is likely that growth factors are elaborated by the infiltrating inflammatory cells which include lymphocytes, monocytes, and macrophages. Such a relationship between astrocytes and these cells has been suggested by others. Thus Fontana et al. (1980) have shown that lymphocytes activated by Concanavalin A will promote DNA synthesis in cultured astrocytes. Interleukin-1 secreted by monocytes and macrophages can also stimulate astrocyte proliferation in culture as shown by Guilian and Lachman (1985). The serum of EAE animals also contains a number of other substances present in abnormal amounts that may stimulate the neural cells which are normally not exposed to these factors. For instance a large increase in apo E is found in plasma of EAE animals (Shore et al., 1987)

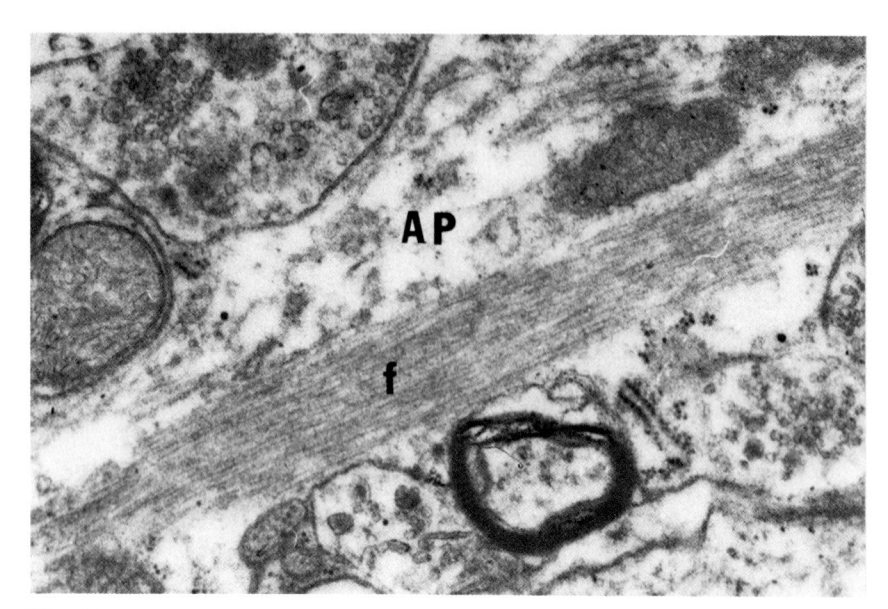

Fig. 5. Electron micrograph of a spinal cord section from a rat immunized with complete Freund's adjuvant alone. The astrocytic process (AP) contains a tight bundle of glial filaments (f) with no glycogen particles (GP) (x 13,000).

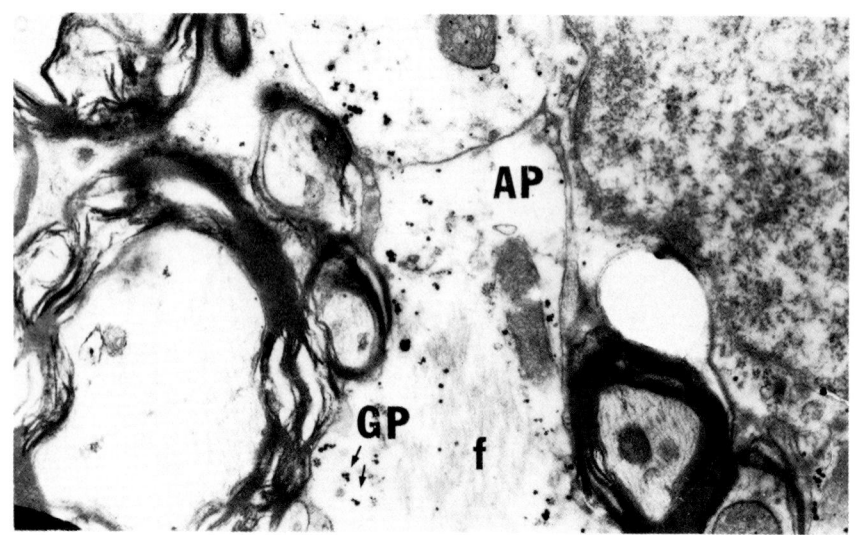

Fig. 6. Electron micrograph of a spinal cord section from a rat with EAE. The edematous astrocytic process (AP) contains dissociated glial filaments (f) and glycogen particles (GP) (x 13,000).

which undoubtedly leaks into the CNS. At present the effects of such factors on the neural cells are unknown.

Whatever the cause, these results indicate that astrocyte division and proliferation are precursor events to the gliosis seen in acute EAE as demonstrated by GFAP staining. Continued astrocyte division and growth of the fibrous processes over a longer time period leads to the development of the gliotic plaques seen in chronic EAE. It is likely that a similar phenomenon is involved in the formation of the dense matrix seen in multiple sclerosis plaques described almost 130 years ago by Charcot.

REFERENCES

Brown AM, McFarlin DE (1981). Relapsing experimental allergic encephalomyelitis in the SJL/J mouse. Lab. Invest. 45:278-284.

Charcot, JM (1877). Disseminated Sclerosis, Pathological Anatomy. In "Lectures on the Diseases of the Nervous System. Delivered at La Salpetriere." Vol. 72. The New Sydenham Society, London, pp. 157-181.

Cutler RWP, Lorenzo AV, and Barlow CF (1967). Brain vascular permeability to I^{125} gamma globulin and leukocytes in allergic encephalomyelitis. J. Neuropathol. Exp. Neurol. 26:558-571.

Eng LF, D'Amelio FE, and Smith ME (1988). Dissociation of GFAP intermediate filaments in EAE. Trans. Am. Soc. Neurochem. 19:in press.

Fontana A, Grieder A, Arrenbrecht St, Grob P (1980). In vitro stimulation of glia cells by a lymphocyte-produced factor. J. Neurol. Sci. 46:55-62.

Guilian D, Lachman LB (1985). Interleukin-1 stimulation of astroglial proliferation after brain injury. Science 288:497-499.

Lumsden CE (1970). The neuropathology of multiple sclerosis. In Vinken PJ, Bruyn GW (eds): "Handbook of Clinical Neurology," Vol. 9, Amsterdam: North Holland Publ., pp. 217-309.

Shore VG, Smith ME, Perret V, and Laskaris MA (1987). Alterations in plasma lipoproteins and apolipoproteins in experimental allergic encephalomyelitis. J. Lipid Res. 28:119-129.

Smith ME, Eng LF (1987). Glial fibrillary acidic protein in chronic relapsing experimental allergic encephalomyelitis in SJL/J mice. J. Neurosci. Res. 18:203-208.

Smith ME, Forno LS, and Eng LF (in press). Astrocyte involvement in chronic relapsing EAE in the SJL/J mouse. In Norenberg M, Hertz L, Schousboe A (ed). "Biochemical Pathology of Astrocytes".New York: Alan R. Liss.

from those of injured-brain extract (Nieto-Sampedro et al.,1985). Furthermore, the postlesion increase in aFGF and

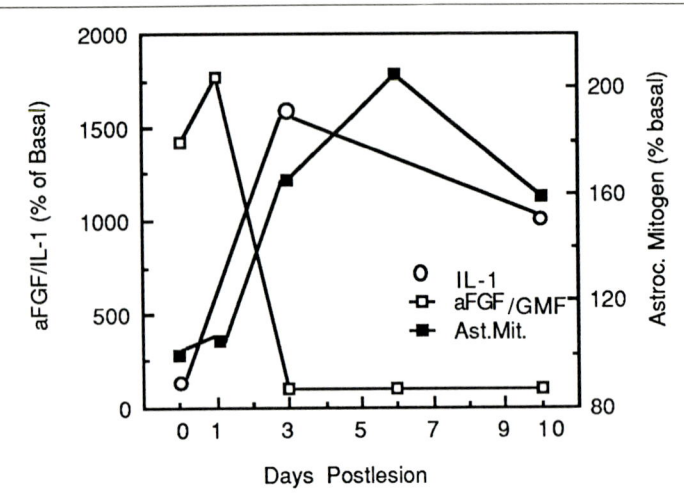

Fig.1. Time-course of the increase in astrocyte mitogenic activity (Ast.Mit.) in injured-brain extract, compared to interleukin-1 (IL-1) and secreted GMF/aFGF.

GMF occurred much earlier than the injury-induced astrocyte mitogenic activity (maximal GMF and aFGF activity 1 hour postlesion vs 6 days; Fig.1). Interleukin-1, also present in brain in comparatively large amounts after injury, differed from the main astrocyte mitogen in fractionation properties and time-course of induction (Fig. 1; Nieto-Sampedro and Berman, 1987). Although the judgement is far from final, we believe that these polypeptides may be involved in the initiation of the CNS injury response but are not likely to be ultimately responsible for astrocyte proliferation after a lesion.

Recently, we have examined the possible role another well known mitogen, epidermal growth factor (EGF; Carpenter and Cohen, 1979). The reports on the presence in brain of EGF-crossreacting material are contradictory (Fallon et al.,1984; Probstmeier and Schachner, 1986) and EGF mRNA is found in brain at very low levels (Rall et al., 1985). However, the discrepancies may arise in part from the fact that the brain EGF-like molecule may not be EGF itself. A cysteine-rich grouping of 40-50 aminoacids, containing all or part of the EGF sequence (EGF domain), occurs in a variety of membrane-bound or secreted proteins, including tumor growth factor, plasminogen activator (PA), low density lipoprotein receptor (LDLR) and the products of genes *notch* and *lin* (Akam, 1986). Some of these systems are present in the CNS. Thus, LDLRs are found in the membranes of microglia and macrophages, and the PA system is a glia mitogen present in developing mammalian CNS (Kalderon, 1982; Moonen.et al., 1985). The problem may be approached by looking at the mediators of the mitogen action, i.e its receptors. If the injury-induced astrocyte mitogenic activity were related to the EGF domain, the appropriate receptors should be present in the CNS.

BRAIN EGF RECEPTORS

The action of EGF is mediated by the EGF receptor (EGFR), a 170-kD trans-membrane glycoprotein presumably located in the physiological targets of the EGF domain. The extracellular domain of the EGFR contains the EGF binding site whereas the intracellular moiety has tyrosine kinase activity (Carpenter, 1987). The EGFR binding site shows high affinity for its ligands but comparatively low specificity. Thus, it binds tumor growth factor with an affinity similar to that for EGF although the homology between both peptides is lower than 25 % (Carpenter, 1987).
In rat brain, EGFR-immunoreactivity was maximal in astroglia at about 19 days postnatal and then became weaker as the animals reached adulthood. In adult animals (30 days and older) glial staining was very weak, whereas a distinct neuronal population in the neocortex (layers IV and V) stained strongly with anti-EGFR (Nieto-Sampedro et al.,1987; Gomez-Pinilla et al., 1987). A brain lesion completely changed this situation. The EGFR-immunoreactivity of the neurons was not affected. However, astrocyte populations adjacent to the injury or in deafferented areas became intensely EGFR positive. EGFR staining appeared first in the cell bodies of the glial cells at 1 day postlesion. It reached maximal intensity 8-12 days after injury, when EGFR immunostaining extended both to the cell body and the astrocytic processes. All EGFR positive cells also stained for Glial Fibrillary Acidic protein (GFAP). However, early after injury the converse was not necessarily true; at one day postlesion, some GFAP positive cells adjacent to the injury site did not stain or stained very weakly for EGFR.

EGFR RELATED MITOGEN INHIBITORS (ERI) AND ASTROCYTE RESPONSE TO INJURY

Glial EGFR immunoreactivity increased dramatically in the proximity of a brain lesion (Nieto-Sampedro et al.,1987). It was possible that the EGF domain/EGFR system was involved in the glial response to injury. Accordingly, we tested the effect of anti-EGFR antibodies on the mitogenic activity for astrocytes of extracts of normal and injured brain. ^{3}H-Thymidine incorporation into astrocytes, promoted by extracts of normal or injured-brain, was dramatically enhanced by both monoclonal and polyclonal antibodies to EGFR (Table 1).

The antibodies may have exerted their mitogenic effect by binding to the EGFR and mimicking EGF action (Carpenter, 1987). However, they had little or no effect when added to astrocyte cultures in the absence of brain extract (Table 1). Alternatively, the antibodies could have acted on the brain extract itself. Pre-treatment of extracts of normal or injured brain with anti-EGFR antibodies immobilized on Protein A-Sepharose had the same effect on the mitogenic activity that the direct antibody addition (Table 1). Therefore, the action of anti-EGFR consisted in removing from the brain extracts an inhibitory molecule that shared epitope/s with the EGFR. I shall call this molecule EGFR related inhibitor (ERI).

Table 1. Removal of EGFR-related mitogen inhibitor (ERI) from brain extracts by soluble anti-EGFR and anti-EGFR bound to protein A- Sepharose*

Experimental Conditions	Thymidine incorporation (cpm/6 h)
Medium (1% serum)	668 ± 37 (n= 6)
+ monoclonal anti-EGFR	625 ± 63 (n= 6)
+ polyclonal anti EGFR	2548 ± 132 (n= 6)
+ BE (2 mg/ml)	760 ± 45 (n= 4)
+ BE + monoclonal anti-EGFR	17,249 ± 2117 (n= 4)
+ BE + polyclonal anti-EGFR	13,183 ± 1054 (n= 4)
+ BE adsorbed with insoluble monoclonal anti-EGFR	16,908 ± 2029 (n= 4)
+ BE adsorbed with insoluble polyclonal anti-EGFR	23,640 ± 2128 (n= 4)

*Brain extract preparation and assay were performed as previously described (Nieto-Sampedro, 1987). Soluble monoclonal antibody was added to the medium to a final IgG concentration of 2 µg/ml and polyclonal antiserum to a final dilution of 1/100. ERI was adsorbed from injured-brain extracts (BE) as follows. Protein A-Sepharose (15 mg) was washed with DMEM/F12 medium and incubated for 1 h at 25 ºC in DMEM/F12 medium (600 µl) containing either 12 µl of polyclonal antiserum or 25 µg of monoclonal IgG. After washing once with medium, the Sepharose-Protein A-antibody complex was treated with BE in DMEM/F12 (2.4 mg protein in 600 µl) for 1 h at 25 ºC, separated by centrifugation and the supernatant used for mitogen assay after supplementation with serum to a final conc.of 1%.

The presence in brain of a *soluble* molecule with the binding properties of the EGFR may have implications regarding the control of astrocyte division. In adult mammals glial cells rarely divide, except following neuronal damage. A possible explanation is that the available mitogens contain the EGF domain and their action is blocked under normal circumstances by soluble EGFR-like inhibitors (ERI). After injury, a decrease in the total amount of ERI would allow dissociation of the ERI-mitogen complex and expression of the mitogenic activity. In order to test this hypothesis, we compared the relative amounts of ERI in the brain of normal animals and at various intervals after injury. Using either an enzyme-linked immunoassay or direct binding of radiolabelled monoclonal anti-EGFR, we found a considerable decrease in the amount of ERI after injury. The concentration of the inhibitor/s in normal brain (about 15 ng/mg protein) decreased in parallel with the increase in astrocyte mitogenic activity (Fig. 2). Minimal levels were observed 6 days postlesion and the values returned to normal by 30 days after injury. Interestingly, injury also caused the appearance of membrane-bound EGFR immunoreactivity in reactive astrocytes (Nieto-Sampedro et al.,1987).

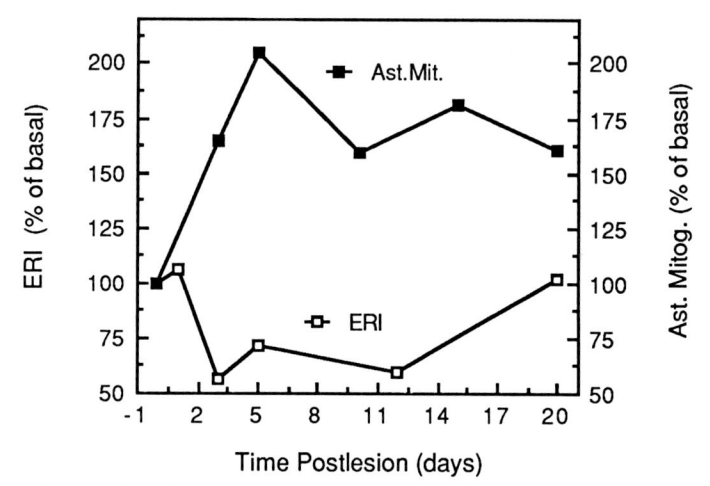

Fig.2 Relationship between the increase in astrocyte mitogenic activity in the tissue adjacent to a brain injury and the decrease in EGFR related inhibitor (ERI).

The existence of mitogen inhibitors in brain was postulated earlier in view of the fact that fractionation of the astrocyte mitogenic activity in brain extracts led to the recovery of more than 100% of the initial activity (Nieto-Sampedro et al., 1985). Subsequently, we observed that the dose-response curves for the mitogenic activity of normal brain extracts had a bell-shape, diagnostic of the simultaneous presence of a growth factor and its inhibitor. This bell-shape was largely lost in extracts of brain tissue adjacent to an injury site, suggesting that the increase in mitogenic activity induced by injury was largely due to the loss of mitogen inhibitor/s (Nieto-Sampedro, 1987; 1988). A similar effect was observed after treating brain extracts with antibody to EGFR. The dose-response curves of antibody-treated brain extracts lost their bell shape and took on a conventional appearance.

RELATIONSHIP BETWEEN EGFR AND ERI

How regulated is the EGFR in astrocyte membranes? Based on the brain response to injury, I hypothesized that the appearance of membrane-bound EGFR was related to the decrease in the amount of extracellular soluble ERI. Under physiological conditions, removal of ERI could be effected by binding to macrophages (that carry the EGF domain on their surface in the form of LDLRs). Experimentally, antibodies to EGFR could also remove ERI and trigger a similar reaction. The hypothesis was tested both *in vitro* and *in vivo*. *In vitro*, purified astrocytes were maintained for 3 days in culture without changing the medium, to permit accumulation of ERI. At this time, one group of cultures was treated for 24 hours with polyclonal antibody to EGFR at a final dilution of 1/100. Control astrocytes were maintained in culture a further 24 hours without any treatment. Both groups of cultures were then fixed and immunostained with anti-EGFR antibody. Control astrocytes stained very weakly with anti-EGFR. Similar cells, treated for 24 hours with anti-EGFR antibody after 3 days in culture showed intense perinuclear and surface EGFR immunoreactivity (Fig. 3A, B).

The experiment *in vivo* was performed by unilaterally injecting antibodies to EGFR in the hippocampus of adult rats. As a control, the same volume of either normal rabbit serum or BSA was injected in the contralateral side. The animals were sacrificed 1, 4, 8 and 15 days after the injection and immunostained with antibodies to EGFR and GFAP. In order to examine the distribution and life time in the brain of the injected anti-EGFR, some sections were directly treated with secondary antibody . The antibody itself diffused through a comparatively large area but was not selectively taken up by astrocytes. One day after anti-EGFR injection, a wide area around the injection site was filled with GFAP positive cells the body of which also stained weakly with anti-EGFR. Between 4 and 8 days after the injection, EGFR staining reached maximal intensity and extended to the astrocytic processes.(Fig. 3C, D). The time course of astrocyte response to anti-EGFR injection was similar to that of the response to injury. The expression of

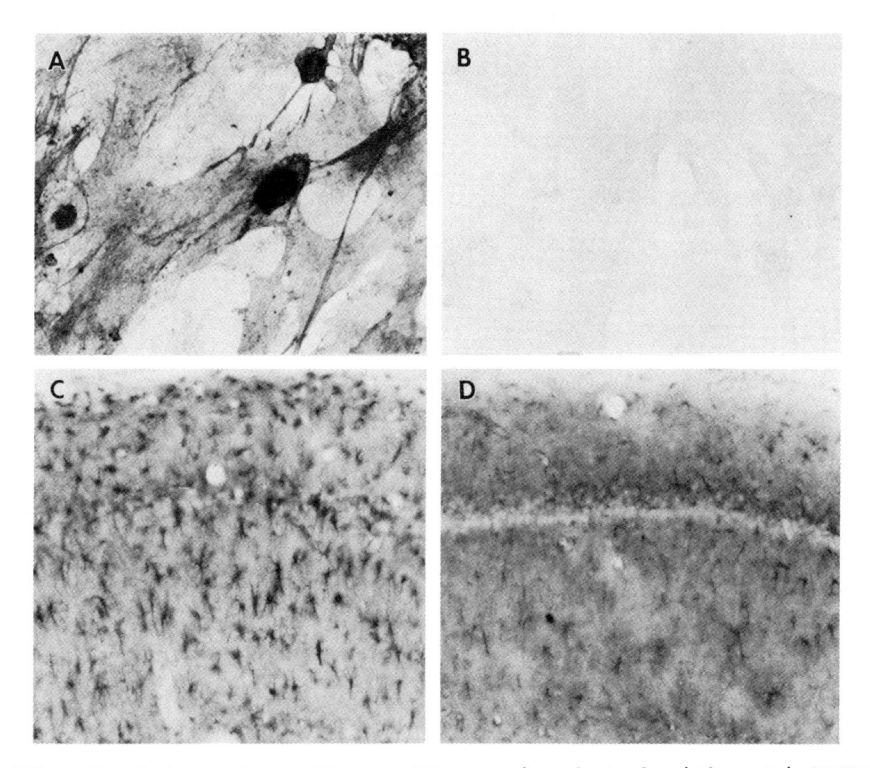

Fig. 3. Astrocyte cultures A) pre-incubated with anti-EGFR, stained much more strongly for EGFR than B) untreated controls. C) EGFR immunoreactive astrocytes in hippocampal CA1 7 days after the injection of 2 µl of anti-EGFR. D) Injection of non-immune serum in the contralateral side did not evoke a comparable response.

membrane EGFR and the loss of soluble ERI seemed to be related. An increase in the expression of membrane-bound EGFR occurred concomitantly with the decrease in ERI concentration. The astrocytes also became intensely GFAP positive, i.e. they underwent a conversion from a resting into a reactive form.

MOLECULAR PROPERTIES OF THE INHIBITORS

The apparent molecular weight of ERI was determined by SDS-polyacrylamide gel electrophoresis followed by immunoblot with polyclonal anti-EGFR and ^{125}I-protein A. Three bands were immunoreactive. The main band (67 %) had an apparent molecular weight of 41 kDalton; minor bands were present at 52 kDalton (25 %) and 69 kDalton (8 %), respectively. Although we cannot exclude the possibility of these molecules arising by proteolysis of the EGFR, this seems unlikely. EGFR, and particularly its extracellular EGF-binding domain, is known to be highly protease resistant. Furthermore, tissue extracts prepared in the presence of inhibitors of the major types of protease, showed similar or higher ERI content than extracts prepared in their absence. Also, ERI content did not decrease by extraction under osmolarity conditions that minimized organelle disruption.

CELLULAR SOURCE OF THE MITOGEN INHIBITORS

What is the cellular source of ERIs? It has been described that cultured astrocytes secrete inhibitors of cell proliferation (Kagen et al., 1982; Aloisi et al., 1987). Accordingly, we examined by ELISA assay (Voller et al.,1978) with anti-EGFR the growth medium conditioned over confluent astrocyte cultures . Similar to the observations of Kagen et al. (1982) on a growth inhibitor, ERIs reached maximal concentration in the conditioned medium after 48 hours. The presence of ERI in astrocyte conditioned medium was further confirmed by examining the effect of anti-EGFR on the incorporation of ^{3}H-Thymidine into astrocytes promoted by EGF. EGF alone was only weakly mitogenic for confluent astrocytes; however, in the presence of anti-EGFR antibodies, its mitogenic activity increased 4 times, becoming comparable to that of injured brain extracts. The most parsimonious interpretation of these results is that an ERI capable of binding EGF was secreted into the culture medium of astroglial cells and partially blocked EGF action. Treatment with anti-EGFR removed the ERI, allowing EGF mitogenic activity to be fully expressed.

EVENTS AFTER CNS INJURY

The results described in this paper can be organized in a simple model to describe the response of astroglial cells to CNS injury (Fig. 4). In normal brain, EGF-like mitogens are inactivated by complex formation with ERI's, present in comparatively large excess. After injury, the CNS tissue is invaded by monocyte/macrophages that carry on their surface low density lipoprotein receptors (LDLR). LDLRs contain the EGF domain and are capable of binding and internalizing excess ERIs. The removal of ERIs from the extracellular space, frees the EGF-like mitogen and triggers the expression of membrane-bound EGFR on astrocytes, which become capable of responding to mitogens containing the EGF domain. This sequence of events is very economical in that a single event, the invasion of the CNS by macrophages, gives rise to the subsequent responses. The model makes testable predictions (i.e. intracerebral injection of macrophages will cause gliosis) and suggests ways of controlling the astrocyte reaction.

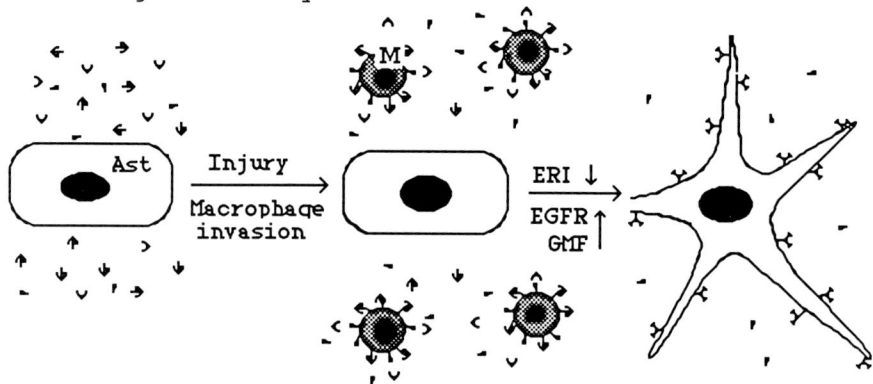

Fig 4. The appearance of EGFR (Y) on the astrocyte (Ast) surface is triggered by the removal of ERI (v) trough binding to macrophages (M) carrying the EGF domain (').

Supported by grants AG 00538-09A from the National Institutes of Aging and TC-87-01 from the American Paralysis Association. I am very grateful to Dr. D.J. Knauer for a generous gift of rabbit anti-EGFR and to Mr. J.T.Broderick for his excellent technical assistance.

REFERENCES

Akam M (1986). Developmental genes. Mediators of cell communication? Nature 319: 447-448.
Aloisi F, Agresti C and Levi G (1987). Glial conditioned media inhibits the proliferation of cultured rat cerebellar astrocytes. Neurochem. Res 12: 189-195
G. Carpenter (1987). Receptors for epidermal growth factor and other polypeptide mitogens. Annu Rev Biochem 56: 881-914.
Carpenter G and Cohen S (1979). Epidermal growth factor. Ann Rev Biochem 48: 193-216.
Fallon JH, Seroogy KB, Loughlin SE, Morrison RS, Bradshaw RA, Knauer DJ and Cunningham DD (1984). Epidermal growth factor immunoreactivity material in the central nervous system: location and development. Science 224: 1107-1109.
Gómez-Pinilla F, Knauer DJ and Nieto-Sampedro M (1987). Epidermal growth factor receptor immunoreactivity in rat brain. Development and cellular localization. Brain Res, in press.

Kagen LJ, Miller SL and Pedrotti M (1982). Glia-derived growth regulator: studies on its production and action. Expt Neurol 78: 517-529.

Kalderon N (1982). Role of the plasmin-generating system in the developing nervous tissue: Proteolysis as a mitogenic signal for the glial cells. J Neurosci Res 8: 509-519

Lim R (1985). Glia maturation factor and other factors acting on glia. In G. Guroff (Ed.), Growth and Maturation Factors, Vol. 3, Wiley, New York, , pp. 119-147.

Moonen G., Grau-Wagemans M.-P., Selak I, Lefebvre PhP, Rogister B, Vasalli JD and Belin D (1985). Plasminogen activator is a mitogen for astrocytes in developing cerebellum. Dev Brain Res 20: 41-48.

Nieto-Sampedro M (1987). Astrocyte mitogenic activity in aged normal and Alzheimer's human brain. Neurobiol Aging 8: 249-252.

Nieto-Sampedro M (1988). Growth factor induction and order of events in CNS repair. In Sabel B and Stein DG (eds): "Pharmacological Approaches to the Treatment of Brain and Spinal Cord Injury," New York: Plenum, in press.

Nieto-Sampedro M and Berman MA (1987). Interleukin-1-like activity in rat brain: sources, targets and effect of injury. J Neurosci Res 17: 214-219.

Nieto-Sampedro M, Gómez-Pinilla F and Knauer DJ (1987). Neuroscience 22: S279

Nieto-Sampedro M, Lim R, Hicklin DJ and Cotman CW (1988). Early release of GMF and aFGF after rat brain injury. Neurosci Lett , in press.

Nieto-Sampedro M, Saneto RP, de Vellis J and Cotman CW(1985). The control of glial populations in brain: Changes in astrocyte mitogenic and morphogenic factors in response to injury. Brain Res. 343: 320-328.

Probstmeier R and Schachner M (1986). Epidermal Growth Factor is not detectable in developing and adult rodent brain by a sensitive double-site enzyme immunoassay. Neurosci. Lett. 63: 290-294.

Rall LB, Scott J, Bell GI, Crawford RJ, Penschow JD Niall HD and Coghlan JP(1985). Mouse prepro-epidermal growth factor synthesis by the kidney and other tissues. Nature 313: 228-231.

Reier, PJ (1986). Astrocytic scar formation following CNS injury: Its microanatomy and effects on axonal elongation. In Fedoroff S and Vernadakis A (eds): "Astrocytes: Cell Biology and Pathology of Astrocytes", Vol. 3, Academic Press, Orlando, pp. 263-324.

Thomas KA and Giménez-Gallego G (1986). Fibroblast growth factors: broad spectrum mitogens with potent angiogenic activity. Trends Biochem Sci 11: 81-84.

Voller A, Bartlett A and Bidwell DE (1978). Enzyme immunoassays with special reference to ELISA techniques, J Clin Pathol 31: 507-520.

INDUCED REGENERATION OF DORSAL ROOT FIBERS INTO THE ADULT
MAMMALIAN SPINAL CORD

M. Kliot, G.M. Smith, J. Siegal, S. Tyrrell and
J. Silver
Dept. of Developmental Genetics, Case Western
Reserve Univ., Cleveland, Ohio and Dept. of
Neurosurgery, Columbia Presbyterian Medical
Center, N.Y.C., N.Y.

INTRODUCTION

It is well known that injured axons regenerate robustly within the peripheral nervous system (PNS) (Cajal, 1928; Guth, 1956). Unfortunately their regrowth within the adult mammalian central nervous system (CNS) is far more limited (Tello, 1907; Cajal, 1928; LeGros Clark, 1943; David and Aguayo, 1981). The lack of CNS regeneration in the mature brain has been attributed, at least in part, to factors in the immediate environment of the injured axon. One such factor is the development of a glial scar at the site of injury (Puchala and Windle, 1977; Reier et al., 1983).

The important and changing role of the astrocyte during development and regeneration has recently become appreciated (Silver and Sidman, 1980; Silver et al., 1982; Smith et al., 1986). Whereas, in the embryo, astrocytes promote the growth and guidance of axons, in the adult they are a major participant in scar formation. An appreciation of this transformation of the astrocyte from "activated" to "reactive" has allowed the development of new strategies for promoting CNS regeneration.

Millipore implants (after Campbell et al., 1957), coated with astrocytes harvested from neonatal brain or embryonic spinal cord, have been shown to reduce scar formation and promote the growth of lesioned adult callosal (Silver and Ogawa, 1983; Smith et al., 1986; Smith and Silver, in press) and corticospinal axons (Schreyer and Jones, 1987). Reducing scar formation by using embryonic astrocytes allowed for better integration of the implant with the surrounding parenchyma and stimulated fiber growth through the original lesion site (Smith et al., 1986). Nevertheless, to date, axonal growth beyond the implant has been negligible for reasons that are still unclear.

The limited ability of adult mammalian neurons to regenerate axons within the CNS is clearly demonstrated by dorsal root sensory fibers that are either crushed or cut and reanastomosed (Moyer et al., 1953; Perkins et al., 1980; Carlstedt, 1983; Liuzzi and Lasek, 1987b). These fibers grow successfully beyond the crush or cut site within the PNS. However, at the cord surface, most of these regenerating axons either make a U-turn and grow back towards the periphery or make stable presynaptic-like endings upon the reactive astrocytes within the dorsal root entry zone (DREZ) (Stensaas et al., 1987; Liuzzi and Lasek, 1987a). A short distance of less than a millimeter separates the DREZ from the dorsal horn. Nonetheless only a few fibers penetrate the DREZ and they fail to make terminal arbors within the spinal grey matter.

Most hypotheses as to why sensory axons fail to regenerate to any significant degree past the DREZ involve the reactive astrocyte population at the root-cord boundary. Although these astrocytes are at a distance from the site of original injury, they nevertheless undergo reactive changes (gliosis), including hyperplasia and proliferation, in response to the degenerating axons (Stensaas et al., 1987). These changes establish a permanent barrier to the passage of regenerating sensory fibers (Reier et al., 1983). In addition, it has recently been suggested that a particular protein component of adult myelin, made by the oligodendroglia, is also a potent inhibitor of axonal elongation (Schwab and Thoenen, 1985; Caroni and Schwab, 1988). It follows, therefore, that the white matter of the posterior columns, as well as the tract of Lissauer, may constitute additional hurdles in the path of regenerating sensory fibers.

In contrast, the crushed dorsal root fibers of newborn rats (Carlstedt et al., 1987), as well as adult amphibians (Peng and Frank, in press), have been shown to regenerate successfully into the cord and form appropriate connections within their target regions. In an attempt to restore this regenerative potential to the adult mammal, we have employed Millipore implants coated with embryonic spinal cord astrocytes

Our results demonstrate that such transplants can promote the growth of adult dorsal root fibers across the DREZ and into the grey matter. Many of these regenerating fibers form axonal terminals with boutons suggesting that there is sufficient synaptic plasticity in the adult mammalian spinal cord to allow for the establishment of new connections. In addition, examples of abortive regeneration of axons passing into but ending abruptly in white matter support the proposed inhibitory action of adult myelin on axonal elongation.

SURGERY AND HRP HISTOCHEMISTRY

Anaesthetized adult male and female albino rats (250-400 gm) underwent bilateral laminectomies of the lower thoracic and upper lumbar levels to expose the caudal part of the spinal cord and nerve roots of the cauda equinae. The fifth lumbar root (L5) on one side was isolated and loosely knotted with a 6-0 silk suture for future reference. The L5 root is the largest, innervating the big and adjacent toes (our behavioural observations), and is therefore readily identified. This root was then crushed with specially designed smooth and rigid forceps approximately 2-3 mm. from its DREZ. The root was squeezed forcefully to the maximal extent possible three times for ten seconds each. This method of crushing has been shown to result in degeneration of all axons distil to the crush site (McQuarrie et al., 1977): Our own EM and HRP studies confirm this observation (unpublished). In some animals the adjacent one or two roots rostral and caudal to the crushed L5 root were cut.

Animals were then divided into several experimental groups. A control group was simply closed and allowed to recover. The other groups were implanted with a Millipore structure in the shape of a pennant. As shown in Fig. 1, the flag portion was inserted along the medial aspect of the L5 DREZ with the pole portion lying just medial and adjacent to the nerve root. One group of animals received "naked" Millipore pennants that had not been coated with any cells. Another group received implants coated with embryonic spinal cord astrocytes as described below. All animals were then closed and allowed to survive for approximately 3 to 4 weeks. During this period their sensory and motor behaviours were tested blindly by ST every three days. Animals were then reanaesthetized and the suture tagged L5 root re-isolated. This root was cut approximately 5 to 6 mm. distal to its

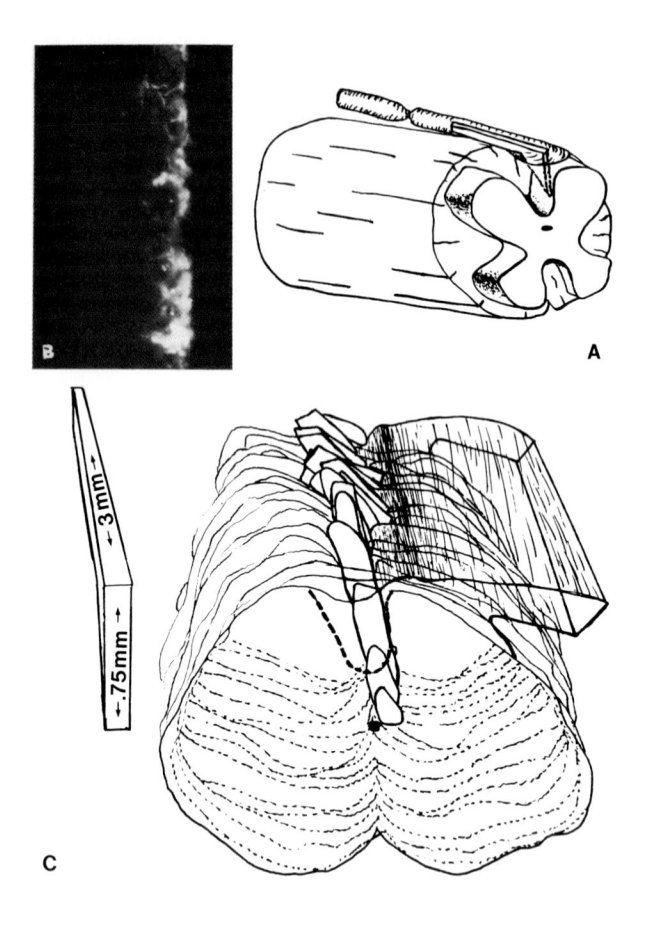

Figure 1. (A) A schematic representation of the 5th lumbar root and the spinal cord showing the placement of the pennant shaped implant. For convenience, anatomical right and left have been transposed in all figures. (B) A fluorescent photomicrograph of a cross section of the implant showing GFAP staining of the astrocytes coating the surface. (C) A three dimensional camera lucida reconstruction of serial sections taken through the full extent of the spinal cord, L5 root, and implant. This reconstruction demonstrates the exact position of the implant within the cord in relation to the dorsal columns (dashed lines), central canal (black dot), and DREZ.

DREZ and a highly concentrated solution of HRP was applied to the proximal cut end of the root for one to two hours. Great care was taken to isolate the viscous HRP from adjacent spinal roots and the underlying cord surface. The excess HRP was removed and the animals allowed to survive for 24 hours. Their sensory and motor behaviours were retested. Animals were then anaesthetized, perfused with fixative, the L5 root-cord removed en bloc and vibratome **sectioned, and** finally processed for HRP histochemistry using DAB with Cobalt Cloride intensification. The sections were examined under the microscope.

ISOLATING THE ASTROCYTES AND COATING THE MILLIPORE IMPLANT

A purified population of astrocytes was isolated from the spinal cords of embryonic day 18 old rat fetuses using a modified method of Cohen (1983). The fetuses were obtained from timed pregnant rats. The spinal cords were removed and stripped free of dura. The cells were then dissociated and incubated in polylysine coated flasks. The astrocytes differentially adhere to the polylysine. Neurons, however, are less adherent and can be removed by intermittently shaking the flasks vigorously and discarding the supernatant. After two days the remaining cells were gently trypsinized, resuspended at a concentration of ten million cells per milliliter, and finally transferred to small wells containing the pennant shaped Millipore implants (Fig. 1). GFAP staining revealed ninety-five percent purity and near total coverage of the implant surface with the astrocytes (Fig. 1B).

RESULTS

Animals having only the L5 root crushed and no Millipore implant show substantial growth of fibers past the crush site. At the DREZ axons either reverse direction and grow back towards the periphery or enter the fringe of the cord where they travel only for a short distance before ending abruptly in a sterile club. Only rarely are fibers seen to proceed past the fringe region and enter the dorsal horn grey matter. These rare fibers take meandering paths.

Animals with naked implants, in addition to the L5 root crush, show a spectrum of changes in response to this form of trauma. At the very least, a significant amount of scar tissue

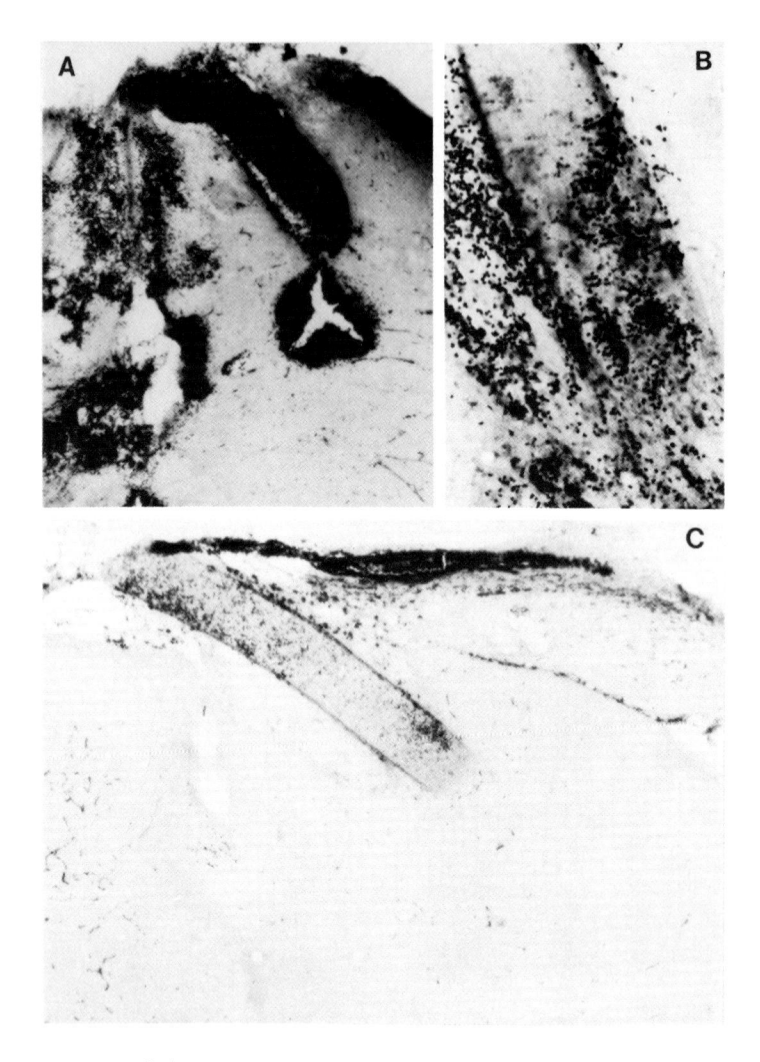

Figure 2. (A) Cross section of the cord in an animal with a naked implant (25X). Note the surrounding regions of chronic hemorrhage and cavitation, particularly along the inferior aspect of the implant and in the dorsal columns. (B) Higher mag. (63X) showing extravasated red blood cells along the implant. (C) Cross section through the cord of an animal with an implant coated with embryonic astrocytes (63X). Note the markedly reduced inflammatory response and the integration of the implant with the surrounding parenchyma.

forms at the interface between Millipore and spinal cord. In several animals a much more severe reaction developed associated with an intense infiltration of phagocytic cells (Fig. 2A,B). Areas of recurrent hemorrhage and caviation occur in the surrounding spinal cord. Animals with naked implants also show reduced ingrowth of axons into the DREZ with none found to extend into the dorsal horn.

Coating the implant with embryonic spinal cord astrocytes (Fig. 1B) gives dramatically different results. The injury response to the implant is greatly reduced and very few instances of hemorrhage or cavitation occur. Instead, in most cases, the implant becomes well integrated with the parenchyma of the spinal cord (Fig. 2C). Of even greater interest, however, is the presence of HRP-labeled axons coursing immediately adjacent to the implant surface (Fig. 3). In these regions the tissue appears to be more loosely organized and infiltrated with large numbers of small phagocytic cells often filled with yellow pigment and other debris (Fig.4).

Successful fiber ingrowth occurs when the pennant-shaped implant is positioned at the interface of dorsal columns medially and the tract of Lissauer laterally. Interestingly, in our best animal, the inserted portion replaces the lateral part of the dorsal columns and lies adjacent to the dorsal horn (Fig. 1C). In this animal the pole portion of the implant indents the surface of the cord. In addition, all along the interface of implant with cord there is intense phagocytic activity (Fig. 4A). Camera lucida reconstructions at multiple levels of this animal reveal the vast majority of axons penetrating the spinal cord immediately adjacent to either the "flag" or pole portion of the implant (Fig. 3A). Fibers entering rostrally appear to course caudally, along the implant surface, before entering appropriate regions of the dorsal horn. Fibers entering subjacent to the pole travel deep along the lateral edge of the dorsal columns before turning into the dorsal horn. Once in the dorsal horn, many of these fibers form normal appearing terminals with boutons (Fig. 5). Of particular interest is a group of fibers that course laterally and superficially immediately after penetrating the DREZ (large arrow in Fig. 5A). These fibers sweep circumferentially arround the dorsal horn and terminate in a variety of bizarrely shaped clusters of densely packed terminal boutons (Fig. 5B,C). To our knowledge, such structures have never been described before (Morgan et al., 1981; Mawe et al., 1986; Smith C, 1983 and personal communication). Some of the fibers along this pathway bypass the clusters and continue on medially (small arrow in Fig. 5A) to make normal appearing terminals in the dorsal horn. Some continue on past the midline above the central canal.

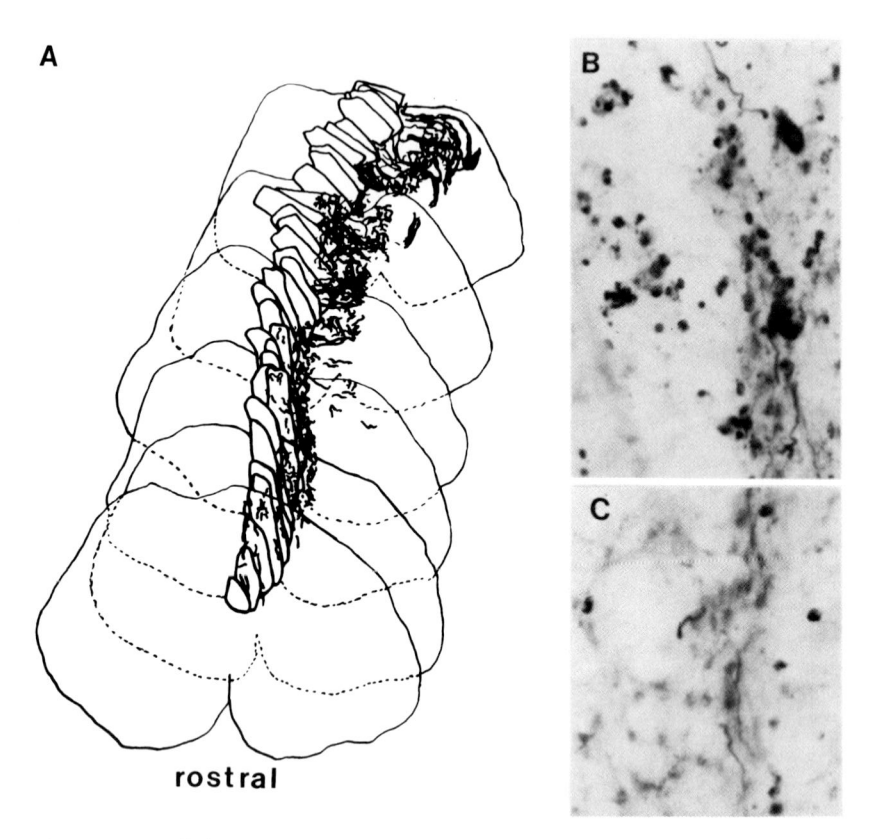

Figure 3. (A) A three dimensional camera lucida reconstruction in an animal with an embryonic astrocyte coated implant. Note the close association of ingrowing HRP-labeled fibers (drawn in black) with the implant surface. (B,C) High power photomicrographs (160X) showing individual labeled axons at two levels. (B) is taken from the third section from the front. (C) shows fibers coursing along the rostral most surface of the implant. Labeled fibers enter the cord within a narrow band of tissue immediately adjacent to only those surfaces of the implant coated with embryonic astrocytes. Note the numerous phagocytes (dark round cells) present in (B). The seperation between the implant (I) and tissue is artifactual.

During their course along the implant surface, many fibers have access to the white matter of the dorsal columns. Large numbers of these fibers enter the myelinated territory but extend only for short distances before ending in either tight spirals or sterile clubs (Fig. 5A). A small contingent of fibers grow into the Millipore implant itself (Fig. 6).

DISCUSSION

In the current study we present evidence that controlling scar formation and providing crushed dorsal root fibers with an embryonic environment, in which to bypass the intervening white matter, markedly enhances regeneration across the DREZ and into the dorsal horn. Evidence that fibers have truly regenerated is the following: 1) a close spatial correlation

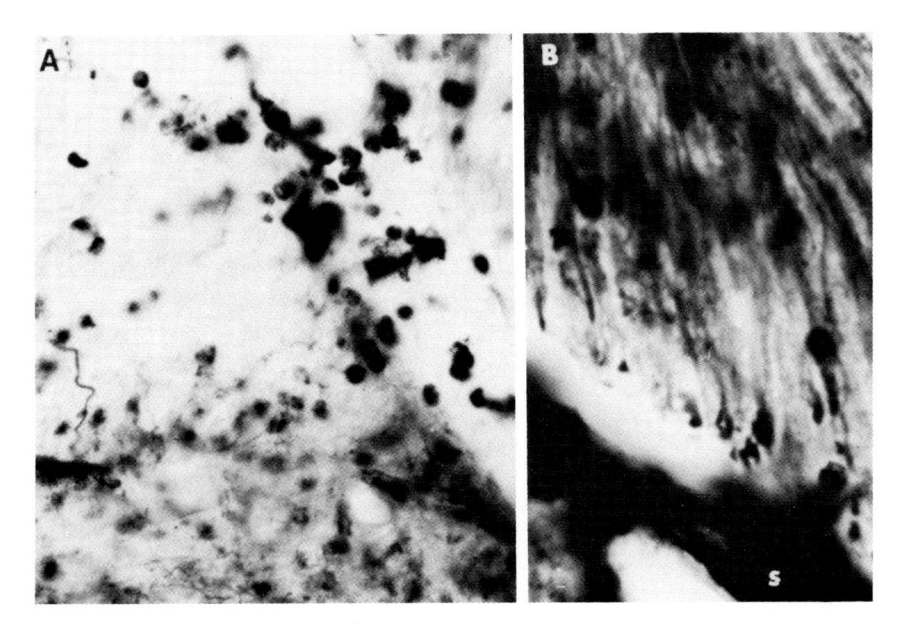

Figure 4. High power photomicrograph (400X) of the Drez immediately adjacent to the implant (A) and further laterally (B). In (A) note the absence of a basal lamina, the loose texture of the tissue, and the presence of numerous phagocytic cells. In (B) note the dense scar (S) which labeled axons are unable to penetrate.

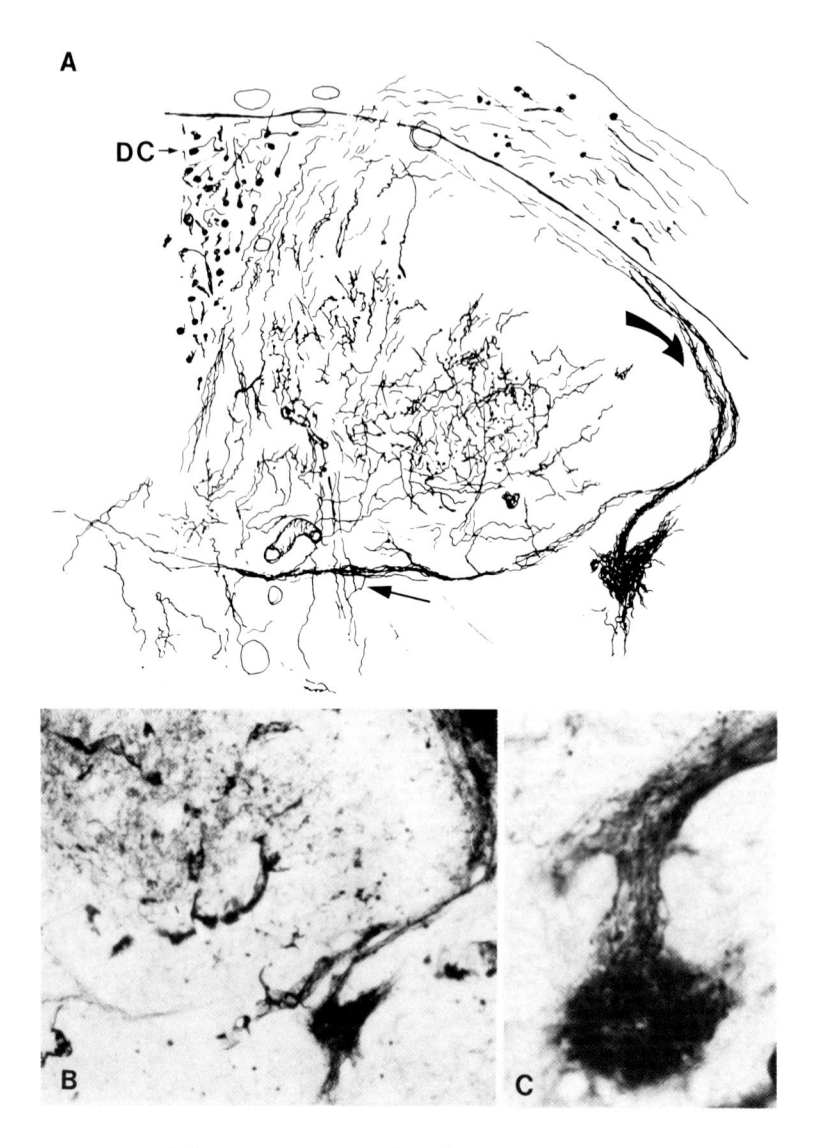

Figure 5. (A) A high mag. (25X) camera lucida drawing of a single caudal section shown in Fig. 3A. After entering the cord, ingrowing labeled fibers take one of three courses. 1) Many fibers enter the dorsal columns (DC) medially but course only for short distances and end in sterile clubs; (legend continued on facing page)

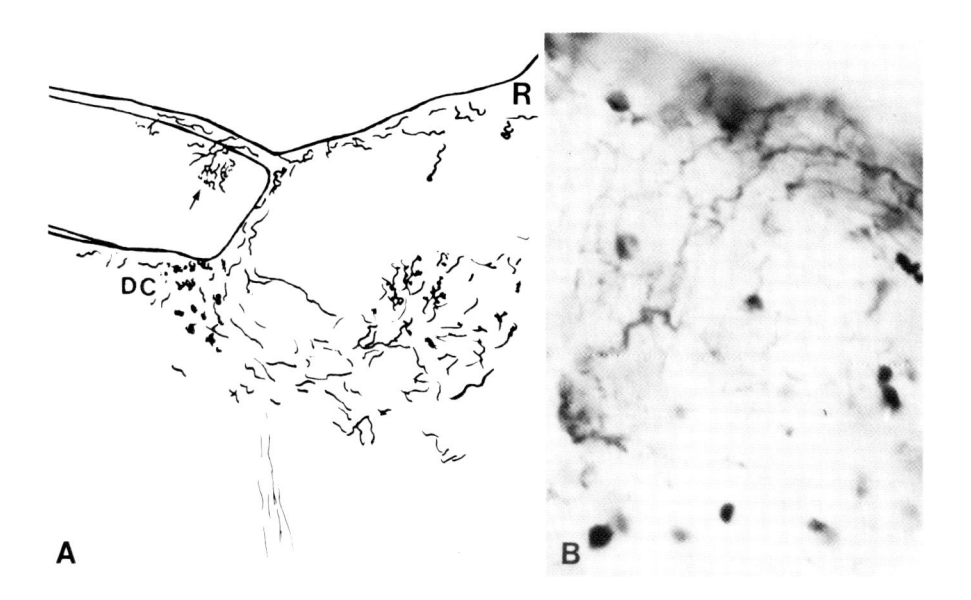

Figure 6. (A) A camera lucida drawing (63X) of a section showing HRP-labeled fibers in the root (R) coursing only along the implant surface. A group of fibers actually arborize within the implant itself (arrow). Some fibers enter the dorsal columns (DC), where they end abruptly, while others bypass the white matter and arborize within the dorsal horn. (B) A high power photomicrograph (400X) of a fiber plexus deep within the implant (I) itself.

2) Other fibers grow directly into the dorsal horn grey matter and form extensive terminal arbors; 3) A small group of fibers turns laterally and travels circumferentially arround the dorsal horn (large arrow). Some of these fibers (small arrow) then turn medially and either arborize in the deep layers of the dorsal horn or continue on across the midline. Of particular interest are a few that end in bizarrely shaped dense clusters of terminals. (B) Photomicrograph (25X) of the section drawn in (A). Note the normal appearing terminal field, in the upper left, and the terminal malformation, in the lower right. (C) High power photomicrograph (63X) of another example of an abnormal terminal cluster.

between the ingrowing fibers and only those surfaces of the implant that are coated with embryonic astrocytes, 2) the presence of highly abnormal terminal arbors, and 3) fiber growth deep within the implant itself. Other potential explanations for the pattern of axonal HRP-labelling are sparing and/or sprouting of axons that would be present regardless of the transplant. Evidence against sparing is the same as that listed above as well as the absence of labelled axons in dorsal columns rostral to the implant. In addition, similar patterns of ingrowth are not seen in any of the control animals. It is difficult to rule out a contribution to the overall axonal pattern in the cord by sprouting from the small number of fibers that normally regenerate (Liuzzi and Lasek, 1987b). However we do not think that this phenomenon is playing a significant role since we do not see extensive proximal branching of axons as they penetrate the DREZ. One of our most striking findings is the capacity of regenerating fibers to arborize extensively over large regions of the dorsal horn. The terminals are within grossly appropriate synaptic territories suggesting that there exists a level of specificity in the adult mammalian CNS similar to that postulated during development (Smith C, 1983; Carlstedt et al., 1987) and also suggested in amphibians that can regenerate spontaneously (Peng and Frank, in press). In addition, these terminals possess boutons suggesting the presence of synapses. This remarkable capacity for reinnervation is supportive of work suggesting ongoing as well as lesion induced synaptic plasticity in the adult mammalian spinal cord (Liu and Chambers, 1958; **Goldberger, 1974; Goldberger and Murray, 1982; Devor and Wall, 1981;** Knyihar-Csillik et al., 1985), peripheral nervous system (Robbins and Polak, 1987; Lichtman et al., 1987), and brain (Merzenich et al., 1987).

Although the great majority of fibers appear to make normal appearing terminals, a small number form extremely unusual configurations. The circumferential route taken by this group of fibers is similar to the arching trajectory of the lateral collateral pathway of sacral autonomic fibers (Morgan et al., 1981; Mawe et al., 1986). This reiteration of axonal pathway formation suggests the presence of spatially organized constraints, either physical or chemical, where axons regrow. In addition, all of the abnormal terminal arbors occupy a stereotyped portion of the dorsal horn. The underlying reasons for their formation at this particular location are not known. However, there are several possi-

bilities: 1) the presence of misplaced axons within this
pathway directed to inappropriate targets, and 2) a change
in the receptivity of normal target neurons in this locale,
possibly induced by denervation (Steward et al., 1988).

Not all fibers arborize after penetrating the DREZ.
Depending on their position on the implant surface, regenerating fibers are confronted with either grey matter of the
dorsal horn or white matter of the dorsal columns. As discussed above, many of the fibers entering the dorsal horn
arborize extensively. Many fibers also enter the white
matter of the dorsal columns adjacent to the implant. In
our most successful example of regeneration, the flag part
of the implant displaces the lateral portion of the dorsal
columns thereby shielding the growing fibers from interacting
with the white matter (Fig. 4). These results demonstrate
that fibers regenerating within the adult CNS can freely
enter myelinated territories. However, once within them
axons grow only for short distances, often in tight spirals,
and usually end in sterile clubs without evidence of boutons.
The in vitro studies of Schwab and colleagues (1985) provide
evidence for the inhibition of axonal growth by adult white
matter and our in vivo studies support this hypothesis.
This inhibition may also explain, at least in part, the
failure of regenerating callosal axons to grow beyond the
astrocyte coated implants and reinnervate the contralateral
hemisphere due to the intervening white matter (Silver:
unpublished observations). Limited reinnervation of target
structures does occur when white matter is bypassed using a
peripheral nerve bridge interposed between retina and tectum
(Vidal-Sanz et al., 1987). One possibility for this limi-
tation is the creation of a scar at the artificially created
PNS/CNS interface. This type of scar may be functionally
equivalent to the reactive astrocytes of the DREZ following
dorsal root crush. We have demonstrated that embryonic
astrocytes reduce the amount of scarring that would have
occurred at the DREZ secondary to placement of the implant.
What are the cellular mechanisms responsible for scar
reduction? In this study we note intense phagocytic activity
in regions immediately adjacent to the astrocyte coated
implant where axons penetrate the cord surface. It is possible that the embryonic astrocyte modulates this phagocytic
response. Recently interactions between astrocytes and
macrophages have been demonstrated (Fierz and Fontana, 1986;
Giulian and Baker, 1985). In addition, an association
between inflammatory cells and limited regeneration of per-

ipheral nerves into the cortex of adult mammals was noted by LeGros Clarke (1943). Interestingly Piromen, a drug modulating the inflammatory response, was also shown to stimulate regeneration (Windle et al., 1952).

It is likely that implants coated with embryonic astrocytes initiate a cascade of cellular interactions which result in the directed growth of dorsal root fibers over widespread areas. Although we do not know precisely which cell type is acting as the substratum for axonal regeneration in this system, the astrocyte is likely to be playing an important role (Smith et al., 1986). It is also conceivable that Schwann cells may be migrating along the implant into the CNS and thereby providing a potential substratum for axonal ingrowth (Richardson and Ebendal, 1982; Bunge, 1987).

In summary, our findings demonstrate the first method for reducing scar formation and promoting the regeneration of dorsal root afferents into appropriate regions of the adult mammalian spinal cord. In a few cases, preliminary evidence suggests that sensory function appears to be mediated through the regenerated root since sensation was reduced following transection of the root for HRP application. These results suggest that the boutons seen at the light level may be functional. However, confirmatory EM-HRP and electrophysiologic studies need to be done. This study provides hope that similar strategies using embryonic astroglia may lead to the repair of damaged intrinsic CNS pathways in animals and perhaps one day in humans.

Acknowledgements: We would like to express our gratitude for outstanding technical assistance by Catherine Doller and Stacey Horn. This work was supported by funds from the Daniel Heumann Fund for Spinal Cord Research, the Brumagin Memorial Fund, the Case Alumni Association, the American Paralysis Association, and the National Eye Institute of the NIH (#EY05952).

REFERENCES

Bunge RP (1987). Tissue culture observations relevant to the study of axon-Schwann cell interactions during peripheral nerve development and repair. J Exp Bio 132: 21.
Cajal SRY (1928). "Degeneration and Regeneration in the Nervous System." New York: Haffner.

Campbell JB, Bassett CAL, Husby J, Noback CR (1957). Regeneration of adult mammalian spinal cord. Science 126: 929.

Campbell JB, Bassett CAL (1957). The surgical application of monomolecular filters (Millipore) to bridge gaps in peripheral nerves and to prevent neuroma formation. Surg Forum 7: 570.

Carlstedt T (1983). Regrowth of anastomosed ventral root nerve fibers in the dorsal roots of rats. Brain Res 272: 162.

Carlstedt T, Dalsgaard C-J, Molander C (1987). Regrowth of lesioned dorsal root nerve fibers into the spinal cord of neonatal rats. Neurosci Letts 74: 14.

Cohen JC (1983). Handbook of Laboratory Methods. From the EMBO course on culturing of neural cells. University College of London.

David S, Aguayo AJ (1981). Axonal elongation into peripheral nervous system "bridges" after central nervous system injury in adult rats. Science 214: 931.

Devor M, Wall PD (1981). Plasticity in the spinal cord sensory map following peripheral nerve injury in rats. J Neurosci 1: 679.

Fierz W, Fontana A (1986). The role of astrocytes in the interaction between the immune and nervous system. In Federoff S, Vernadakis A (eds): "ASTROCYTES Cell Biology and Pathology" Vol 3, Orlando: Academic Press, p 203.

Giulian D, Baker TJ (1985). Peptides released by ameboid microglia regulate astroglial proliferation. J Cell Biology 101: 2411.

Goldberger ME (1974). Recovery of movement after CNS lesions in monkeys. In Stein D (ed): "Recovery of Function After Neural Lesions," New York: Academic Press, p 265.

Goldberger ME, Murray M (1982). Lack of sprouting and its presence after lesions of the cat spinal cord. Brain Res 241: 227.

Guth, L (1956). Regeneration in the mammalian peripheral nervous system. Physiol Rev 36: 441.

Knyihar-Csillik E, Rakic P, Csillik B (1985). Fine structure of growth cones in the upper dorsal horn of the adult primate spinal cord in the course of reactive synaptoneogenesis. Cell and Tissue Res 239: 633.

LeGros Clark W (1943). The problem of neuronal regeneration in the central nervous system. II. The insertion of peripheral nerve stumps into the brain. J Anat 77: 251.

Lichtman JW, Magrassi L, Purves D (1987). Visualization of neuromuscular junctions over periods of several months in living mice. J Neurosci 4: 1215.

Liu CN, Chambers WW (1958). Intraspinal sprouting of dorsal root axons. Arch Neurol Psychiat 79: 46.

Liuzzi FJ, Lasek RJ (1987). Astrocytes block axonal regeneration in mammals by activating the physiological stop pathway. Science 237: 642.

Liuzzi FJ, Lasek RJ (1987). Some dorsal root axons regenerate into the adult rat spinal cord. An HRP study. Soc Neurosci Abstr 13: 395.

Mawe GM, Bresnahan JC, Beattie MS (1986). A light and electron microscopic analysis of the sacral parasympathetic nucleus after labeling primary afferent and efferent elements with HRP. J Comp Neurol 250: 33.

Merzenich MM, Nelson RJ, Kaas JH, Stryker MP, Jenkins WM, Zook JM, Cynader MS, Schoppmann A (1987). Variability in hand surface representations in Areas 3b and 1 in adult Owl and Squirrel monkeys. J Comp Neurol 258: 281.

Morgan C, Nadelhaft I, de Groot WC (1981). The distribution of visceral primary afferents from the pelvic nerve to Lissauer's tract and the spinal grey matter and its relationship to the sacral parasympathetic nucleus. J Comp Neurol 201: 415.

Moyer EK, Kimmel DL, Winborne LW (1953). Regeneration of sensory spinal nerve roots in young and in senile rats. J Comp Neurol 98: 283.

Mcquarrie IG, Grafstein B, Gershon MD (1977). Axonal regeneration in the sciatic nerve: Effect of a conditioning lesion and of dbcAMP. Brain Res 132: 443.

Peng YY, Frank E (1988). Anatomical specificity of regenerating muscle sensory afferents in the spinal cord of the Bullfrog. J Neurobiology (in press).

Perkins S, Carlstedt T, Mizuno K, Aguayo AJ (1980). Failure of regenerating dorsal root axons to regrow into the spinal cord. Can J Neurol Sci 7: 323.

Puchala E, Windle WF (1977). The possibility of structural and functional restitution after spinal cord injury. A review. Exp Neurol 55: 1.

Reier PJ, Stensaas LJ, Guth L (1983). The astrocytic scar as an impediment to regeneration in the central nervous system. In Kao CC, Bunge RP, Reier PJ (eds): "Spinal Cord Reconstruction," New York: Raven Press, p 163.

Richardson PM, Ebendal T (1982). Nerve growth activities in the rat peripheral nerve. Brain Res 246: 57.

Robbins N, Polak J (1987). Forms of growth and retraction

at mouse neuromuscular junctions revealed by a new nerve terminal stain and correlative electron microscopy. Soc Neurosci Abstr 13: 2007.

Schreyer DJ, Jones EG (1987). Growth of corticospinal axons on prosthetic substrates introduced into the spinal cord of neonatal rats. Dev Brain Res 35: 291.

Schwab ME, Theonen H (1985). Dissociated neurons regenerate into sciatic but not optic nerve explants in culture irrespective of neurotrophic factors. J Neurosci 5: 2415.

Silver J, Sidman RL (1980). A mechanism for the guidance and topographic patterning of retinal ganglion cell axons. J Comp Neurol 189: 101.

Silver J, Lorenz SE, Wahlsten D, Coughlin J (1982). Axonal guidance during development of the great cerebral commissures: Descriptive and experimental studies in vivo on the role of preformed glial pathways. J Comp Neurol 210: 10.

Silver J, Ogawa M (1983). Postnatally induced formation of the corpus callosum in acallosal mice on glia-coated cellulose bridges. Science 220: 1067.

Smith C (1983). The development and postnatal organization of primary afferent projections to the rat thoracic spinal cord. J Comp Neurol 220: 29.

Smith GM, Miller RH, Silver J (1986). Changing role of forebrain astrocytes during development, regenerative failure, and induced regeneration upon transplantation. J Comp Neurol 251: 23.

Smith GM, Silver J (1988). Transplantation of immature and mature astrocytes and their effect on scar formation in the lesioned CNS. Prog in Brain Res (in press).

Stensaas LJ, Partlow LM, Burgess PR, Horch KW (1987). Inhibition of regeneration: The ultrastructure of reactive astrocytes and abortive axon terminals in the transition zone of the dorsal root. In Seil FJ, Herbert E, Carlson BM (eds): "Neural Regeneration," Amsterdam, Elsevier, p 457.

Steward O, Caceres AO, Reeves TM (1988). Rebuilding synapses after injury; remodelling the postsynaptic cell's receptive surface during reinnervation. In Petit TL, Ivy GO (eds): "Neural Plasticity: A Lifespan Approach," Neurology and Neurobiology Vol 36, New York, Alan R Liss, p 143.

Tello F (1907). La regeneration des voies optiques. Trab Lab Invest Biol 5: 237.

Vidal-Sanz M, Bray GM, Villegas-Perez MP, Thanos S, Aguayo AJ (1987). Axonal regeneration and synapse formation in the superior colliculus by retinal ganglion cells in the adult rat. J Neurosci 7: 2894.

Windle WF, Clemente CD, Chambers WW (1952). Inhibition of formation of a glial barrier as a means of permitting a peripheral nerve to grow into the brain. J Comp Neurol 96: 359.

Caroni P, Schwab ME (1988). Two membrane protein fractions from rat central myelin with inhibitory properties for neurite growth and fibroblast spreading. J Cell Biol 106:1281-1288.

NEURAL STRUCTURAL REPAIR AND FUNCTIONAL RESTORATION

SUCCESSFUL SPINAL CORD REGENERATION: KNOWN BIOLOGICAL STRATEGIES

Jerald J. Bernstein

Laboratory of Central Nervous System Injury and Regeneration, VA Medical Center and Departments of Neurosurgery and Physiology, The George Washington University School of Medicine, Washington, D.C.

The regenerative capacity of the vertebrate spinal cord is nonexistent if the classical definition of regeneration ["the renewal or repair of lost tissue or parts"] is invoked. This is due to the fact that the classical definition implies that there must be duplication of the organ or tissue involved. This is not the case in regeneration of the spinal cord. In lower vertebrates that can regenerate their spinal cord, return of function occurs in the absence of normal prelesion anatomy and physiology. This ability to regenerate the spinal cord should be termed *regenerative capacity*. This capacity is studied reductionistically in modern biological science and the most minuscule phenomena in the regenerative process are being studied. However, the regenerative capacity of the spinal cord will only be defined by the holistic phenomenon of the return of function, such as walking.

Since lower vertebrates show considerable regenerative capacity in the absence of restitution of normal anatomy and physiology, medical science can be optimistic about the possibility for spinal cord regeneration in humans utilizing the return of function as the definition for spinal cord regeneration. The study of lower vertebrate biological strategies for the restitution of function are a valuable scientific tool for understanding interventions to restore function in human para- and quadraplegics.

The absence of restitution of normal anatomy of the spinal cord with the return of function occurs in the primitive adult fish, the lamprey (Cohen and Hall, 1986; Mackler et al, 1986; Mackler and Selzer, 1985; Yin and Selzer, 1983; Buchanan and Cohen, 1982), bony fish (Bernstein et al, 1978; Bernstein and Geldered, 1973; Bernstein and Geldered, 1970; Bernstein, 1970; Bernstein and Bernstein, 1969; Bernstein and Bernstein, 1967; Bernstein, 1964) and adult salamander (Piatt, 1955). After spinal cord regeneration in the adult lamprey and bony fish there are aberrant terminations of the regenerated axons neurons rostral to the transection and the normal diameter axons were local or did not pass the site of the original transection. After the second spinal transection the fish were again paraplegic and lay on their sides on the bottom of the aquarium (Bernstein et al, 1978; Bernstein and Geldered, 1973). These data show that the large regenerated axons were necessary for the return of function although they constituted only approximately 30-44% of the original compliment of axons.

The next question that arose was: did the large axons regenerate to the original sites of termination and restore the original synaptic map as in the visual system of the fish. The answer was no. There was no point-for-point (Sperry, 1965; Attardi and Sperry, 1963) anatomical regeneration of axons or reconstitution of physiological regeneration in the fish or any regenerating spinal cord. What ocurred was the regeneration of long descending tract axons into the locomotor generator neuronal circuit (Grillner, 1985; Grillner and Wallen, 1985; Grillner, 1973) in the ventral horn of the spinal cord and a loss of direct long tract innervation of the motoneurons.

The evidence for spinal cord axon regeneration in the young of the year goldfish comes from a series of experiments which utilized a modified silver stain for the visualization of synaptic terminals (Bernstein et al, 1978; Bernstein and Geldered, 1973). Using coded counts, the numbers of terminals [two cm from the transection] were determined for normal numbers of synaptic terminals on intermediate gray matter neurons, ventral horn interneuron [locomotor generator neurons] somata and ventral horn motoneuron somata and motoneuron dendrite. The number of terminals on these neurons were determined over a 60 day period after transection of the spinal cord just rostral to the dorsal fin [Figs 2-5]. In order to determine the termination of the regenerated axons, a group of animals had their spinal cord retransected

---

Fig. 1. A. 60 days after spinal cord transection 4X8 times larger than normal axons [arrows] were observed in the regenerated ventral tract 2.0 cm from the transection [protargol X 1200] (Bernstein and Geldered, 1970).

B. Nine days after retransection [at 60 days] the large axons [arrows] degenerated whereas the normal diameter axons did not [silver stain for degenerating axons X 975] (Bernstein and Geldered, 1970).

Fig. 2. Number of synaptic terminals on neurons in the intermediate gray, 2.0 cm from the site of a spinal cord transection [over 60 days]. Square represents spinal retransection in a separate group of animals. The retransection data is represented as 65 days (Bernstein and Geldered, 1973).

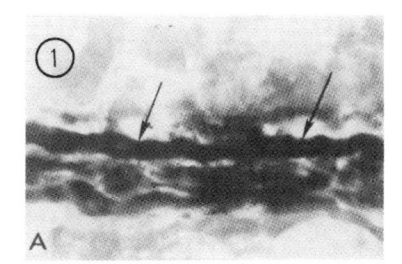

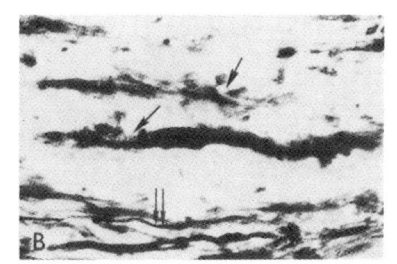

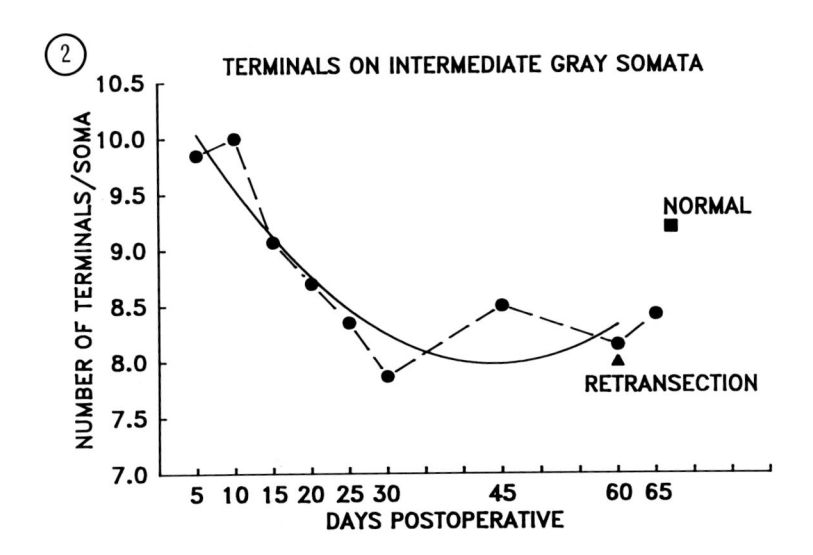

Spinal Cord Regeneration / 335

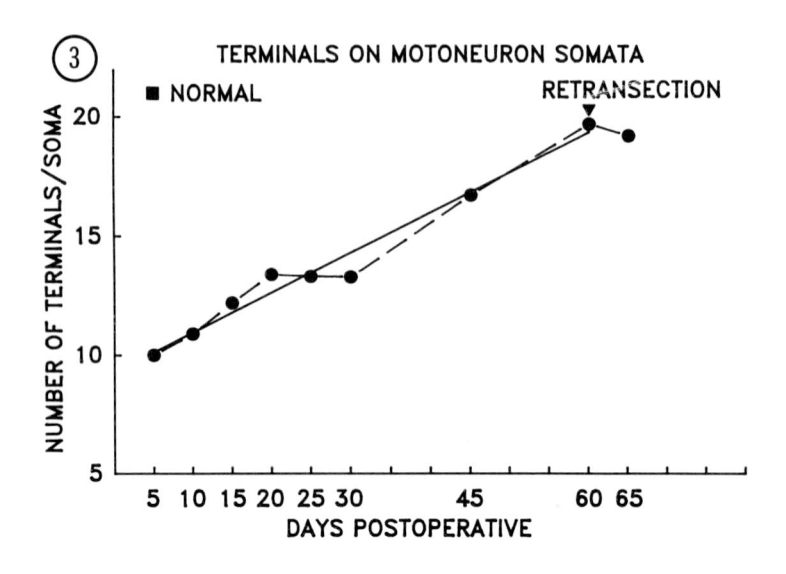

3 TERMINALS ON MOTONEURON SOMATA

Figure 3.

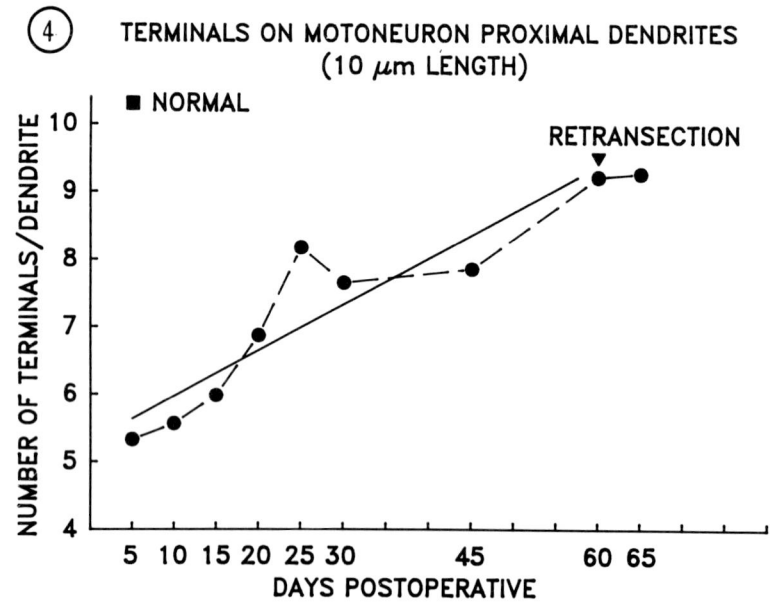

4 TERMINALS ON MOTONEURON PROXIMAL DENDRITES (10 μm LENGTH)

Figure 4.

[one segment rostral to the original transection] 60 days later. These animals spinal cords were examined 5 days later when it is known that the degenerating and degenerated synaptic terminals would not take up silver (Bernstein et al, 1978; Bernstein and Geldered, 1973).

Neurons in the intermediate gray matter were slowly deafferented over 30 days and then remained chronically deafferented to 60 days [Fig. 2]. Retransection of the spinal cord did not effect the number of synaptic terminals on these neurons. These data show that the regenerated descending long tract axons did not reinnervate intermediate gray neurons. In addition, the slow decline in synaptic terminal number suggests that the intermediate gray neurons were polysynaptically innervated.

Motoneuron soma [Fig. 3] and dendrites [Fig. 4] were directly innervated by the axons of the long descending tracts. Spinal cord transection resulted in an immediate loss of about 50% of the terminals on both the soma and dendrite of the motoneuron. This was followed by a slow increase in the number of terminals to near normal or normal numbers of terminals by 60 days. Interestingly, retransection of the spinal cord did not result in an immediate loss of terminals on the dendrite or soma of the motoneuron although the retransected fish were paraplegic. These data show that the regenerated descending long tract axons did not reinnervate the motoneuron. The regenerating axons which restored 50% of the normal complement of synaptic terminals for motoneurons were derived derived from local axon sprouting.

The neuron that was reinnervated by the descending long tract axons was the ventral horn interneuron which is the locomotor generator neuron [Fig. 5]. This neuron was normally innervated by the long descending spinal tracts since the initial spinal transection of the spinal cord resulted in partial denervation of the soma. This was followed by a return to normal numbers at 20-30 days [normal swimming also returned]. From 45 to 60 days the locomotor generator

---

Fig. 3. Number of synaptic terminals on motoneuron soma as in Fig. 2.

Fig. 4. Number of synaptic terminals on motoneuron dendrites as in Fig. 2.

5 TERMINALS ON VENTRAL HORN INTERNEURON SOMATA

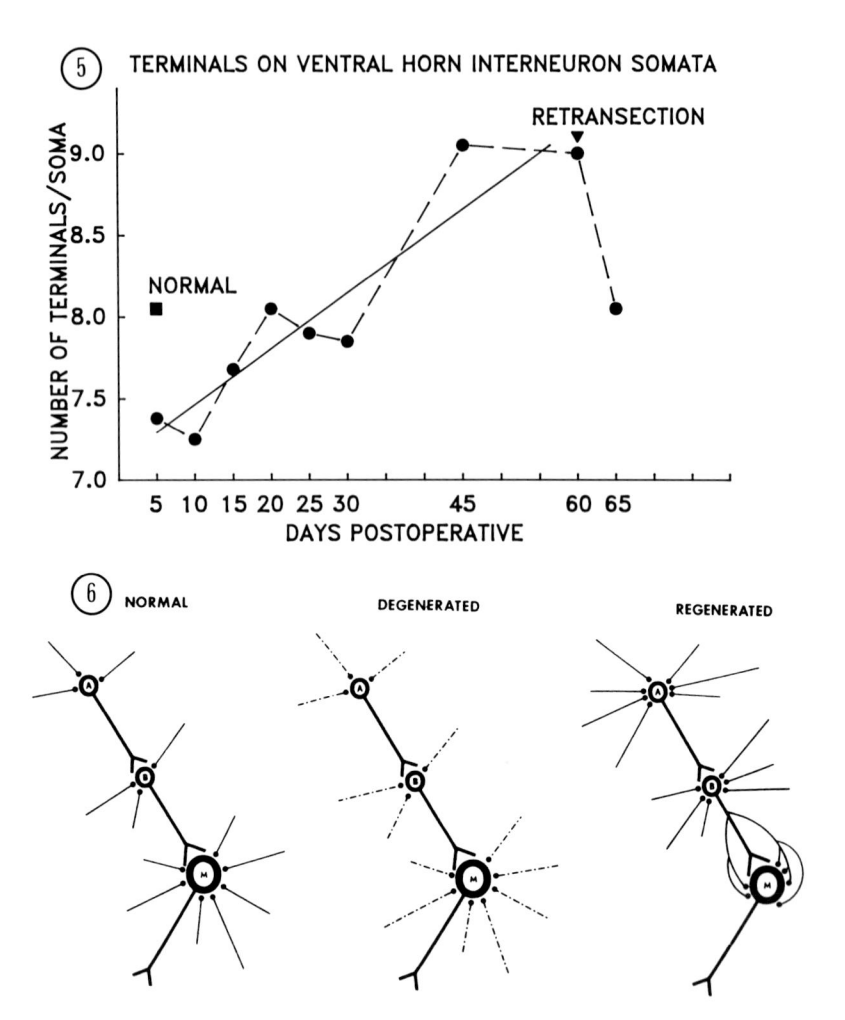

Fig. 5. Number of synaptic terminals on ventral horn interneurons [locomotor generator neurons] as in Fig. 2.

Fig. 6. Schematic of alteration of the locomotor generator circuit in the regenerated spinal cord of the goldfish. The locomotor generator neurons [A,B] and motoneurons [B] normally receive long tract and local innervation [left]. After spinal cord transection the long tracts degenerated [middle, dashed line]. After regeneration the long tracts soley terminate on/ and hyperinnervate the locomotor generator neurons which sprout and reinnervate the motoneuron, restoring the locomotor generator circuit [right] (Bernstein et al, 1978).

neurons were hyperinnervated. Retransection of the spinal cord at 60 days resulted an immediate decrease to normal numbers of synaptic terminals on soma with a concomitant return of paraplegia. These data show that these cells were innervated by the regenerated descending long tracts [because of loss of swimming and terminals after retransection] and were the only recipients of direct long tract descending regenerated axons.

The return of the upright posture at 12 days after the first transection was probably due to local sprouting since there was not enough time to regenerate the long tacts. The initiation of swimming appeared to be the result of the arrival of early regenerating long tract fibers on the locomotor generator neurons at 20-25 days. The retransection data of the spinal cord at 60 days shows that the locomotor generator neurons were hyperinnervated by the descending regenerated long tract axons. The motoneurons were reinnervated by local sprouting most probably derived from the hyperinnervated locomotor generator neurons since the number of synaptic terminals increased from 30-60 days on motoneuron soma and dendrite [Schematic Fig. 6].

The spinal cord regenerative strategy utilized by the goldfish was reinnervation of only the locomotor generator neuron. This strategy was the most efficient regenerative mechanism since the neuronal locomotor generator circuit appeared to be reinnervated at the most plastic part of the neuronal circuit and resulted in functional regeneration.

There was a remarkable degree of recovery after transection of the spinal cord of young weanling rats whereas this did not occur after transection of the adult rat spinal cord (Bernstein, 1987; Bryz-Gornia and Stelzner, 1986; Bernstein and Stelzner, 1983; Cummings et al, 1981; Stelzner and Weber, 1979; Prendergast and Stelzner, 1976a,b). This could be due to the retention of the primitive local spinal locomotor generator circuit in spinal transected young weanling rats [less than 5 days postnatal (Prendergast and Stelzner, 1976a,b)]. This is of interest since the pyramidal or corticospinal system had not grown to the lower thoracic and lumbar spinal cord by that time. There was never any descending pyramidal system control to modify the primitive circuit. This could be the basis for the young-old dichotomy in the recovery of function in vertebrates, the presence and influence of the extrapyramidal system in lower vertebrates and the presence and influence of the pyramidal system in mammals.

This regenerative strategy of reinnervation of the locomotor pattern generator neuron probably evolved from the primative chordates. The pattern generator was an early vertebrate nervous system mechanism adopted for locomotion which is present in developing and adult mammalian tetrapods (Grillner, 1985; Grillner and Wallen, 1985; Grillner, 1973), developing bipeds and bipeds after injury or diseases of the nervous system. Activation of this repressed primitive locomotor circuit might be the basis for the alternate leg stepping spastic response seen in human para- and quadraplegics. If this was the case then the numbers of axons from selected descending tracts necessary for the return of walking might be less than previously thought.

The author thanks Ms. M.F. Bernstein for her many years of hard work and critical thinking. The topic of this chapter was based on the symposium presentations [J.B. chairman] of Drs. A. Cohen, M. Selzer and D. Stelzner who have chapters in this volume.

REFERENCES

Attardi D, Sperry R (1963): Prefential selection of central pathways by regenerating optic fibers. Exp Neurol 9:161-174.
Bernstein D, Stelzner D (1983): Plasticity of corticospinal tract following midthoracic spinal injury in the postnatal rat. J Comp Neurol 221:382-400.
Bernstein JJ (1987): Spinal Cord Regeneration. Davidoff RA (ed.): "Handbook of the Spinal Cord. Vol 4." New York, Marcel Dekker, pp 97-118.
Bernstein JJ (1970): Anatomy and physiology of the central nervous system. Hoar W, Randall D (eds.): "Fish Physiology, Vol.4." New York, Academic Press, pp 1-90.
Bernstein JJ (1964): Relation of spinal cord regeneration to age in adult goldfish. Brain Res 9:161-174.
Bernstein JJ, Bernstein ME (1969): Ultrastructure of normal regeneration and loss of regenerative capacity following teflon blockage of goldfish spinal cord. Exp Neurol 24:538-557.
Bernstein JJ, Bernstein ME (1967): Effects of glial-ependymal scar and teflon arrest on the regenerative capacity of goldfish spinal cord. Exp Neurol 19:25-32.
Bernstein JJ, Geldered J (1973): Synaptic reorganization following regeneration of goldfish spinal cord. Experimental Neurology 41:402-410.
Bernstein JJ, Geldered J (1970): Regeneration of the long spinal tracts in the goldfish. Brain Res 20:33-38.
Bernstein JJ, Wells M, Bernstein ME (1978): Spinal cord regeneration: Synaptic renewal and neurochemistry. Cotman C (ed.): "Neuronal Plasticity." New York, Raven Press, pp 49-71.
Bryz-Gornia W, Stelzner D (1986): Ascending tract neurons survive spinal cord transection in the neonatal rat. Exp Neurol 93:195-210.
Buchanan J, Cohen A (1982): Activities of identified interneurons, motoneurons, and muscle fibers during fictive swimming in the lamprey and effects of reticulospinal and dorsal cell stimulation. J Neurophysiol 47:948-960.
Cohen MJ, Hall GF (1986): Control of neuron shape during development and regeneration. Neurochem Pathol 5:331-343.
Cohen A, Mackler S, Selzer M (1986): Functional regeneration following

spinal transection in the isolated spinal cord of the larval sea lamprey. PNAS 83:2763-2766.

Cohen A, Wallen P (1980): The neuronal correlate of locomotion in fish. "Fictive swimming: induced in an in vitro preparation of the lamprey spinal cord". Exp Brain Res 41:11-18.

Cummings J, Bernstein D, Stelzner D (1981): Further evidence that sparing of function after spinal cord transection in the neonatal rat is not due to axonal generation or regeneration. Exp Neurol 74:615-620.

Grillner S (1985): Neurobiological bases of rhythmic motor acts in vertebrates. Science 228:143-149.

Grillner S (1973): Locomotion in the spinal cat. Adv Behav Biol 7:515-535.

Grillner S, Wallen P (1985): Central pattern generators for locomotion with special reference to vertebrates. Ann Rev Neurosci 8:380-386.

Mackler S, Selzer M (1987): Specificity of synaptic regeneration in the spinal cord of the larval sea lamprey. J Physiol (Lond) 388:183-198.

Mackler S, Selzer M (1985): Regeneration of functional syapses between individual recognizable neurons in the lamprey spinal cord. Science 229:774-776.

Mackler S, Yin H, Selzer M (1986): Determinants of directional specificity in the regeneration of lamprey spinal axons. J Neurosci 6:1814-1821.

Piatt J (1955): Regeneration of the spinal cord of the salamander. J Exp Zool 129:177-207.

Prendergast J, Stelzner D (1976a): Increases in collateral axon growth rostral to a thoracic hemisection in neonatal and weanling rat. J Comp Neurol 166:145-162.

Prendergast J, Stelzner D (1976b): Changes in the magnocellular portion of the red nucleus following thoracic hemisection in the neonatal and adult rat. J Comp Neurol 166:163-172.

Sperry R (1965): Embryogenesis of behavioral nerve nets. Dehaan D, Ursprung H (eds.): "Organogenesis." New York, Holt, Rhineland and Winston, pp 161-186.

Sperry R (1963): Chemoaffinity in the orderly growth of nerve fiber patterns and connections. PNAS 50:703-710.

Stelzner DJ, Weber ED (1979): A comparison of the effect of mid-thoracic spinal hemisection in neonatal and weanling rats on the distribution and density of dorsal root axons in the lumbosacral spinal cord of the adult. Brain Res 172:407-426.

Windle W (1955): "Regeneration in the Central Nervous System." Springfield, Ill., Charles C. Thomas.

Yin H, Selzer M (1983): Axonal regeneration in lamprey spinal cord. J Neurosci 3:1135-1144.

PLASTICITY AND RECOVERY OF FUNCTION AFTER INJURY TO THE
DEVELOPING SPINAL CORD OF THE RAT

Dennis J. Stelzner and James M. Cullen

Department of Anatomy and Cell Biology, SUNY
Health Science Center, Syracuse, New York 13210

INTRODUCTION

The development and recovery of function which occurs after injury to the developing mammalian central nervous system (CNS) is often greater than the amount of recovery seen in an adult animal after the same injury. This phenomenon is often referred to as sparing of function or the infant lesion effect (Johnson and Almli, 1978; Schneider et al., 1985). In various situations, different mechanisms are responsible for this effect. For instance, learning plays a role. An animal growing up with a damaged nervous system may learn strategies that allow it to solve problems with parts of the nervous system not used for this purpose in the normal animal. It may be more difficult for the adult animal to learn new strategies with its established habits. With long postoperative survival times or with special training of operated adult animals, differences between them and infant operates sometimes disappear (Beck and Chambers, 1970; Goldberger, 1972; Kennard, 1942).

Besides behavioral adaptations, other changes occuring within the substrate of the CNS may also be responsible for sparing of function. It is this type of plasticity that our laboratory has been investigating. Sparing of function does not occur uniformly throughout the CNS (Goldman, 1974; Johnson and Almli, 1978). The state of maturation of a system at the time it is damaged is an important factor related to the degree of sparing seen. The clearest type of CNS plasticity which is responsible for sparing of function occurs when a lesion which damages a pathway responsible for a particular behavior in the adult animal does not actually cut this pathway in the developing animal. For instance, the corticospinal tract (CST) is still elongating and forming connections in altricial mammalian species. After pyramidotomy or partial spinal cord injury which cuts the region through which the CST normally grows, developing CST axons are able to grow around the region of damage (Bernstein and Stelzner, 1983; Bregman and Goldberger, 1983; Kalil and Reh, 1979, 1982; Schreyer and Jones, 1983). Connections are formed controlling behaviors which are lost when this pathway is then cut or is cut in normal adult animals (Bregman and Goldberger, 1983; Reh and Kalil, 1982). Another form of CNS plasticity is the retention of exuberant projections which would normally be lost during development. These "saved" projections can then subserve the spared behavior (Leonard and Goldberger, 1987). The anatomical substrate for a different type of developmental CNS plasticity is more difficult to discern. When the midthoracic spinal cord is completely transected in the neonate, isolating the lumbosacral enlargement from all descending influences, the development and recovery of hindlimb behaviors is much greater than when the same lesion is made in the adult animal. In this case, regeneration or continued growth of developing axons across the lesion site does not occur. Therefore, the plasticity must take place within the isolated cord, itself. It is this form of plasticity which concerns most of the discussion of this paper.

THE EFFECT OF SPINAL TRANSECTION DURING POSTNATAL DEVELOPMENT.

A number of laboratories, including our own, have studied the postnatal development and recovery of hindlimb responses after neonatal midthoracic spinal cord transection in several different altricial species (Forssberg, 1979; Forssberg et al., 1974; Goldberger, 1986; Robinson and Goldberger, 1986a; Shurrager and Dykman, 1951; Smith et al, 1982; Stelzner et al, 1975; Viala et al, 1986; Weber and Stelzner, 1977). Although special training or therapy did foster the appearance of certain behaviors (Kozak and Westerman, 1966; Shurrager and Dykman, 1951; Viala et al, 1986) sparing of function was also seen in cases where neonatal operates received no conditioning or special handling. All of these studies have a number of findings in common. In the neonate, behavioral responses in the hindlimbs show much greater autonomy and are much less influenced by supraspinal sources than in the adult. Many responses seen prior to midthoracic spinal transection in the neonatal operate are apparent immediately after recovery from anesthesia. The response depression always seen in the immediate postoperative period in adult operates (spinal shock, diaschisis) is minimal in neonates. In general, the appearance of responses in the hindlimbs follows the same sequence as normal response ontogeny. However, certain neonatal reflexes that normally disappear as supraspinal control predominates remain permanent in neonatal operates. In addition, the development of certain locomotor and supporting reactions appear earlier in neonatal operates than in unoperated littermates. Apparently, these behaviors are already programmed in the spinal cord at birth but are under inhibition from descending sources. The behavioral repertoire of the chronic neonatal operate is complete near the time of normal response maturation. Therefore, the development of the circuitry underlying these behaviors appears programmed to continue to develop at a normal rate within the isolated spinal cord. Even though responses seldom attain all of the characteristics of the fully mature response in normal animals, responses such as hindlimb supporting reactions and locomotor responses are consistently seen in chronic neonatal operates. These responses are never seen in the spinally transected adult rat (Stelzner et al., 1975; ; Stelzner et al., 1986; Stelzner, 1986; Weber and Stelzner, 1977) and, in the spinally transected adult cat are seen inconsistently, at long postoperative survival periods, and never to the degree seen in the neonatal operates (Goldberger, 1986; Robinson and Goldberger, 1986a; Rossignol et al, 1986; Smith et al., 1986). The hindlimbs of neonatal operates are more responsive to various stimuli than adult operates. Even low threshold contact or "tactile" placing is seen although it is more variable than in the unoperated animal (Forssberg et al, 1974; Goldberger, 1986; Weber and Stelzner, 1980). In the adult mammal, tactile placing is dependent on the cerebral cortex and is permanently lost when the sensorimotor cortex is ablated. Table 1 summarizes the behavioral differences seen in rats chronically surviving midthoracic spinal transection made at the neonatal or at the weanling/adult stage.

Table 1

Chronic Hindlimb Behaviors of Rats
Spinally Transected at Different Ages

Neonatal Operates	Weanling/Adult Operates
1. Spinal shock minimal	1. Spinal shock pronounced
2. Wriggling, long lasting	2. Wriggling, brief
3. Spontaneous responses common: scratch, flexion reflexes, few spasms	3. Spasms and choreoathetoid movements common: scratch, flexion reflexes present
4. Hindlimb support	4. not present
5. Locomotor responses: stepping, hopping	5. " "
6. Hindlimb replacement	6. " "
7. Hindlimb palpitations	7. " "
8. Extensor thrust responses	8. " "
9. "Tactile placing"	9. " "

The age or stage of development at which sparing of function is no longer demonstrable after midthoracic spinal transection has been most clearly defined in the rat (Weber and Stelzner, 1977). The period between 12 and 15 days of age appears to be critical in this species. Twelve day operates recover or develop many of the same hindlimb behaviors seen in chronic neonatal operates. Twelve day operates initially lose many of the hindlimb responses that had developed by this age showing that these responses had been influenced by supraspinal sources. However, spinal shock is not as marked as in the adult operate. Instead, the responses in the immediate postoperative period are similar to those seen during this postoperative period in neonatal operates. Many of the responses initially lost in 12 day operates recover by the end of the first postoperative week. These same responses have not yet developed by 7 days of age in normal animals or in newborn operates. The ultimate amount of recovery seen in 15 day operates is much less and the amount of response depression is much greater when compared with that seen in 12 day operates. In most respects, the initial level of spinal shock and final paraplegic state are equivalent to that seen in the adult operate.

It is surprising that the critical period for sparing of function ends between 12 and 15 days of age in the rat for all of the different categories of behavior tested. Since various responses appear at different times over the first two to three postnatal weeks, something in addition to the time of first appearance of a behavior is important for its subsequent recovery. Data show that the final maturation of connections from descending sources and the completion of synaptogenesis within the lumbosacral gray matter are, at least, temporally related to sparing of function. Other than the corticospinal tract, which innervates the gray matter of the lumbosacral enlargement at the end of the second postnatal week (Donatelle, 1977), other nerve tracts descending to the lumbosacral enlargement are already present during the neonatal period (Bregman, 1987; Leong et al, 1984; Shieh et al, 1983). However, although these pathways are present, innervation of the lumbosacral gray by these pathways is incomplete until relatively late in development. For instance, the innervation by serotonergic descending reticulospinal projections does not become mature until the third postnatal week even though these pathways are present in the lumbosacral spinal cord at birth (Bregman, 1987). Probably not off the point, locomotor centers in the upper brainstem which project to these reticulospinal neurons, also show large maturational changes at the beginning of the third postnatal week (Conrad et al, 1987). Even the overall distribution of descending axons within the gray matter remains incomplete until the beginning of the third postnatal week using a degeneration method to show these projections (Gilbert and Stelzner, 1979). In addition, degenerating synaptic endings can not be identified in the intermediate gray matter after cutting all descending nerve tracts until animals are 12-18 days of age at the time of injury, a time when behavioral maturation is also nearing completion. At least using the degeneration method as a criterion, few mature connections from descending nerve tracts are present in the lumbosacral spinal cord until the end of the critical period for sparing of function. Moreover, the growth of the gray matter in the L6 segment of the normal animal, and after midthoracic spinal transection at birth, increases rapidly during the first two postnatal weeks nearing completion by 15 days of age (Stelzner et al, 1986; Weber and Stelzner, 1980). Synaptogenesis in the intermediate gray matter also appears to near completion in the early part of the third postnatal week (Weber and Stelzner, 1980).

Taken together, all of the data discussed in the above paragraph suggest that the maturation of descending and intrinsic connections are closely linked with the end of sparing of function. Clearly, the amount of supraspinal influence on spinal circuitry also increases as these circuits mature. The increased amount of response depression or spinal shock seen after spinal cord transection beginning at 15 days of age reflects this maturation (Chambers et al, 1973). Prior to this time, spinal reflexes and the intrinsic functioning of the spinal cord can operate independently after spinal transection. After this time, the spinal circuitry appears to be permanently modified so that certain circuits are unable to operate without supraspinal connections. The loss of supraspinal influences may cause a physiological or anatomical rearrangement of the circuitry in the mature isolated spinal cord, thereby suppressing the normal functioning of these circuits (reviewed in Stelzner, 1982). Spinal transection prior to 15 days of age may have a less deleterious affect on the spinal circuits controlling the spared behaviors and the developmental plasticity seen may, in essence, be an escape from the pathology found in the mature animal. However, it may be that blocking the growth of descending connections prior to the time synaptogenesis is complete may allow intrinsic connections to remain or be formed unlike the normal animal or adult operate. Competition may normally occur between descending and segmental connections leading to the elimination of many local connections that subserve the spared behaviors that are found after neonatal spinal transection. Synaptic reorganization of this type has been seen in the isolated spinal cord of the neonatal operate. In the rat, the dorsal root projection is increased in the neonatal but not the weanling operate (Hulsebosch and Coggeshall, 1983; Stelzner et al, 1979). Such an increase in dorsal root input could increase the amount of facilitation driving the spinal circuitry underlying the spared behaviors. In the cat, a change in the distribution of glutamic acid decarboxylase (GAD) immunoreactivity, a marker of gamma-aminobutryric acid (GABA), an inhibitory neurotransmitter contained in intrinsic spinal neurons, was seen only in the dorsal horn of neonatal operates. GAD immunoreactivity was reduced in lamina II compared to normal animals or adult operates (Robinson and Goldberger, 1986b). This suggests that removal of descending projections during development has allowed intrinsic inhibitory synapses to be reorganized in the kitten. A difference in the amount of inhibition of spinal circuitry between adult and neonatal operates was also shown in this experiment by the enhanced locomotor behavior seen in only adult operates when they were given bicuculline, a GABA antagonist.

THE EFFECTS OF BILATERAL THORACIC SPINAL HEMISECTIONS IN THE NEWBORN AND WEANLING RAT.

A number of experiments have been done in the adult mammal where hemisection lesions are made several segments apart on opposite sides of the spinal cord (Basbaum, 1973; Kato et al, 1985; Lassek and Anderson, 1961; Ingebritsen, 1933; Jane et al, 1964)). In this way an attempt is made to cut all long ascending and descending tracts on both sides of the spinal cord but leave an intact area of spinal cord between the lesions. Normal propriospinal connections terminating in the zone between the two lesions and neurons within this zone which project out of it could serve as a functional bridge connecting the spinal tissue rostral and caudal to the double hemisection lesions. In addition, nerve tracts damaged by the lesions could terminate anomalously within this region either forming new connections or increasing the number of connections made within this zone by regenerative or collateral sprouts (Prendergast and Stelzner, 1976). These experiments have shown a variable amount of recovery including, in most instances, recovery of locomotor and supporting reactions. However, the majority of the reconstructed lesion sites showed some sparing, particularly in the ventral or ventrolateral funiculi. This region is especially important for locomotion (Eidelberg, 1981). A small number of spared axons in this region results in considerable behavioral recovery. Modern neuroanatomical tract tracing methods have not been used in these experiments to evaluate sparing or potential growth of pathways within the region between the lesions. We felt that this double hemisection model would be another way to evaluate the different types of anatomical and behavioral plasticity seen in the developing rat spinal cord.

Hemisection lesions were made on opposite sides of the spinal cord and were intended to slightly overlap the midline and be separated by 1-2 spinal segments (T5-T6; double hemisection, DH operates). Hindlimb motor behavior was then assessed at regular intervals for 6 p.o. months. Our analysis included the same behavioral tests used previously to document the development and recovery of function after midthoracic spinal cord transection of neonatal and weanling operates (Weber and Stelzner, 1977). A rating scale was used to quantitate behavioral development and recovery. A score of 0 was equal to the hindlimb responses seen in the acute spinally transected adult rat and a score of 75 was equal to the hindlimb responses seen in the chronic spinally transected newborn rat. One month old female rats (N=18) and newborn rats of both sexes (less than 24 hrs old; N=16) survived these lesions for the full postoperative period. Lumbar injections of 3H-proline were made 6 days prior to sacrifice to anterogradely label ascending nerve tracts arising from this region and multiple injections of HRP were made two spinal segments below the caudal hemisection 2 days prior to sacrifice to retrogradely label neurons having axons either terminating in this area or damaged by the injections. These methods and reconstructions of each lesion site were used to evaluate lesion completeness.

In all cases, Nissl staining of the longitudinally sectioned tissue as well as the axonal tracing methods show that the spinal tissue remaining between the two lesions is viable and neuronal morphology appears normal. The anatomical tracing methods have been particularly informative for understanding the behavioral findings in weanling operates (Cullen and Stelzner, 1986a; In preparation). Behavioral differences between animals are marked, some animals having differences in amount of recovery between the hindlimbs, some animals showing only moderate impairments of balance and coordination, and some having only the minimal behavioral recovery previously seen in the spinally transected adult or weanling rat. Ascending nerve tracts terminate unilaterally in the interlesion zone, mainly in the intermediate gray matter contralateral to the caudal hemisection. Many retrogradely labeled neurons are apparent bilaterally within this region, mainly within the intermediate gray, laminae VII-VIII of Rexed. Larger numbers of labeled neurons are seen in the gray matter contralateral to the caudal hemisection but the labeling appears symmetrical. Only the three animals showing behavioral deficits similar to spinally transected weanling operates (Fig. 1) have two complete spinal hemisection lesions. The remaining animals show evidence of fiber sparing confined to either the ventral part of the lateral funiculus or the medial portion of the ventral funiculus. In these cases, neurons are retrogradely labeled in the brainstem, particularly in reticular nuclei that project to the spinal cord. We conclude from the results in the three weanling operates with complete bilateral hemisection lesions that when all long tract axons are cut, propriospinal connections from the spared tissue between the two lesions have no obvious behavioral effect on recovery of hindlimb responses. This is true even though descending axons terminate in the region between the two lesions and neurons within it descend out of this zone into the caudal spinal tissue. Electrophysiological data and further anatomical results are needed to determine if an actual functional circuit is present and further behavioral experiments are needed to determine if this potential functional circuit can be enhanced by training.

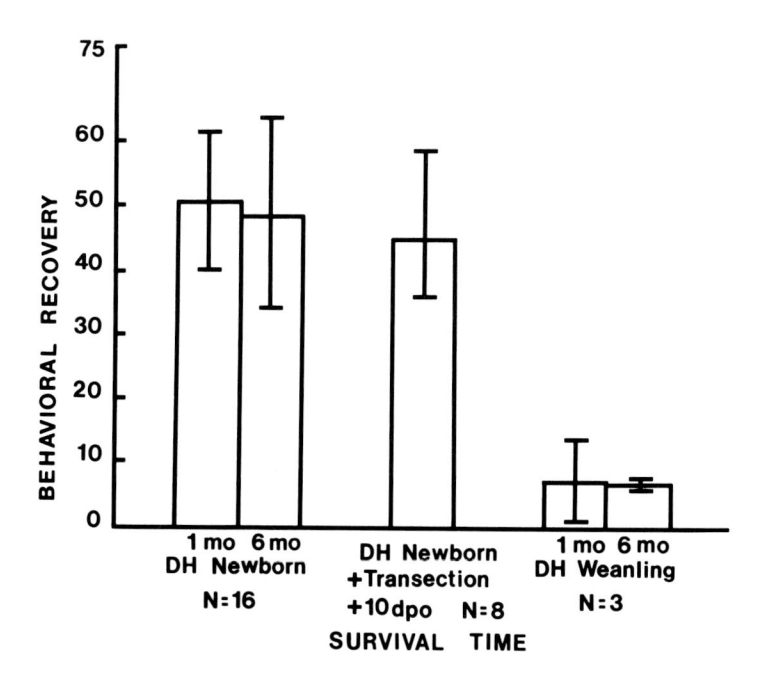

Figure 1. Behavioral development and recovery of hindlimb responses was assessed (Weber and Stelzner, 1977) in newborn double hemisected (DH) operates and in weanling DH operates at one and six mo. p.o. Using a semiquantitative (legend continued on page 352)

There was much less variability in the development and recovery of function of hindlimb behaviors in newborn double hemisection operates (Cullen and Stelzner, 1986b; In preparation). All newborn operates have hindlimb supporting reactions, stepping and hopping responses, a reciprocal locomotor gait of the hindlimbs not in phase with the forelimbs, spontaneous motor activity, and a contact or tactile placing response. These animals also never vocalize or react to noxious stimuli although a strong wriggling response occurs in the hindquarters. Thus, newborn DH operates have the same hindlimb behaviors spared in rats spinally transected at the same age (Fig 1).

The anatomical results have also been more consistent in the newborn double hemisection operates. The double hemisection lesion sites are complete and are longer in length probably due to greater neuronal loss than seen in weanling operates (Fig. 2D). No neurons are retrogradely labeled above the rostral hemisection lesion and anterogradely labeled axons do not project beyond the rostral lesion. However, the distribution of anterogradely labeled axons and retrogradely labeled neurons found between the bilateral hemisection lesions is similar to that seen in weanling operates (Fig. 2D,E). Again, the substrate for a propriospinal circuit bridging the spinal cord rostral and caudal to the bilateral hemisection lesions remains intact.

In 8 additional newborn double hemisection operates, an attempt has been made to determine if the potential propriospinal circuit remaining after this surgery is related to the sparing of function seen in this group of animals. At one month of age, these rats received a high thoracic spinal transection, several segments rostral to

---

rating scale for assessing hindlimb responses, there is much greater behavioral development and recovery for all seven different classes of behavior tested in newborn DH compared with weanling DH operates. The middle bar indicates that there is little behavioral effect if newborn DH operates receive a spinal cord transection rostral to the DH lesions when animals are 1 month of age. The range of recovery in individual animals is shown by the error bar for each group.

Sparing of Function / 353

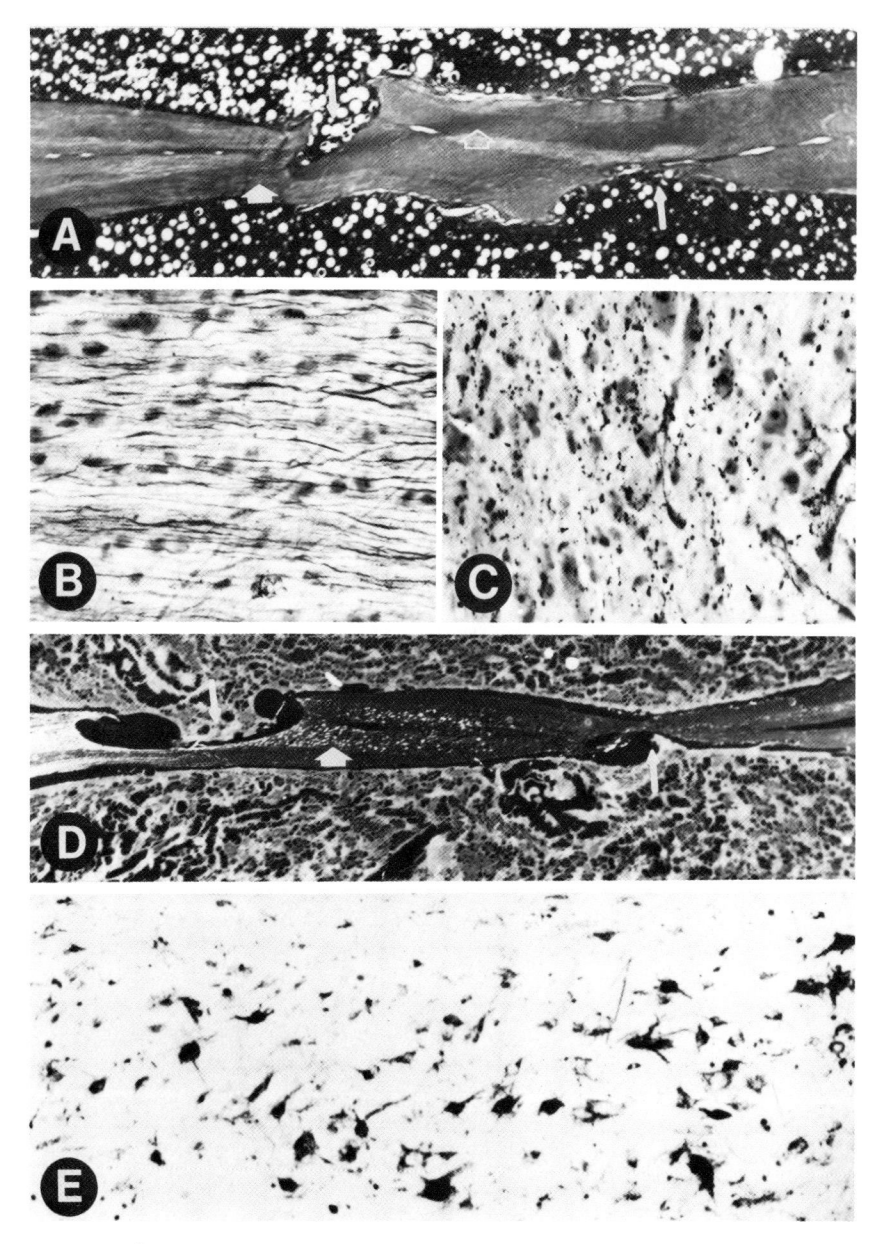

Figure 2. Newborn DH operates. A. and D. show DH lesion sites (long arrows) in longitudinal sections from two different animals. Caudal is to the left in each case. (legend continued on page 354)

the bilateral hemisection lesions. Immediately after recovery from anesthesia, all the behavioral responses seen prior to this lesion return (Fig. 1). The urinary bladder remains reflexic, and locomotor and supporting reactions return immediately. The pronounced spinal shock and minimal recovery of the hindlimbs seen in control animals of the same age receiving the same type of spinal transection lesion does not occur. However, the overall activity level of the double hemisection newborn operates did decrease somewhat for the first p.o. week following the spinal transection suggesting that a propriospinal pathway could have made a small contribution to hindlimb behaviors in the newborn operate. Further experiments are needed to test this possiblity.

The double hemisected newborn operates survived for 10 days after receiving the rostral spinal transection at 1 mo. of age. The spinal cords from these operates were then stained using the Fink-Heimer method for degenerating axons (Fig.2 A-C). Since axonal degeneration resulting from the neonatal double hemisection lesions clears by 3 days p.o. (Gilbert and Stelzner, 1979), any Fink-Heimer degeneration argyrophilia within and below the bilateral hemisection lesions is a result of the rostral spinal transection cutting supraspinal and propriospinal descending pathways. Fink-Heimer degeneration fills the gray matter bilaterally in the interlesion zone (Fig 2 A,C). The degeneration is in greatest density within laminae V-VIII, with only scattered degeneration apparent in the

---

A. has been stained by the Fink-Heimer method 10 days after a rostral spinal transection was made at 30 days of age. B. is from the area marked by the filled short arrow and shows the lack of degenerating axons passing caudal to the DH lesions. Only normal fibers are stained. Degeneration bilaterally fills the region between the DH lesions as indicated in C., from the area marked by the open short arrow in A. D. has been reacted using TMB histochemistry, two days after injecting the spinal cord caudal to the DH lesions with HRP. Many retrogradely labeled neurons are seen in the zone between the DH lesions but none are found rostral to these lesions (dark field micrograph). A number of retrogradely labeled neurons are shown at higher power in E., from the zone indicated by the filled short arrow in D.

upper laminae of the dorsal horn. Degeneration is distributed symmetrically but heavier contralateral to the rostral hemisection lesion. No degeneration is seen caudal to the hemisection lesions (Fig. 2B) even though the zone between the two lesions is filled with degenerating axons and terminals. Thus, there is no evidence that descending long tract axons normally passing through the white matter cut by the double hemisections lesions are able to grow around these lesions to enter the spinal cord distal to them.

Summary

Our results in both newborn and weanling double hemisection operates indicate that a viable propriospinal circuit exists in the zone between these lesions connecting the rostral and caudal spinal cord. Further experiments are needed to determine whether different connections have been formed in this interlesion zone in either age group of operate, either by regenerative sprouting, collateral sprouting, or exuberant growth in the newborn animal which may remain subsequent to the spinal surgery. However, even if such connections have formed, in neither case does this circuit appear to contribute to the recovery and development of the hindlimb behaviors tested in this study. The sparing of function in newborn operates is due, just as after complete spinal transection, to the isolated spinal cord controlling behaviors autonomously which, in the adult, are under supraspinal control. Additionally, no long tract axons appear able to grow around these lesions in newborn operates, at least when tested using the degeneration method for this analysis. Clearly, there is a limit to this type of developmental plasticity in the newborn rat spinal cord.

The present study shows that propriospinal pathways projecting from the intact spinal tissue between bilateral midthoracic hemisection lesions of spinal cord in the newborn and weanling rats does not substantially contribute to behavioral recovery of the hindlimbs. A number of different laboratories are using implants of embryonic brain and spinal cord to try to amelioriate the devastating behavioral affects of spinal cord injury in the adult and developing mammal, and with some success (Bregman,

1986; Buchanan and Nornes, 1986; Kunkel-Bagden and Bregman, 1987; Privat, et al., 1987; Reier et al., 1986). One hypothesis is that damaged axons growing into a CNS implant and embryonic axons growing out of the implant can form a new circuit contributing to behavioral recovery (Reier et al, 1986). It must be emphasized that the present experiment does not address that hypothesis. Certainly, the formation of new connections within and out of embryonic CNS tissue could give a very different anatomical and behavioral outcome from the present experiment which uses surviving newborn or weanling spinal tissue as a substrate for potential CNS plasticity.

REFERENCES

Basbaum AI (1973). Conduction of the effects of noxious stimulation by short fiber multisynaptic systems of the spinal cord in the rat. Exp Neurol 40:699-716.
Beck CH, Chambers WW (1970). Speed, accuracy and strength of forelimb movement after unilateral pyramidotomy in rhesus monkeys. J Comp Physiol Psychol 70:1-22.
Bernstein DR, Stelzner DJ (1983). Plasticity of the corticospinal tract following midthoracic spinal injury in the postnatal rat. J Comp Neurol. 221:382-400.
Bregman BS (1986). Neural tissue transplants modify central neurons' responses to damage. In Goldberger ME, Gorio A, Murry M (eds): "Development and Plasticity of the Mammalian Spinal Cord," New York: Springer-Verlag, pp 271-291.
Bregman BS (1987). Development of serotonin immunoreactivity in the rat spnal cord and its plasticity after neonatal spinal cord lesions. Dev Brain Res 34:245-263.
Bregman BS, Goldberger ME (1983). Infant lesion effect. III. Anatomical correlates of sparing and recovery of function after spinal cord damage in newborn and adult cats. Dev Brain Res 9:137-154.
Buchanan JT, Nornes HO (1986). Transplants of embryonic brainstem containing the locus coeruleus into spinal cord enhance the hindlimb flexion reflex in adult rats. Brain Res 381:225-236.
Chambers WW, Liu CN, McCouch GP (1973). Anatomical and physiological correlates of plasticity in the central nervous system. Brain Behav Evol 8:5-27.

Cullen JM, Stelzner DJ (1986a). A spinal cord injury model via bilateral throacic hemisection. Anat Rec 214:27A.
Cullen JM, Stelzner DJ (1986b). Sparing of function after bilateral hemisections of the midthoracic spinal cord in neonatal rats is not due to descending connections. Neurosci Abstr 12:1510.
Conrad C, Henderson V, Skinner RD, Abraham P, Garcia-Rill E (1987). Development of the pedunculopontine nucleus. Neurosci Abstr 13:1176.
Donatelle JM (1977). Growth of the corticospinal tract and the development of placing reactions in the postnatal rat. J Comp Neurol 175:207-232.
Eidelberg E (1981). Consequences of spinal cord lesions upon motor function with special reference to locomotor activity. Prog Neurobiol 17:185-202.
Forssberg H (1979) On integrative motor function in the cat's spinal cord. Acta Physiol Scand (Suppl) 474:2-56.
Forssberg H, Grillner S, Sjostrom A (1974). Tactile placing in chronic spinal kittens. Acta Physiol Scand 92:114-120.
Gilbert M, Stelzner DJ (1979). The development of descending and dorsal root connections in the lumbosacral spinal cord of the postnatal rat. J Comp Neurol 184:821-838.
Goldberger ME (1972). Restitution of function in the CNS: the pathological grasp in *Macaca mulatta*. Exp Brain Res 15:79-96.
Goldberger ME (1986). Autonomous spinal motor function and the infant lesion effect. In Goldberger ME, Gorio A, Murray M (eds): "Development and Plasticity of the Mammalian Spinal Cord," New York: Springer-Verlag, pp 363-381.
Goldman PS (1974). An alternative to developmental plasticity: Heterology of CNS structures in infants and adults. In Stein DG, Rosen JJ, Butters N (eds): "Plasticity and Recovery of Function in the Central Nervous System," New York: Academic Press, pp 149-174.
Hulsebosch CE, Coggeshall, RE (1983). A comparision of axonal numbers in dorsal root following spinal cord hemisection in neonate and adult rats. Brain Res 265:187-197.
Ingebritsen OC (1933). Coordinating mechanisms of the spinal cord. Genet Psychol Monogr 13:483-553.
Jane JA, Evans JP, Fisher LE (1964). An investigation concerning the restitution of motor function following

injury to the spinal cord. J Neurosurg 21:167-171.
Johnson DA, Almli CR (1978). Age, brain damage, and performance. In Finger S (ed): "Recovery from brain damage: Research and theory," New York: Plenum, pp 115-134.
Kalil K, Reh T (1979). Regrowth of severed axons in the neonatal CNS. Science 205:1158-1161.
Kalil K, Reh T (1982). A light and electron microscopic study of regrowing pyramidal tract fibers. J Comp Neurol 211:265-276.
Kato M, Murakami S, Hirayama H, Hikino K (1985). Recovery of postural control following chronic bilateral hemisections at different spinal cord levels in adult cats. Exp Neurol 90:350-364.
Kennard, MA (1942). Cortical reorganization of motor function. Studies of series of monkeys of various ages from infancy to maturity. Arch Neurol Psychiat 48:227-240.
Kozak W, Westerman R (1966). Basic patterns of plastic change in the mammalian nervous system. Symp Soc Exp Biol 20:509-544.
Kunkel-Bagden E, Bregman BS (1987). Transplants enhance recovery of locomotor function after spinal cord lesions in newborn rats. Neurosci Abstr 13:1504.
Lassek AM, Anderson PA (1961). Motor function after spaced contralateral hemisections in the spinal cord. Neurol 11:362-365.
Leonard CT, Goldberger ME (1987). Consequences of damage to the sensorimotor cortex in neonatal and adult cats. II. Maintenance of exuberant projections. Dev Brain Res 32:15-30.
Leong SK, Shieh JY, Wong WC (1984). Localizing spinal-cord-projecting neurons in neonatal and immature albino rats. J Comp Neurol 228:18-23.
Prendergast J, Stelzner DJ (1976). Increases in collateral axonal growth rostral to a thoracic hemisection in neonatal and weanling rat. J Comp Neurol 166:145-162.
Privat A, Mansour H, Sandillon F (1987). Interactions between grafted monoaminergic cells and the host spinal cord. In Gash DM, Sladek JR (eds): "Schmitt Neurological Sciences Symposium, Transplantation into the Mammalian CNS," Rochester: Abstracts.
Reh T, Kalil, K (1982). Functional role of regrowing pyramidal tract fibers. J Comp Neurol 211:276-283.
Reier PJ, Bregman BS, Wujek JR, Tessler A (1986). Intraspinal transplantation of fetal spinal cord tissue:

an approach toward functional repair of the injured spinal cord. In Goldberger ME, Gorio A, Murray M (eds): "Development and Plasticity of the Mammalian Spinal Cord," New York: Springer-Verlag, pp 251-271.

Robinson GA, Goldberger ME (1986a). The development and recovery of motor function in spinal cats. I. The infant lesion effect. Exp Brain Res 62:373-386.

Robinson GA, Goldberger ME (1986b). The development and recovery of motor function in spinal cats. II. Pharmacological enhancement of recovery. Exp Brain Res 62:387-400.

Rossignol S, Barbeau H, Julien C (1986). Locomotion of the adult chronic spinal cat and its modification by monoaminergic agonists and autogonists. In Goldberger ME, Gorio A, Murray M (eds): "Development and Plasticity of the Mammalian Spinal Cord," New York: Springer-Verlag, pp 323-347.

Schneider GE, Jhaveri S, Edwards MA, So KF (1985). Regeneration, re-routing, and redistribution of axons after early lesions: changes with age, and functional impact. In Eccles JC, Dimitrijevic M (eds): "Recent Achievements in Restorative Neurology 1," Basel: Karger, pp 291-310.

Schreyer DJ, Jones EG (1983). Growing corticospinal axons by-pass lesions of neonatal rat spinal cord. Neurosci 9:31-40.

Shieh JY, Leong SK, Wong WC (1983). Origin of the rubrospinal tract in neonatal, developing and mature rats. J Comp Neurol 214:79-86.

Shurrager PS, Dykman RA (1951). Walking spinal carnivores. J Comp Physiol Psychol 44:252-262.

Smith JL, Bradley NS, Carter MC, Giuliani CA, Hoy MG, Koshland GF, Zernicke RF (1986). Rhythmical movements of the hindlimbs in spinal cat: considerations for a controlling network. In Goldberger ME, Gorio A, Murray M (eds): "Development and Plasticity of the Mammalian Spinal Cord," New York: Springer-Verlag, pp 347-363.

Smith JL, Smith LA, Zernicke RF, Hoy MG (1982). Locomotion in exercised and non-excerised cats cordotomized at two or twelve weeks of age. Exp Neurol 76:393-413.

Stelzner DJ, Ershler, WB, Weber ED (1975). Effects of spinal transection in neonatal and weanling rat: Survival of function. Exp Neurol 46: 156-177.

Stelzner DJ, Weber ED, Prendergast J (1979). A comparison of the effect of mid-thoracic spinal hemisection in the neonatal or weanling rat on the distribution and density of dorsal root axons in the lumbosacral spinal cord of the adult. Brain Res 172:407-426.

Stelzner DJ (1982). The role of descending systems in maintaining intrinsic spinal function: A developmental approach. In Sjolund B, Bjorklund A (eds): "Brain Stem Control of Spinal Mechanisms," Amsterdam: Elsevier, pp 297-321.

Stelzner DJ (1986). Ontogeny of the encephalization process. In Greenough WT, Juraska JM (eds): "Developmental NeuroPyschobiology," New York: Academic Press, pp 241-270.

Stelzner DJ, Weber ED, BryzGornia WF (1986). Sparing of function in developing spinal cord: Anatomical substrate. In Goldberger ME, Gorio A, Murray M (eds): "Development and Plasticity of the Mammalian Spinal Cord," New York: Springer-Verlag, pp 81-101.

Viala D, Viala G, Fayein N (1986). Plasticity of locomotor organization in infant rabbits spinalized shortly after birth. In Goldberger ME, Gorio A, Murray M (eds): "Development and Plasticity of the Mammalian Spinal Cord," New York: Springer-Verlag, pp 301-311.

Weber ED, Stelzner DJ (1977). Behavioral effects of spinal cord transection in the developing rat. Brain Res 125:241-255.

Weber ED, Stelzner DJ (1980). Synaptogenesis in the intermediate gray region of the lumbar spinal cord in the postnatal rat. Brain Res 185:17-37.

SHORTENING OF THE RAT SPINAL COLUMN: A METHOD FOR
STUDYING COAPTATION OF CORD STUMPS

Luis de Medinaceli, M.D.

Microsurgical Research Center, Medical College
of Hampton Roads, Norfolk, VA 23507

INTRODUCTION

Grafts are sometimes introduced in the central nervous system, for example in order to bridge or by-pass a spinal cord lesion (Woolsey et al.,1944; Winialski et al., 1987). Systematic analysis of the physiopathologic events occurring at the site of coaptation of the tissues, i.e. at the junction host/graft, is indispensable to determine conditions necessary for graft survival and neurotization. The simplest and most satisfactory interface for studying nervous tissue "repair" should be a host/host junction, i.e. the site of coaptation of a given central nervous tissue with itself. However this type of interface has rarely been analyzed because, for anatomical reasons, it is very difficult to obtain such apposition without inflicting trauma on the fragile nervous tissue. As far as the spinal cord is concerned, a satisfactory cord/cord apposition can be obtained only by shortening of the spinal column.

Elaborate procedures on spine and spinal cord of experimental animals are usually made on large laboratory mammals. The draw-back is that experiments are then limited to a few subjects by financial costs and difficulty in postoperative care. What is desirable is a small inexpensive mammal like the rat. I here describe a simple surgical technique allowing an operator to perform, unaided, complete spondylectomies on the rat at the thoracic level (T8-T9), with a satisfactory survival rate. The procedure has several experimental applications. When the cord is not transected, functional recovery is usually complete; it is then possible to study recovery from spinal shock, and eventual modifications such as development of edema. When the cord is intentionally transected, the spondylectomy allows intimate abutment of the cord stumps without mechanical stress. This is especially useful to study the factors that might influence scar formation in the cord such as surface adhesion, trapping or ingrowth of foreign elements, edema and hemorrhage. In this preliminary study, the cord was not injured. The fact that this procedure was not in itself harmful to the nervous system was demonstrated by conservation of cord function.

MATERIAL AND METHODS

Preliminary Studies and their Results

All pilot studies were made on Sprague-Dawley rats of either sex, anesthetized with pentobarbital and chloral hydrate i.p. The location of the animals' center of gravity was determined on seven rats, and found to be on a line passing by L2. Evaluation of mass distribution around this center indicated that during normal activity the mid-thoracic column was submitted to mechanical stress two to three times smaller than the lumbar column. Therefore, the chances of secondary displacements should be minimized after thoracic spondylectomy.

Thirty-nine animals were then used to determine the most appropriate technique and level for extensive laminectomies. This preliminary study confirmed that the mid-thoracic level was appropriate: when extensive laminectomies were performed at low-thoracic or thoracolumbar level, they were sometimes followed by spontaneous fracture, indicating excessive mechanical stress; on the other hand, when laminectomies were performed at high thoracic level, the animal could not lift its head to drink or feed for several days.

In another group of 44 animals, the exposed cord was transected at various thoracic levels; the width of the gap created by retraction of the cord stumps was measured and several methods for bringing these stumps back together were tested. Passing stitches through the cord (Fowler, 1905; Harte and Stewart, 1902), suturing pia or dura (Babbini, 1956; Derlon et al., 1983; Lortat-Jacob et al., 1915), modifying the flexion-extension of the spine (Breig, 1978), or pulling the structure by the roots (Zhia, 1980) proved ineffectual. It was concluded that removal of a length of bone equal to 1 or 1.5 vertebral segment was indispensable and sufficient to suppress the gap created by a simple transection, in agreement with Murray's observations (Murray et al., 1965).

Experimental Protocols

Thirteen Sprague-Dawley female rats weighing approximately 350 g at the beginning of the experiment were used. The animals were laid ventrally and an incision was made over the thoracic spinous processes. The level was determined with the help of the large vein which is a landmark of the fifth thoracic vertebra (Fig. 1).

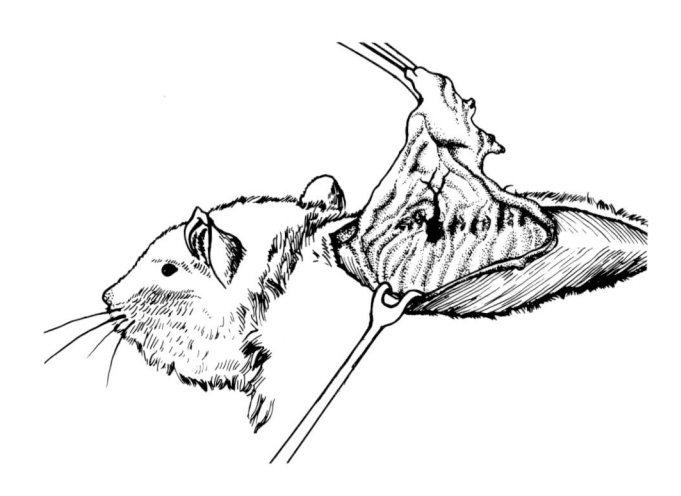

Figure 1. Extra-thoracic portion of the vein. The vessel, strictly median, drains the hibernating gland and disappears between the laterovertebral muscular masses. It is a reliable landmark of the fifth spinous process (Reprinted from de Medinaceli, 1986, with permission).

On both sides, the pleura was dissected from the 8th, 9th and 10th ribs, and the 9th rib was cut at the posterior costal angle. Pleura and mediastinal organs were dissected from the vertebral bodies. The laminae of T9 and the caudal half of the laminae of T8 were removed. The right side of the vertebral bodies was removed. A small "rod" made from the shaft of a 23 gauge needle was placed alongside the column and fixed with non-absorbable thread (Fig. 2).

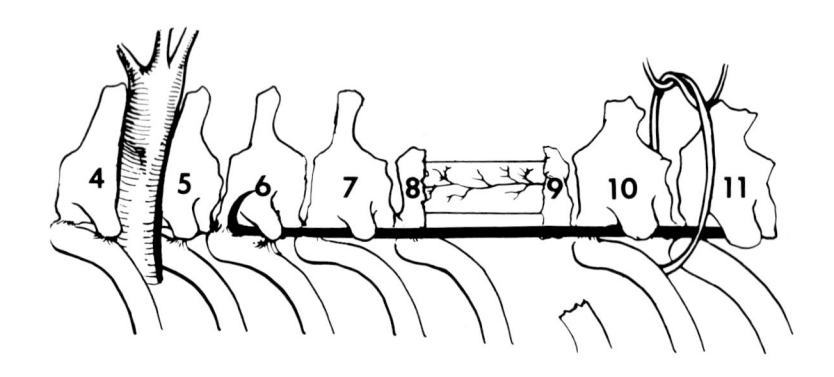

Figure 2. Schematic representation of spine stabilization. A small rod is hooked around the transverse process of T6 and lain along the spine. Tying the knot then applies it firmly against the column.

These steps were repeated on the left side. The column stumps were then brought into contact by sliding along the rods and held by an "approximating" stitch. At the end of this maneuver, the cord was almost invisible, hidden in the reconstituted bone canal. Muscles and skin layers were closed. The animals were caged separately on soft beddings for one month and then housed under ordinary conditions. They were observed for a period of six months. No special postoperative care, such as regular bladder expression, was found necessary.

RESULTS

Immediately after the procedure, all animals had a marked impairment of function. Four rats died (shortly after the procedure). Nine animals survived until the end of the experiment. In these nine rats, improvement from the postoperative deficit was observed between the 2nd and the 25th day. The final result was satisfactory in eight animals and mediocre in one rat. A detailed analysis of behavioral and histologic results is in preparation (Fig. 3).

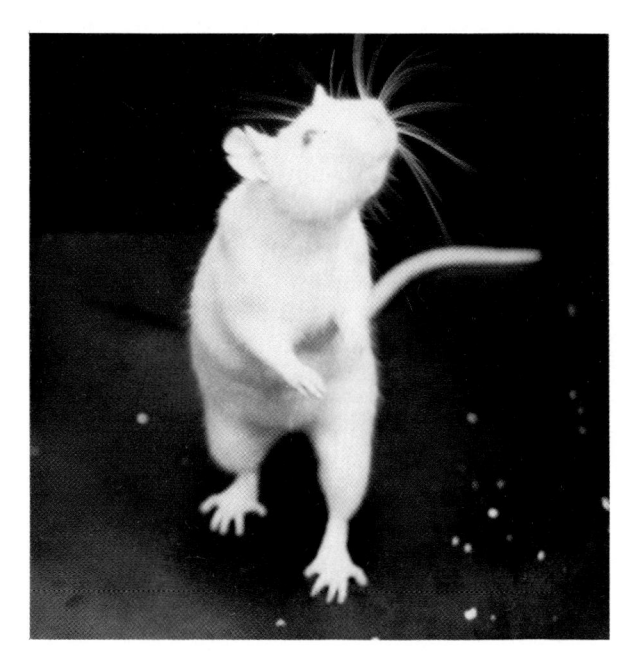

Figure 3. Spontaneous activity of a rat, four months after the shortening procedure. In this preliminary study, no injury was inflicted on the cord.

DISCUSSION

The first attempt to obtain a satisfactory cord/cord coaptation is almost one century old. Suturing the cord tissue itself was quickly abandoned because of the fragility of the structure (Fowler, 1905; Harte and Stewart, 1902). Attempts to bring the stumps together by suturing the dura showed that although dura suturing can be achieved without tearing, the cord itself does not move with the sheath and the gap remains (Lortat-Jacob et al., 1915; Babbini, 1956; Derlon et al., 1983). A recent attempt by Zhia to pull the stumps by the roots of the spinal nerves was not successful (Zhia, 1980). The roots are sufficiently strong (Tarlov, 1937) and do not rupture, but the cord does not follow the movement and the stumps do not come into contact. Furthermore, pulling on the roots probably does damage of its own. Breig showed that by modifying the flexion-extension of the spine, it is possible to change the position of the cord stumps within the canal and to bring these stumps into contact (Breig, 1978). This works well on cadavers if the gap is not too wide, but not on a living cord: the stumps do not come close to each other (de Medinaceli, unpublished observations).

If abutment of cord stumps is sought, shortening the spine is the only way to obtain it. Bone removal creates a slack and the stumps come into contact. This observation triggered a few studies (Babbini, 1956; Murray et al., 1965; Street, 1967; Yturraspe and Lumb, 1973; Lumb and Nornes, 1983; Derlon at al., 1983). In reality, reunion of cord stumps through spondylectomy has never been thoroughly tested, probably because of the technical difficulties and the cost involved. In the rare publications dealing with the technique of spondylectomy, few animals were successfully operated upon. The present study demonstrated that shortening the thoracic spine of inexpensive laboratory animals could be achieved without excessive difficulties, thus making the procedure practical on a large scale. This will render possible in-depth studies of various local factors that might influence the outcome of spinal cord injuries.

REFERENCES

Babbini RJ (1956). Suture medullaire. Neuro-Chirurgie 2:168-179.
Breig A (1978). "Adverse mechanical tension in the central nervous system. An analysis of cause and

effect. Relief by functional neurosurgery." New York: Wiley & Sons.
de Medinaceli L (1986). An anatomical landmark for procedures on rat thoracic spinal cord. Exp Neurol 91:404-488.
Derlon JM, Roy-Camille R, Lechevalier B, Bisserie M, Coston A (1983). Delayed spinal cord anastomosis. In Kao CC, Bunge RP, Reier PJ (eds): "Spinal cord reconstruction," New York: Raven Press, pp. 223-234.
Fowler GR (1905). A case of suture of the spinal cord, following a gunshot injury involving complete severance of the structure. Ann Surg 42:507-513.
Harte RH, Stewart FT (1902). A case of severed spinal cord in which myelorraphy was followed by partial return of function. Trans Am Surg Ass 20:28-38.
Lortat-Jacob, Girou, Ferrand (1915). Suture de la moelle epiniere. Bull Acad Nat Med Paris 74:423-427.
Lumb WV, Nornes HO (1983). Vertebral resection and spinal cord reapposition. In Kao CC, Bunge RP, Reier PJ (eds): "Spinal cord reconstruction," New York: Raven Press, pp. 223-234.
Murray G, Ugray E, Graves A. (1965). Regeneration in injured spinal cord. Am J Surg 109:406-409.
Street DM (1967). Traumatic paraplegia treated by vertebral resection, excision of spinal cord lesion, suture of the spinal cord and interbody fusion. In "Proceedings of Veterans Administration Annual Spinal Cord Injury Conference, pp. 92-102.
Tarlov IM (1937). Structure of the nerve root I. Nature of the junction between the central and peripheral nervous system. Arch Neurol Psychiat (Chicago) 37:555-583.
Winialski D, Houle J, Jakeman L, Reier P (1987). Transplantation of fetal rat spinal cord into longstanding contusion injuries of adult rat spinal cord. Soc Neurosci Abstr 207,11.
Woolsey D, Minckler J, Rezende N, Klemme R (1944). Human spinal cord transplant. Exp Med Surg 2:93-102.
Yturraspe DJ, Lumb WV (1973). Second lumbar spondylectomy and shortening of the spinal column of the dog. J Am Vet Med Assoc 161:1651-1657.
Zhia YC (1980). "Anastomosis of the spinal cord" (In Chinese). Chung Hua Shan Ching Ching Shen Ko Tsa Chih 13:178-179.

PATHFINDING BY REGENERATING AXONS IN THE LAMPREY SPINAL CORD

Diana Lurie and Michael E. Selzer

The Department of Neurology, and The David Mahoney Institute of Neurological Sciences, University of Pennsylvania School of Medicine, Philadelphia Pennsylvania 19104-4283

INTRODUCTION

An important goal in spinal cord injury research is the regeneration of severed axons through or around the site of injury. Recent advances in the technology of tissue grafting and implantation (David and Aguayo, 1981; Reier, 1985; Bregman, 1987) suggest that this goal may be achieved but this in itself might not lead to functional recovery if the regrowth is chaotic. It may be that useful function can be achieved only through an orderly regeneration of appropriate neuronal connections. Is there reason to believe that the cellular elements of injured CNS can re-express the specificity cues which guided the original development? One approach to this question is to determine, in an animal that does recover functionally from spinal transection, whether regenerating axons are guided selectively along their normal pathways and form synapses specifically with their normal target neurons.

The large larval sea lamprey (Petromyzon marinus) recovers normal appearing swimming and crawling movements from six to twelve weeks following complete spinal transection (Rovainen, 1976; Selzer, 1978; Park et al., 1986; Currie and Ayers, 1987). These animals are four to five years old and in a stable phase of neurological development. Preliminary observations by A. Tangoren in our laboratory suggest that there are few, if any, dividing cells in the CNS at this stage. Synaptic connections previously demonstrated among several types of large neurons in the brain and spinal cord of the adult (Rovainen, 1974a,b) are already present at this stage of development (Mackler and Selzer, 1987) as are the major axon tracts. Thus, spinal transection in the large larval lamprey interrupts known patterns of previously established axonal projection and synaptic connectivity. Adult lampreys also recover from spinal transection and show axonal regeneration (unpublished data). They have larger neurons than the larval form, which simplifies cellular analysis. However, larvae are much more available and have been used almost exclusively in these studies.

FUNCTIONAL RECOVERY INVOLVES AXONAL REGENERATION

An advantage of the lamprey is that it has large reticulospinal axons (Muller and Mauthner axons) which extend unbranched almost the entire length of the spinal cord (Rovainen, 1967a,b). These fibers have been traced in serial sections through the scar in animals which had recovered from spinal transection (Rovainen, 1976; Selzer, 1978). Moreover, axons labeled by intracellular injection of tracer such as horseradish peroxidase (HRP) can be examined in spinal cord wholemounts and their regenerated processes viewed directly (Wood and Cohen, 1979; Yin and Selzer, 1983). In such preparations, the maximum distance of regeneration was estimated to be of the order of 5 mm beyond the scar (Yin and Selzer, 1983). Subsequently we have traced some fibers as far as 21 mm. This view of a limited distance of regeneration has been confirmed by retrograde tracing techniques (Croop et al., 1987) and electrophysiological methods (Yin and Selzer, 1983). Nevertheless, within those few mm regenerated neurites form vesicle containing junctions with as yet unidentified postsynaptic neurons (Wood and Cohen, 1979; 1981). Evidence from our laboratory and others suggests that the axonal and synaptic regeneration can account, at least in part, for the functional recovery (reviewed in Cohen et al., <u>in press</u>).

SPECIFICITY IN SYNAPTIC REGENERATION

Simultaneous recordings from pairs of visible, recognizable neurons on opposite sides of a healed transection have demonstrated that regenerating neurites in the lamprey spinal cord form electrophysiologically active synapses (Mackler and Selzer, 1985). In fact, there appears to be specificity in the synaptic regeneration. Types of neurons which are synaptically linked in unlesioned animals can become reconnected following spinal transection and regeneration, while types of neurons which are not normally linked fail to establish such regenerated connections (Mackler and Selzer, 1987). A similar specificity has been described in the regeneration of synaptic contacts between lesioned dorsal root axons and their appropriate motoneurons in the frog spinal cord (Sah and Frank, 1984).

Several lines of evidence suggest that the behavioral recovery derives at least in part from the regenerated connections. Retransection eliminates the recovered behavior (Borgens et al., 1981; Park et al., 1986). Stimulation of the head elicits tail movements and vice versa in previously transected animals in which the body wall had been removed for several cm rostral and caudal to the scar, leaving a long portion of isolated cord which included the original lesion (Selzer, 1978). Similarly, with the body wall removed rostral to a healed transection, stimulation of the floor of the fourth ventrical elicits undulatory movements of the body and tail caudal to the healed transection (Currie and Ayers, 1983). Finally, in the isolated spinal cord, ventral root discharges from segments on opposite sides of a healed transection can become time locked during "fictive locomotion" (Cohen et al., 1986).

Thus, the large larval sea lamprey recovers behaviorally from complete spinal transection by a process which involves regeneration of axons across the site of injury and the formation of synapses with appropriate neurons distal to the scar. The factors which govern the correctness of regeneration are currently under investigation. One theoretical contributor to the reestablishment of correct synaptic connections is the mechanosensory feedback which results from attempts of the animal to acquire useful behaviors. This hypothesis has been tested recently by allowing animals to recover from spinal transection ensheathed in tubular restraints, which prevented them from performing the behaviors which they ultimately reacquired (Park et al., 1986). The restrained animals recovered swimming speed and coordination as quickly as animals allowed to recover unrestrained (Fig. 1A). This was also true for crawling on a dry surface (Fig. 1B) and for forward and backward escape from an open glass tube. Experiments in developing frog embryos have shown that apparently normal behavior and anatomical connectivity results even though neuronal activity is suppressed by the addition of local anesthetics to the bathing medium (Harrison, 1904; Carmichael, 1926; 1927; 1928; Mathews and Detwiler, 1926; Haverkamp and Oppenheim, 1986; Haverkamp, 1986). Although the observations on immobilized lampreys do not rule out a role for neuronal activity in the reestablishment of correct neuronal connections following spinal transection, they do show that the animals do not require a trial and error type of mechanosensory feedback in establishing such connections. Instead they suggest that intrinsic mechanisms may be important in regeneration of synaptic circuitry involved in locomotor behavior.

SPECIFICITY IN AXONAL PATHFINDING

A prerequisite for specificity in synaptic regeneration is that axons must grow processes back to their appropriate postsynaptic target neurons. Observations on several classes of neurons suggest that there is considerable specificity in the direction of neurite regeneration (Yin et al., 1984). The most compelling data comes from experiments on the giant interneurons. These are second order mechanosensory neurons which number 12-25 per animal and are located in the caudal half to two thirds of the spinal cord (Rovainen, 1967a,b; Selzer, 1979). Their axons originate from anteromedial wall of the perikaryon and decussate below the central canal, projecting in the contralateral white matter to the brainstem (Fig. 2A). Following spinal transection at the level of the cloaca, the original axon dies back completely in about 20% of giant interneurons caudal to the lesion and can no longer be identified in intracellularly labeled preparations. Instead, long axon-like neurites extend from anomalous locations on the dendritic tree. Although these neurites are initially misoriented, the majority cross the midline in the ventral commissure and loop anteriorly to assume

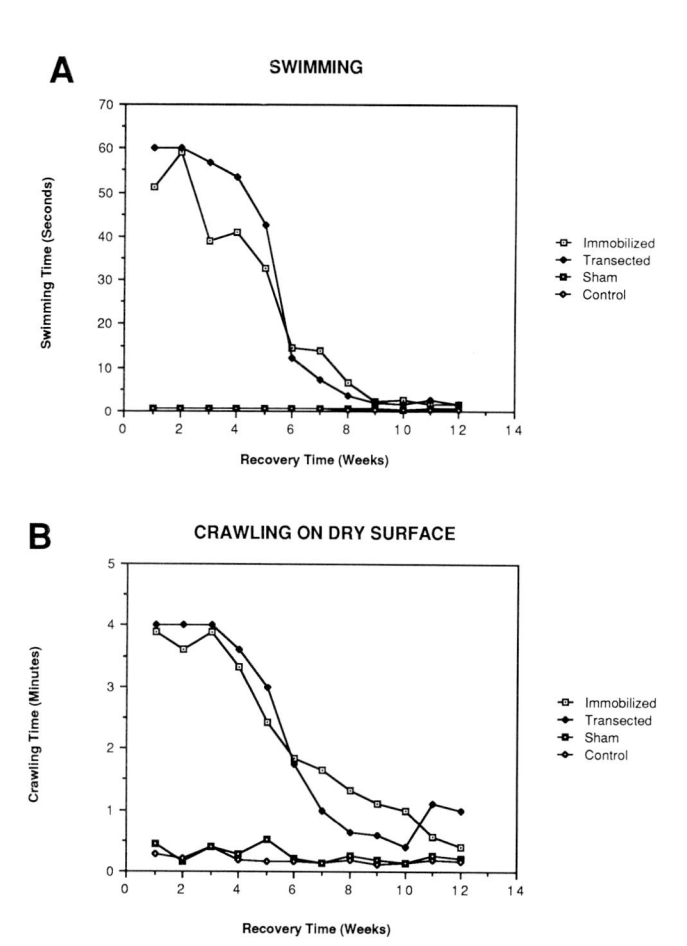

Fig. 1. Lack of effect of physical restraint on behavioral recovery (Park et al., 1986). A, Comparison of time course of recovery of swimming speed for larval sea lampreys recuperating in glass sheaths and lampreys allowed to swim freely. Animals were placed in a rectangular aquarium and the time to swim 20 cm was measured at weekly intervals. Standard error bars and animal numbers are omitted for graphic clarity, but there were at least 6 animals in each group at each time period and the recovery time courses were not significantly different. The graphs for sham and control overlap entirely. B, there was also no significant difference between the recovery of restrained and freely moving recuperants in time to crawl 15 cm on a dry board.

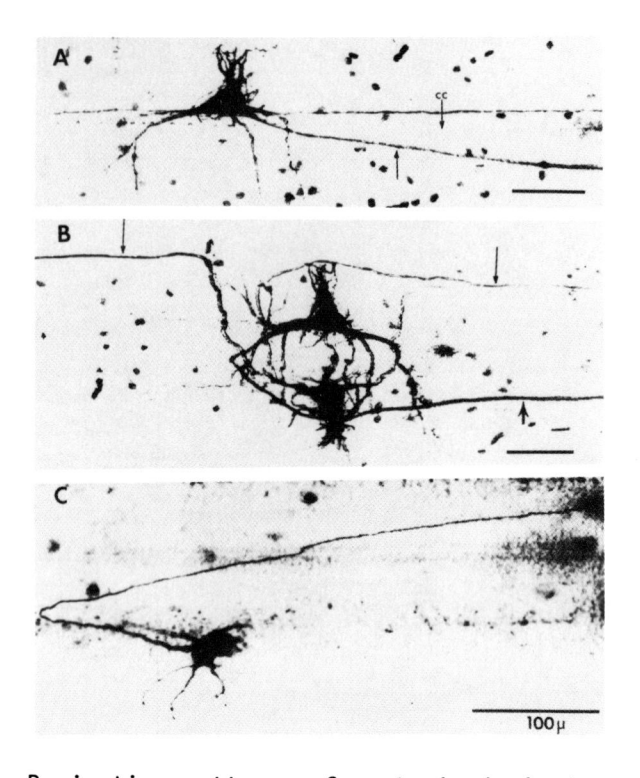

Fig. 2. Projection patterns of axotomized giant interneurons (A) Normal axon origin from the anterior end of the cell body. The axon (arrow) projects rostrally and contralaterally. Abbreviation: CC, central canal. (B) Two giant interneurons located approximately 1.2 mm caudal to a transection performed 20 days earlier. Their original axons have undergone complete retrograde degeneration. Two neurites (small arrows) grow from a caudal dendrite of the cell on the bottom. One neurite (large arrow) extends from a caudal dendrite of the top cell. Two of the three long neurites that initially project caudally reverse direction and grow rostrally and contralaterally in their normal projection path. (C) A giant interneuron in an island formed by double transection 60 days earlier. This cell was located 6.5 mm below the rostral cut and 1.5 mm above the caudal cut. Despite the proximity to the more caudal scar, a long neurite that initially grew posteriorly loops to project rostrally on the contralateral side. A second neurite (not in plane of focus) originating medially also projects rostrally. Scale, 100 m. (Figure reproduced with permission. From Yin, Mackler, and Selzer, "Directional Specificity in the Regeneration of Lamprey Spinal Axons", Science, 224 (1984) 894-896.)

their normal projection path (Fig. 2B). The behavior of neurites belonging to cells located between two transections was similar (Fig. 2C). Thus it is unlikely that the tendency of giant interneuron axons to regenerate rostralward is due to a trophic influence of the zone of injury. Nor did removal of a one cm length of spinal cord affect the direction of regeneration of neurites from giant interneurons caudal to the lesion (Mackler et al., 1986). It is therefore unlikely that the potential target neurons distal to a lesion are the source of a remote trophic effect on the regenerating fibers.

The directional specificity was not a consequence of initial random outgrowth of long axon-like neurites with subsequent retraction of inappropriately directed fibers. Even at the earliest times of neurite outgrowth (2-4 weeks after transection), both regenerating axons and axon-like neurites with anomalous origins were oriented in the normal trajectory for axons of unlesioned giant interneurons (Mackler et al., 1986). Moreover, when axon-like neurites did grow in an incorrect orientation (either posteriorally or ipsilateral to the cell body or both), their average distance of regeneration was half that of correctly oriented neurites (Fig. 3).

The above observations suggest that the directional specificity of regenerating neurites cannot be explained by a tendency of axons to grow in an already established direction, nor by a process of pruning following random outgrowth, nor by a concentration gradient of a trophic factor released by remote targets such as the scar. Thus it seems likely that the neurites are following guidance cues in their local enviroment and it becomes important to examine this enviroment in more detail in order to determine where those guidance cues might be. Studies of the ultrastructural environment of regenerating reticulospinal axon growth cones are under way and preliminary results will be described later.

ROLE OF THE SCAR

If the scar is not determining the direction of axon growth by a remote effect, at least it is behaving very differently from the glial scar in transected mammalian

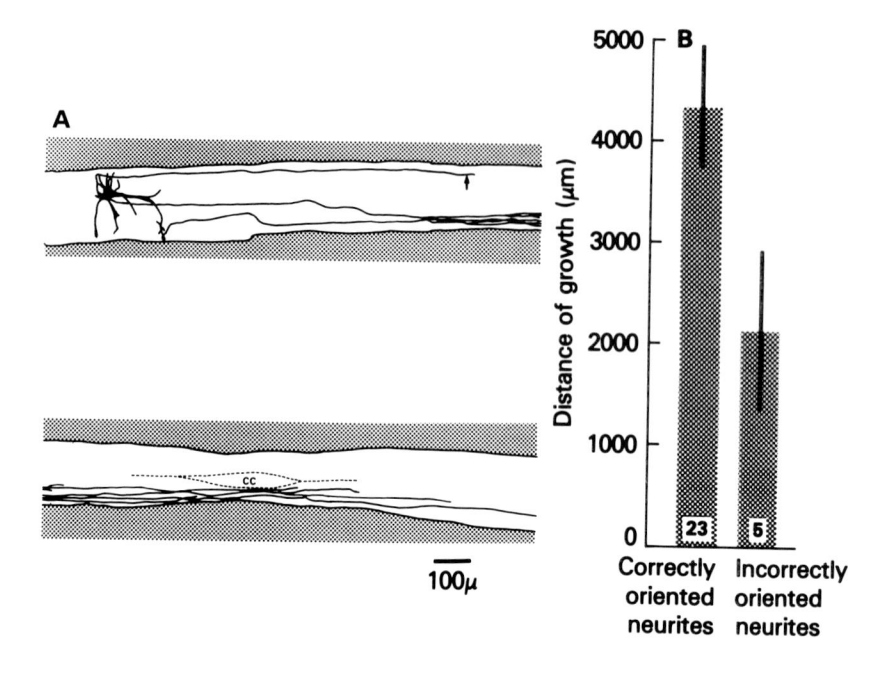

Fig. 3. GI neurites positioned in correct pathways grow further than incorrectly projecting neurites. A, A GI 64 d after single transection. The neurite projecting ipsilaterally and rostralward (small arrow) terminates about 1 mm from the cell. Another neurite arising from a contralateral dendrite sends 2 branches in the correct projection. These fibers grow beyond the scar located where the central canal (cc) widens . A third fiber (probably the original axon) gives rise to several branches. These branches also remain correctly positioned and grow beyond the scar. Because they may arise from the original axon, these branches are not included in the bar graph in B. cc, Central canal. B, In 28 GIs, the distance of growth of properly oriented neurites is more than double that of incorrectly oriented neurites (p 0.05). From Mackler et al., 1986.

spinal cord, which appears to be an absolute barrier to regeneration. The collateral sprouting of dorsal root fibers in partially deafferented and hemisected mammalian spinal cord shows that neurites can grow within the CNS parenchyma (Liu and Chambers, 1958; Goldberger and Murray, 1974; Murray and Goldberger, 1974). Thus the scar in the mammal provides a barrier which is much more intractable than the spinal cord extracellular space. Does the lamprey scar actively support regeneration or is it also a deterrent, albeit not an absolute one? This question has been approached by performing spinal hemisections and observing the pathways taken by the regenerating neurites of cut Muller and Mauthner axons. If the scar is a relative impediment to regeneration, then the neurites should grow around rather than through it, as do developing corticospinal axons in hemisected neonatal cats (Bregman and Goldberger, 1983). On the other hand, if the scar provides a supportive environment for regeneration, neurites should grow preferentially through the scar in order to remain in their correct orientation.

Spinal cords were hemisected at the level of the third gill and the animals allowed to recover for ten weeks. The CNS was isolated and transilluminated in a perfusion chamber. Individual Muller and Mauthner axons were injected with HRP, either by direct impalement or by impaling their cell bodies in the brainstem. In ten hemisected animals, thirty axons were labeled. They gave rise to eighty-two neurites, of which 55% regenerated beyond the level of the scar. Of these, 80% regenerated through the scar and remained on the same side as their parent axons (Fig. 4B). The remaining 20% (all from a single animal) decussated at the level of the scar and did not recross (Fig. 4C). In a control group of 5 animals, complete spinal transection at the level of the third gill was followed by regeneration of 56% of labeled neurites, of which 86% remained on the correct side (Fig. 4A). We conclude that the probability of regeneration for an injured axon in a partially transected cord is not significantly different from that in a complete transection and that neurites will grow through the scar rather than around it.

One possible explanation for this preferential growth of axons through the scar is that the lesioned

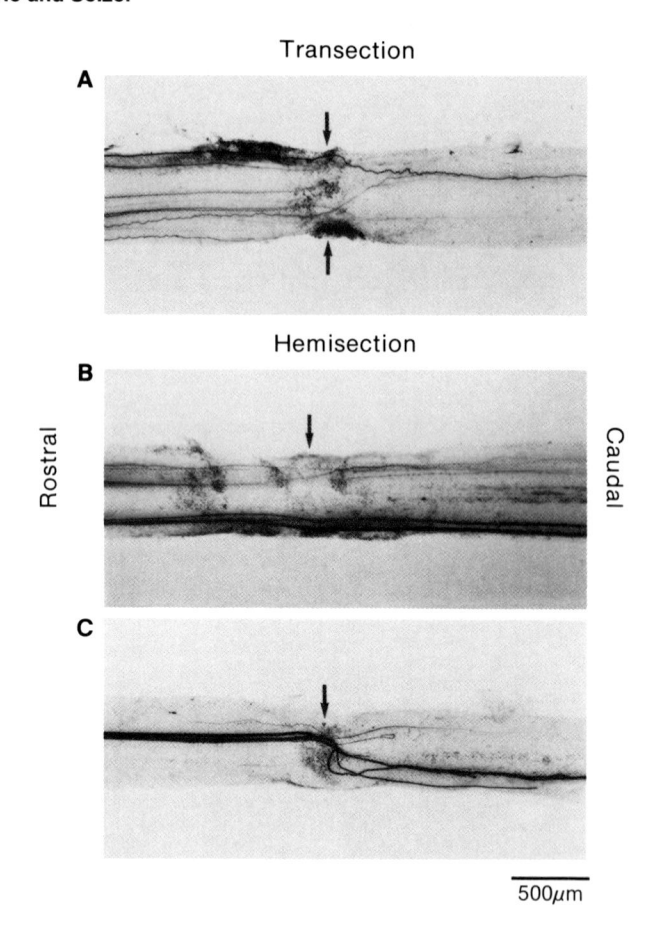

Fig. 4. Preferential regeneration of neurites from giant reticulospinal axons (RAs) through the scar in hemisected spinal cords. A, ten weeks after complete transection at the level of the third gill (arrows), most neurites have regenerated across the scar and continued on the same side of the cord. One axon decussated anomalously and another looped rostralward before crossing the scar. B, ten week hemisection at the level of the third gill (arrow). Neurites of axons cut by the lesion are attenuated in caliber but regenerate through the scar and remain ipsilateral to their parent axon. For comparison, untransected RAs have also been injected with HRP (bottom). C, in only one hemisected animal, several regenerating RA neurites decussated at the level of the scar (arrow) and remained contralateral to their parent axon. Some neurites in this cord grew through the scar (top). From Selzer et al., 1987.

side of the cord contains more empty spaces and axonal debris as a result of Wallerian degeneration. This was ruled out by performing a second simultaneous hemisection contralateral and 10 mm caudal to the first. In this case both sides of the cord have similar amounts of Wallerian degeneration. The trajectory of regeneration was determined for axons on both sides of the cord. In ten double hemisected animals, forty axons were labeled. They gave rise to one hundred thiry-two neurites, of which 60% regenerated beyond the level of the lesion. Despite the presence of large amounts of Wallerian degeneration on the contralateral side, all of these neurites grew through their respective scars rather than around them (Fig. 5).

We conclude from these experiments that the transection scar in the large larval lamprey is not a relative impediment to regeneration, but in fact presents a preferential pathway of growth for regenerating fibers compared to normal spinal cord parenchyma and spinal cord with axonal debris and empty spaces resulting from Wallerian degeneration. The origin of the cells of the scar is not known with certainty but the histological appearance suggests that it derives in large part from ependymal cells rather than from glial cells.

ULTRASTRUCTURAL ENVIRONMENT OF GIANT AXONS

During the first one to two weeks following transection, the Muller and Mauthner axons die back varying distances up to 2 cm. Thereafter, they begin to regenerate toward the scar, which has already been formed. Between two and five weeks most cut axons are elongating within the proximal stump. After five weeks many axons have crossed the scar, with peak distances achieved by seven to nine weeks (Yin and Selzer, 1983). A study of the growth cone during each of these epocs is currently under way. At present, observations have been made only on untransected axons and on axons four weeks post-transection in the proximal (rostral) stump of spinal cord. Axons have been injected with HRP and the spinal cords kept at 4 C for 24 hours to allow for transport into the growth cones. As illustrated in figure 7, Muller axons are surrounded by glial fibers except at points of en passant synapses with unidentified

Double Hemisection

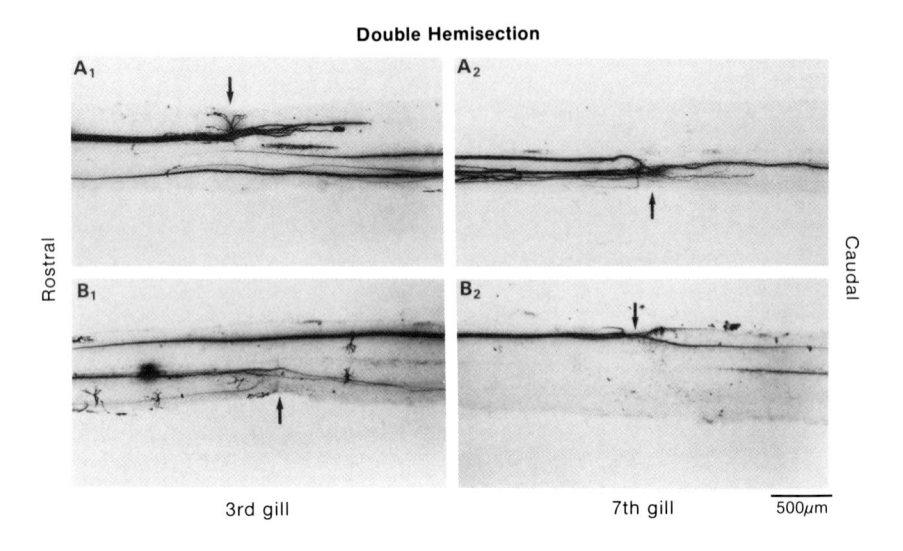

Rostral — 3rd gill — 7th gill — Caudal — 500μm

Fig. 5. Preferential regeneration through the scars of double hemisected spinal cords. Spinal wholemounts of 10 week double hemisected animals. A_1 and B_1, third gill (rostral) hemisections (arrows). Even though some axons terminated at the level of the scar and begin to loop rostrally, those neurites which regenerated past the level of the hemisection remained on the correct side of the cord. Axons at the bottom of A1 and the top of B1 were not cut at this level but were lesioned by the caudal hemisection (7th gill) shown in A2 and B2 (arrows). The behavior of neurites at the caudal hemisection was similar. From Selzer et al. in press.

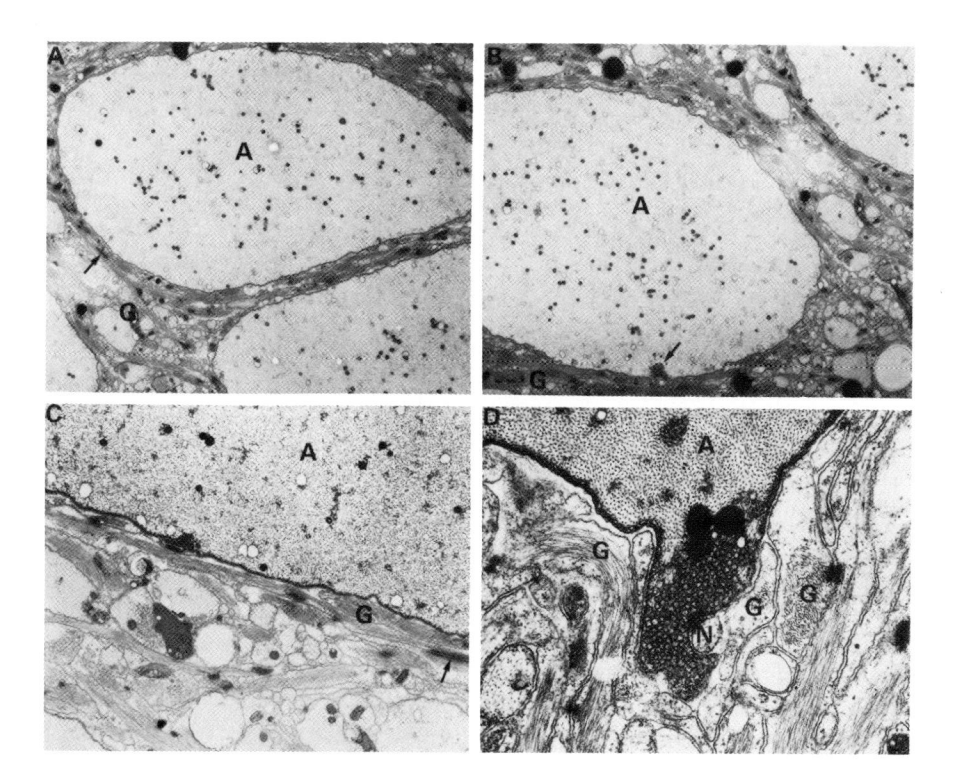

Fig. 6. Investment of control Muller axons by glial processes. A, an unlabeled giant axon (A) completely surrounded by glial processes (G). The latter can be identified by their densely packed, longitudinally oriented glial filaments or by contiguity with parts of the cell containing such filaments. X4,400. B, a Muller axon making en passant synapse (arrow) with a neural process. X4,400. C, a higher magnification electron-micrograph of an axon lightly labeled with HRP, showing its contacts with glial processes. Note desmosomal junctions (arrow) which are seen frequently between glial processes. X19,300. D, a lightly labeled axon showing a short vesicle-containing projection forming an en passant synapse with an unidentified neural process (N). Except at this contact, the axon is surrounded by glial processes. X33,950.

neural elements. Observations on regenerating material are still preliminary. It will be important to determine whether a similar pattern of glial investment characterizes the elongating growth cone.

SUMMARY AND CONCLUSIONS

The large larval sea lamprey recovers behaviorally from complete spinal transection. This is dependent on regeneration of axons for relatively short distances beyond the site of the lesion. Within this range, however, neurites grow selectively in the directions appropriate to the original axon of the injured neurons and form synaptic contacts only with their normal target neuron types. Thus, it is likely that axon guidance and synaptic target recognition cues which determined the original pattern of neuronal connectivity during development can be at least partially expressed during regeneration. This gives hope that if axons can be induced to regenerate beyond the site of injury in the mammalian spinal cord, they would make appropriate synaptic connections rather than random contacts with neurons distal to the lesion and that some functional recovery might result.

ADKNOWLEDGEMENTS

This work was supported by National Institutes of Health Grant NS14837 and the American Paralysis Association Grant RC 87-01.

REFERENCES

Borgens RB, Roederer E, Cohen MJ (1981). Enhanced spinal cord regeneration in lamprey by applied electrical fields. Science 213:611-617.
Bregman BS, Goldberger ME (1983). Infant lesion effect: III. Anatomical correlates of sparing and recovery of function after spinal cord damage in newborn and adult cats. Devel Brain Res 9:137-154.

Bregman BS (1987). Spinal cord transplants permit the growth of serotonergic axons across the site of neonatal spinal cord transection. Dev Brain Res 34:265-279.

Carmichael L (1926). The development of behavior in vertebrates experimentally removed from the influence of external stimulation. Psychol Rev 33:51-58.

Carmichael L (1927). A further study of the development of behavior in vertebrates experimentally removed the from influence of external stimulation. Psychol Rev 34:34-47.

Carmichael L (1928). A further study of the development of behavior in vertebrates experimentally removed the from influence of external stimulation. Psychol Rev 35:253-260.

Cohen AH, Mackler SA, Selzer ME (1986). Functional regeneration following spinal transection demonstrated in the isolated spinal cord of the larval sea lamprey. Proc Natl Acad Sci 83:2763-2766.

Cohen A, Mackler SA, Selzer ME (1988). Functional regeneration in the lamprey spinal cord. TINS 11:227-231.

Croop RS, Snedeker JA, Selzer ME (1987). Distance of axonal regeneration in spinal transected sea lamprey. Neurology 37 (Suppl 1):234.

Currie SN, Ayers J (1983). Regeneration of locomotor command systems in the sea lamprey. Brain Res 279:23-240.

Currie SN, Ayers, J (1987). Plasticity of fin command system function following spinal transection in larval sea lamprey. Brain Res 415:337-341.

David S, Aguayo AJ (1981). Axonal elongation into peripheral nervous system "bridges" after central nervous system injury in adult rats. Science 214:931-933.

Goldberger ME, Murray M (1974). Restitution of function and collateral sprouting in the cat spinal cord: The deafferented animal. J Comp Neurol 158:37-54.

Harrison RG (1904). An experimental study of the relation of the nervous system to the developing musculature in the embryo of the frog. Am J Anat 3:197-220.

Haverkamp LJ (1986). Anatomical and physiological development of the Xenopus embryonic motor system in the absence of neural activity. J Neurosci 6:1338-1348.
Haverkamp LJ, Oppenheim RW (1986). Behavioral development in the absence of neural activity: Effects of chronic immobilization on amphibian embryos. J Neurosci 6:1332-1337.
Liu CN, Chambers WW (1958). Intraspinal sprouting of dorsal root axons. Arch Neurol Psychiat 79:46-61.
Mackler SA, Selzer ME (1985). Regeneration of functional synapses between individual recognizable neurons in the lamprey spinal cord. Science 229:774-776.
Mackler SA, Yin HS, Selzer ME (1986). Determinants of directional specificity in the regeneration of lamprey spinal axons. J Neurosci 6:1814-1821.
Mackler SA, Selzer ME (1987). Specificity of synaptic regeneration in the spinal cord of the larval sea lamprey. J Physiol (Lond.) 388:183-198.
Mathews SA, Detwiler SR (1926). The reaction of amblystoma embryos following prolonged treatment with chloretone. J Exp Zool 45:279-292, 1926.
Murray M, Goldberger ME (1974). Restitution of function and collateral sprouting in the cat spinal cord: The partial hemisected animal[1]. J Comp Neurol 158:19-36.
Park S, Snedeker JA, Selzer ME (1986). Behavioral recovery in spinal transected lamprey does not require specific behavioral feedback. Soc Neurosci Abstr 12, 425.6.
Reier P (1985). Neural tissue grafts and repair of the injured spinal cord. Neuropath and Applied Neurobiol 11:81-104.
Rovainen CM (1967a). Physiological and anatomical studies on large neurons of the central nervous system of the sea lamprey (Petromyzon marinus): I. Muller and Mauthner cells. J Neurophysiol 30:1000-1023.
Rovainen CM (1967b). Physiological and anatomical studies on large neurons of central nervous system of the sea lamprey (Petromyzon marinus). II. Dorsal cells and giant interneurons. J. Neurophysiol 30:1024-1042.
Rovainen CM (1974a). Synaptic interactions of identified nerve cells in the spinal cord of the sea lamprey. J Comp Neurol 154:184-206.

Rovainen CM (1974b). Synaptic interactions of reticulospinal neurons and nerve cells in the spinal cord of the sea lamprey. J Comp Neurol 154:207-224.

Rovainen CM (1976). Regeneration of Muller and Mauthner axons after spinal transection in larval lampreys. J Comp Neurol 168:545-554.

Sah DWY, Frank E (1984). Regeneration of sensory-motor synapses in the spinal cord of the bullfrog. J Neurosci 4:2784-2791.

Selzer ME (1978). Mechanisms of functional recovery and regeneration after spinal cord transection in larval sea lamprey. J Physiol 277:395-408.

Selzer ME (1979). Variability in maps of identified neurons in the sea lamprey spinal cord examined by a wholemount technique. Brain Res 163:181-193.

Selzer ME, Lurie D, Mackler SA (in press). Pathfinding and synaptic specificity of regenerating spinal axons in the lamprey. Post Lesion Neural Plasticity Flohr, Springer-Verlag.

Wood MR, Cohen MJ (1979). Synaptic regeneration in identified neurons of the lamprey spinal cord. Science 206:344-347.

Wood MR, Cohen MJ (1981). Synaptic regeneration and glial reactions in the transected spinal cord of the lamprey. J Neurocytol 10:57-79.

Yin HS, Selzer ME (1983). Axonal regeneration in the lamprey spinal cord. J Neurosci 3:1135-1144.

Yin HS, Mackler SA, Selzer ME (1984). Directional specificity in the regeneration of lamprey spinal axons. Science 224:894-896.

FUNCTIONAL AND NON-FUNCTIONAL REGENERATION IN THE SPINAL CORD OF ADULT LAMPREYS

Avis H. Cohen and Margaret T. Baker

Section of Neurobiology and Behavior,
Seeley G. Mudd Hall, Cornell University
Ithaca, NY 14853

INTRODUCTION

To study functional regeneration after central nervous system damage, one would like a system in which the function of the regenerated neuronal tissue can be assessed directly during the execution of a behavior. When this is impossible, it is difficult to separate the contributions of other factors. These factors can include either reflexes activated via sensory inputs, or alternative neuronal pathways that circumvent the lesion site, or passive movements mechanically produced. There can also be problems separating local synaptic actions from diffuse release mechanisms. For example, it is often possible for diffusely released neurotransmitters to elicit or modulate behavior. While function at the level of behavioral initiation or modulation may indeed be restored in such cases, diffuse transmitter release is not an adequate mechanism for many of the more precisely controlled functions of the nervous system, and it is important to distinguish between the two forms of recovery.

The lamprey provides an ideal model for the direct assessment of functional regeneration after spinal injury. The animals are known to recover behaviorally from spinal transection (Rovainen,1976; Selzer, 1978; Wood and Cohen, 1981; Currie and Ayers, 1983), and fibers are known to regenerate and reconnect across the lesion site (Mackler and Selzer, 1987; Wood and Cohen, 1981). To test that the fibers have restored a functional neural circuit, the activity of the spinal pattern generator for locomotion can be assessed (Cohen et al., 1986). It is this final step we will discuss here.

The central pattern generator (CPG) for locomotion is the spinal circuit which produces the motor output pattern which underlies swimming. The lamprey CPG is a distributed network; each segment, or small group of segments, has the necessary circuitry to produce a locomotor-type bursting pattern (Cohen and Wallén, 1980). Such "fictive swimming" can be elicited by the bath application of excitatory amino acids such as D-glutamate (Cohen and Wallén, 1980) and N-methyl-D-aspartate (NMDA)(Grillner et al.,1981b). Unlesioned adult spinal cords generate a periodic ventral root discharge pattern of about 1 Hz which travels along the segments fairly uniformly so that bursts of more rostral segments temporally lead the activity in more caudal ventral roots by a constant *phase* delay (as distinguished from a constant *time* delay. The phase delay is defined as the rostral to caudal delay divided by the cycle period of the rostral segment). The phase delay approximates 1% of the cycle period per segment. In control cords this discharge pattern is remarkably stable and reproducable within and between animals (Cohen, 1987). Larval lamprey cords differ from adults in their behavior somewhat (Cohen et al., 1986), but the differences are unimportant here.

Since any small group of spinal cord segments can generate this pattern, a lesion to the cord should not interfere with fictive locomotion in unlesioned segments. Functional reconnection of regenerated fibers can then be assessed how well the fibers restore coordination of fictive swimming across the lesioned segment.

DEMONSTRATION OF FUNCTIONAL REGENERATION IN LARVAL LAMPREYS

This method of demonstrating functional regeneration

was used in larval lamprey spinal cords (Cohen et al., 1986). The original demonstration did not include the use of any neuromuscular blocker because there was no movement observed in the small amount of muscle which remained attached to the notochord. However, the possibility remained (Hill et al., 1987) that there were residual movements which could produce reflex entrainment through periodic activation of spinal mechanoreceptors in the spinal cord (Grillner et al., 1981a). To rule out this possibility, the experiments were repeated in the presence of curare (Cohen, in press).

Larval *Petromyzon marinus* were transected and allowed to recover. Spinal cords and supporting notochord were removed and placed in a dish. D-glutamate (0.25mM) and D-tubocurarine (15mg/l) were superfused over the cords while bipolar suction electrodes monitored the motor nerve discharge in a conventional manner. Activity began with a slow often irregular discharge pattern which could continue for some time. This was followed by unpatterned activity with little evidence for coordinated bursting across the lesion site. During this time the rostral and caudal segments could burst for brief **episodes**® with two different rhythms. However, after as long as 45 minutes, a rapid burst pattern (>1Hz) was seen with the bursting well coordinated across the injured segment.
Coordinated bursting was seen with excitatory amino acid and was always preserved in the presence of both excitatory amino acid and curare.

This evidence adds further confirmation that in the larval lamprey the fibers can form connections capable of restoring some behaviorally important functions. It should also be stressed that by assessment in isolated cord preparations all larval animals which had had adequate recovery time exhibited some degree of restored coordination. However, in the regenerated spinal cords coordination was severely degraded even though the animals swam normally before their cords were tested. Therefore, although the functional recovery was not to full capacity or even nearly full **capacity,** with the spinal cord in place, the animal was using sensory inputs and mechanical factors to augment its coordination to achieve normal swimming movements.

ADULT MODELS FOR STUDIES OF FUNCTIONAL REGENERATION

It seems likely that the adult central nervous system will be more limited than the larval in its capacity to recover function. It is true that the larval lamprey is a relatively stable life phase. Nevertheless, the nervous system must be equipped to restructure itself to accomodate the behavioral and anatomical changes it will undergo during metamorphosis. The adult has no such need. Comparison of larval and adult nervous systems might give clues as to the factors which limit recovery should such

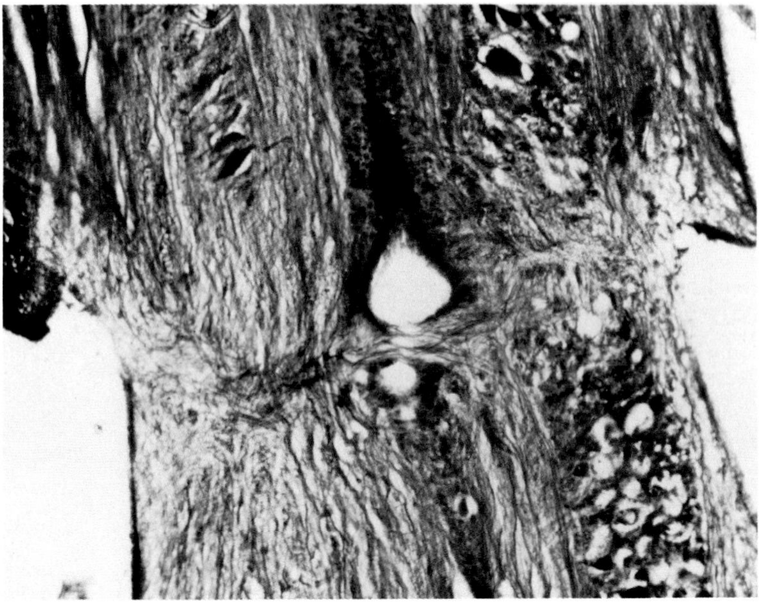

Figure 1: Lesioned cord showing tangled regenerated fibers in the medial tracts and cellular regions. The lateral tracts were cut in the dish during testing (note lateral cuts to regenerted region). Rostral (above) and caudal to the lesion site normal somata and axons can be seen for comparison.

limits be found. However, adult lampreys require a recovery time which is so long and a temperature that is so high that the animals must feed to survive.

Because of this, we now provide prey fish and make partial lesions in the mid-body region to help the animals to maintain their full behavioral repertoire needed for prey catching. It has now become possible to keep the animals healthy for the extended times needed to observe functional regeneration. It should be noted that we have see fibers crossing the lesion site much earlier, but such times seem to be inadequate for coordination to reappear. There is no question that adults can regrow fibers across a lesion site (fig. 1); the problem is, as in the larval cords, to prove that the fibers are making functional synapses. The work described here will prove that the synapses can be functional, although not as often as are the larval fibers. We will also demonstrate that the adult lamprey cord can serve as a model for comparing regrowth that is and is not functional.

Another advantage of using adult cords is that a great deal is known about its intersegmental coordinating

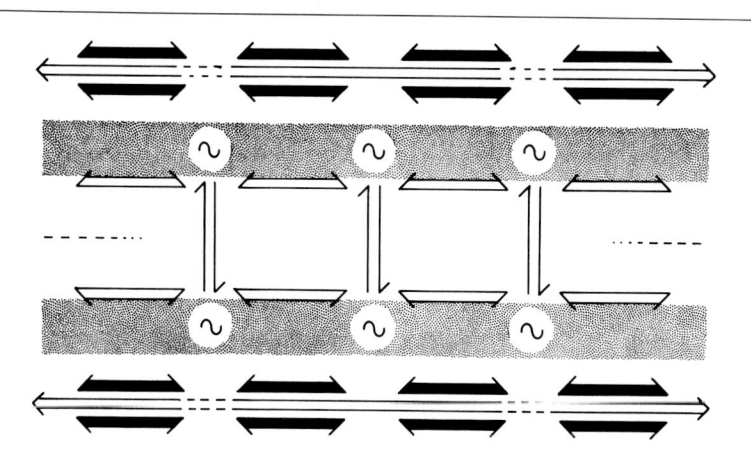

Figure 2: Organization of CPG superimposed on a diagram of medial and lateral tracts and cellular gray region (stipples). Segmental burst generators (circles) are coupled across and up and down the cord.

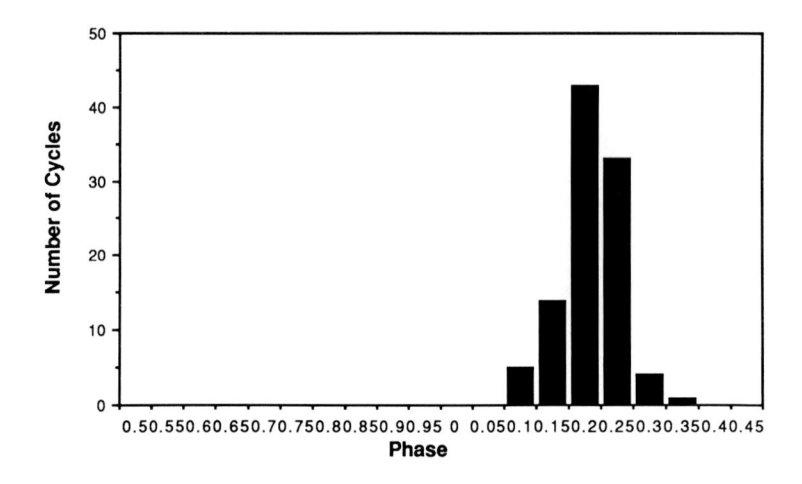

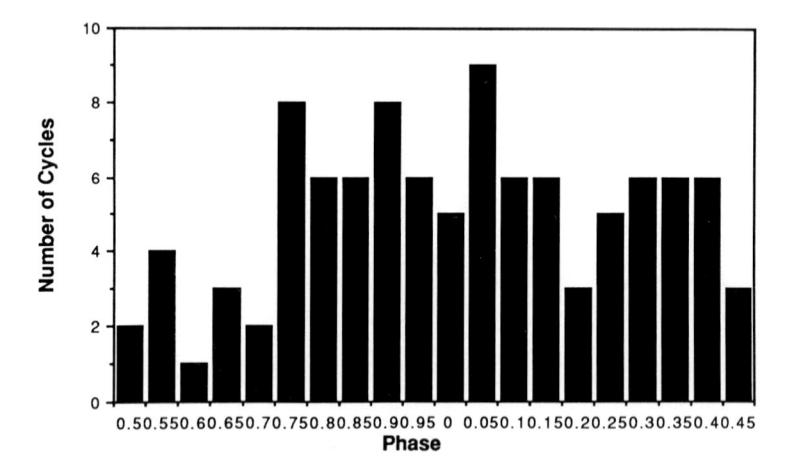

Figure 3: (Upper) Histogram of phase delays between motor nerves 12 segments apart separated by an acute lesion sparing only the lateral tracts. By Chi square test, the distribution is highly non-random (p << .001). (Lower) Phase delays between two motor nerves 20 segments apart connected across regenerated lateral tracts. The distribution of phases does not differ from random.

system (Cohen, 1987). Three paired sub-divisions can visually be distinguished, the lateral and medial tracts and the cellular gray region. There are apparently at least three major anatomical subdivisions of the coordinating system, two short fiber subsystems and one long fiber subsystem(fig. 2). The two short fiber subsystems are in the medial and lateral tracts. The long fibers are almost all restricted to the lateral tracts. To date, definition of long and short have been limited to greater than or less than 10 segments long. Each of these subsystems can sustain stable coordination when the others have been removed. However, the most effective appear to be the short fibers of the lateral tracts.

Eleven lampreys were tested after having been subjected to hemisections (n=4) or lesions of their lateral (n=3) or medial (n=4) tracts 8-9 months earlier. If made acutely in an isolated adult spinal cord preparation none of these lesions normally would cause disruption of coordination (Cohen, 1987; cf.fig. 3, upper). The cords were dissected out, the spared regions of the cord cut acutely leaving only the regenerated fibers intact,and the cords were examined for coordinated bursting which spanned the lesioned segment.

Unlike the larval lampreys, most adults did not exhibit bursting coordinated across the injured segment. In the majority of the cords the segments on either side of the lesion could be induced to stable activity, but the activity was not well coordinated. Only in 3 cords did the bursting achieve a non-random degree of coordination (fig. 4). Even in these, while the coordination was clear it was not tight. There were always episodes in which the two regions would drift apart from one another.

Even though control studies indicate many coordinating fibers in the lateral tracts (Cohen, 1987) regenerated lateral tracts did not sustain coordination in those animals tested (fig. 3,lower). The hemisected animals also did not exhibit coordinated activity. The animals with lateral lesions displayed some interaction but it was very weak and unstable. By contrast, lesions of medial tracts and gray cellular regions were, at least to date, much more successful in leading to restored function (fig. 4). All 3 cords that produced significantly coordinated bursting had had medial lesions.

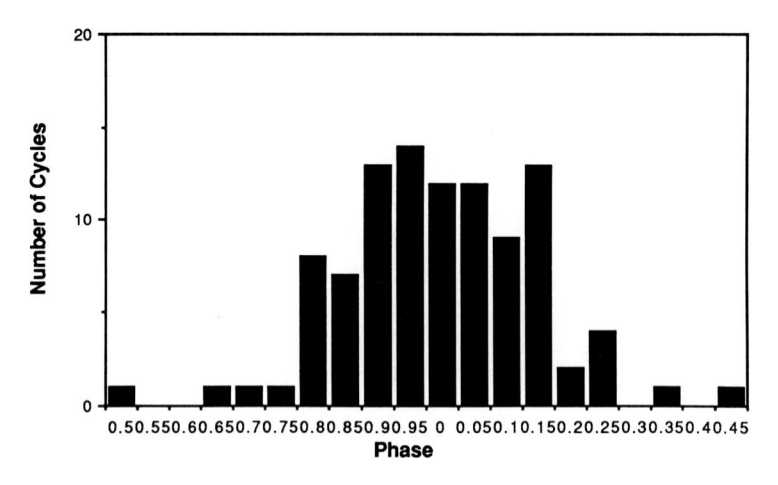

Figure 4: Phase delays of motor nerves 11 segments apart separated by regenerated medial tracts. Distribution of phase delays is significantly different from random (p << .001).

From the histology, it is clear that adult lamprey spinal axons have the capacity to regenerate after transection (fig. 1), but with the partial lesion protocol they are less likely to restore function than are larval stage lampreys. It appears that medial tract fibers are more apt to be successful than are lateral tract fibers, but this conclusion must be viewed as preliminary. If true, one possible explanation could relate to the lengths of the fibers in the different tracts, as it is known that long fibers are less likely to regenerate following axotomy (Yin and Selzer, 1983). Moreover, even if long fibers do regenerate, they are not likely to grow the required distance to reconnect appropriately (Yin and Selzer, 1983). It is known that the lateral tract fibers include almost all the long coordinating fibers (Cohen, 1987). But we know little about the lengths of the short fiber components of the coordinating system. It is entirely possible that the lateral tract short fiber system is composed of fibers which extend over several segments while the more medial coordinating fibers are local interneurons. However, this remains to be proven.

However, another explanation must be found to explain the difference between larval and adult lampreys. Unfortunately, larval spinal cords are difficult to work with and little is known about the immature coordinating system. Preliminary experiments indicated that the coordinating system was similarly organized with respect to the distribution of its fibers, but the relative lengths of the components of the anatomical subsystems were not examined. We do not know, for example, if the larval lamprey simply has fewer long coordinating fibers and therefore has fewer problems regenerating and reconnecting them. Thus, we cannot distinguish between a simple extension of the fiber length argument and another more developmentally oriented explanation for their greater success. For example, is the system more able to adapt to incorrect connections than is the adult system? Are the fibers more apt to search out their correct targets than are the adult fibers? It also remains uncertain how adults with complete transections will compare with larval animals. The preparation should **offer us** good opportunities to answer such questions and to unravel the mechanisms for the successful and unsuccessful regeneration of spinal neurons.

Acknowledgments: This work was supported by NIH grant NS16803 (to AHC) and AFOSR contract no. F49620-87-C-0013 to Northeastern University.

LITERATURE CITED

Cohen, A. H., The structure and function of the intersegmental coordinating system in the lamprey spinal cord., J. Comp. Physiol.,A, 160(1987)181-193.

Cohen, A. H., Regenerated fibers of the lamprey spinal cord can coordinate fictive swimming in the presence of curare, J. Neurobiol., in press.

Cohen, A. H., Mackler, S. A. and Selzer, M. E., Functional regeneration following spinal transection demonstrated in the isolated spinal cord of the larval sea lamprey, Proc. Nat. Acad. Sci., 83(1986)2763-2766.

Cohen, A. H. and Wallén, P., The neuronal correlate of locomotion in fish: "Fictive swimming" induced in an in vitro preparation of the lamprey spinal cord, Exp. Brain Res., 41(1980)11-18.

Currie, S. N. and Ayers, J., Regeneration of locomotor command systems in the sea lamprey, Brain Res., 279(1983)238-240.

Grillner, S., McClellan, A., and Perret, C., Entrainment of the spinal pattern generators for swimming by mechanosensitive elements in the lamprey spinal cord in vitro, Brain Res.. 217(1981a)380-386.

Grillner, S., McClellan, A., Sigvardt, K., Wallén, P., Wilén, M., Activation of NMDA-receptors elicits "fictive locomotion" in lamprey spinal cord in vitro, Acta Physiol. Scan., 113(1981b)549-551.

Hill, R. H., Wallén, P., Carlstedt, T., Grillner, S., and Aguayo, A. J., A re-examination of regeneration and recovery of swimming after spinal transection in lamprey, Acta Physiol. Scan., 129(1987)28A.

Mackler, S. A. and Selzer, M. E., Specificity of synaptic regeneration in the spinal cord of the larval sea lamprey, J. Physiol. (Lond.), 388(1987)183-198.

Rovainen, C. M., Regeneration of Müller and Mauthner axons after spinal transection in larval lampreys, J. Comp. Neurol., 168(1976)545-554.

Selzer, MN. E., Mechanisms of functional recovery and regeneration after spinal cord transection in larval sea lampreys, J. Physiol. (London), 277(1978)395-408.

Wood, M. R. and Cohen, M. J., Synaptic regeneration and glial reactions in the transected spinal cord of the lamprey, J. Neurocytol., 10(1981)57-79.

Yin, H. S. and Selzer, M. E., Axonal regeneration in lamprey spinal cord, J. Neurosci., 3(1983)1135-1144.

Index

A23187, 202
3A3 antigen, PC 12 cells, 152
Acetylcholine, 202
Acetylcholinesterase
    axon terminals at synaptic sites, maintenance in absence of muscle fibers, frog NMJ, 170, 175
    nerve growth factor in partial fimbrial transected rats, 106, 107, 111
    neuron rescue, CNS lesions, 69, 72
ACTH, 202
Actin, 215
    α-, 17–19
    cytoskeleton, regenerating motoneuron axon, 13–20, 24–28, 30
    microfilamints, 149, 154
    see also Cytoskeleton, regenerating motoneuron axon
α-Actinin, 215
Action potentials, neuron response to injury, 4–8
    ion channels, 4–5
Adenosine, astrocyte responses to, 258
Adhesion
    cell-to-cell, 147
    cell-to-matrix, 147, 148
    molecules
        F11, 212
        on glia (AMOG), 220–221
    see also Cell adhesion molecules *entries*
β-Adrenergic agonists, astrocyte responses to, early molecular events, 258
Afferent synaptic efficiency, spinal motoneurons, target-dependence, 60–61
Age and spinal cord regenerative capacity, 333
Aldolase, 24
Alzheimer's disease, 105, 112
    reactive astrogliosis, 248
4-Aminopyridine, 4, 6, 7

Ankyrin, 215
Apo E, 297
Arachidonic acid metabolites, mononuclear phagocytes in acute CNS injury, 283
AraC, mononuclear phagocytes in acute CNS injury, 285
Arborization, axon terminals at synaptic sites, maintenance in absence of muscle fibers, frog NMJ, 167, 168
Arg-Gly-Asp (RGDS) sequence, 139–143, 151
Astrocyte(s), 151, 184
    activation, EAE, gliotic plaque, 292
    adhesion, 210
    dorsal root fiber regeneration into adult mammalian spinal cord, 311
    functions, 247–248
    injury, EGF receptors in rat brain, 301–309
    types, 247
Astrocyte and plasminogen activator, rat, 271–279, 302
    astrocyte maturity and reactivity, 271, 273–276, 278
    plasminogen activator inhibitors, 276–278
Astrocyte-coated Millipore implants, embryonic, dorsal root fiber regeneration into spinal cord, 311, 313, 315–319, 322
Astrocytes, responses to GFs and hormones, early molecular events, 257–267
    β-adrenergic agonists, 258
    cyclic AMP, 258, 260, 265
        forskolin, 265
    fibroblast growth factor
        acidic, 258, 301–302
        basic, 258, 259, 301
    glial fibrillary acidic protein, 258–260

glutamine synthetase, 258–260, 265
hydrocortisone, 259, 265
insulin, 258, 259, 265
interleukin-1, 258, 302
stellate-process bearing, 258, 259, 265
transiently-induced sequences (TIS) genes, 260–267
  cf. c-fos, 261–263
  TPA-induction, 260, 262–264
vimentin, 258, 259
VIP, 258
Astroglia and plasminogen activator, rat, 271–279, 302
  astrocyte maturity and reactivity, 271, 273–276, 278
  and PA inhibitors, 276–278
Astrogliosis, reactive, 248–251, 311
Axon(s)
  elongation, raphe spinal projection, target-specific requirements, immature axotomized CNS neurons, rats, 82–83
  growth, substratum organization, two-dimensional neural network, insect wing graft experiments, 127–129
  long, vertebrate spinal cord, regenerative capacity, 338, 339
  regrowth, cytoskeleton, neuron response to injury, 3–5
  supernumerary, 49
  see also Cytoskeleton, regenerating motoneuron axon
Axon terminals at synaptic sites, maintenance in absence of muscle fibers, frog NMJ, 167–175
  acetylcholinesterase, 170, 175
  basal lamina sheaths, 167–172, 175
  cutaneous pectoral muscle, removal, 168–169
  cf. development, 175
  freeze-fracture, fine structure, 171–173
  Schwann cells, 173–174
Axotomy and transport changes, cytoskeleton, regenerating motoneuron axon, 24–25; see also Ganglioside GM$_1$ effect on rat rubral neuron axotomy response; Target-specific requirements, immature axotomized CNS neurons, rat

Bands of Bungner, 180
Basal lamina sheaths, axon terminals at synaptic sites, maintenance in absence of muscle fibers, frog NMJ, 167–172, 175
Bicuculline, 349
Blood-brain barrier, 257, 282
Brain, spectrin (fodrin), 215
Brainstem, spinal cord injury, rat, plasticity, 351
Broca's band, 105, 108

E-Cadherin, 218
N-Cadherin, 121, 123
P-Cadherin, 218
Calcium-calmodulin dependent protein kinase, growth cone regulation, 200–201
Calcium channels, voltage-dependent, 271
Calcium-dependent cell-cell adhesion mechanisms, 229–230, 232
Calcium-dependent protease, 162
Calcium-independence, N-CAM, 229
Calcium-phospholipid-dependent protein kinase, growth cone regulation, 200–201
Calmodulin, cytoskeleton, regenerating motoneuron axon, 24, 26, 28, 29
Cell adhesion molecule(s), 163, 229
  L1. See L1 antigen
  Ng-CAM, 191, 213
  see also Adhesion; specific molecules
Cell adhesion molecule, neural (N-CAM), 121, 189–191, 209, 212, 213, 218, 220, 229–234, 237–242
  and calcium-dependent cell-cell adhesion mechanisms, 229–230, 232
  calcium-independence, 229
  components/fragments
    115 kDa, 237, 239
    120 kDa, 193–194, 215–216
    140 kDa, 215, 237, 239
    180 kDa, 214, 215

190 kDa, 237, 239
growth cones, 230–231
heparin binding domain, 219
and L1 antigen, 214–217, 237–242
  molecular genetics, 237–238
  post-translational modifications, 238–239
  NCAM-NCAM binding, 232, 233
  permissive hierarchies, 234
  polysialic acid (PSA) content, 229–234, 239, 240
  regulatory mechanism, proposed, 232–233
Cell body reaction, 13–16, 24
Cell migration, plasminogen activator production, 277, 278
Cell surface affinity hierarchies, two-dimensional neural network, insect wing graft experiments, 128–129; *see also* Extracellular matrix–cell surface interactions in regeneration
Cell-to-cell adhesion, 147
Cell-to-matrix adhesion, 147, 148
Central cf. peripheral nervous system
  extracellular matrix, 148, 153
  –cell surface interactions in regeneration, 119
  fibronectin–neuronal growth interactions, chick embryo, 138–139, 143
Central pattern generator for locomotion, spinal cord transection recovery, *Petromyzon marinus* (lamprey), 388, 391
Cerebellar granule cells, 213, 220
Chalones, 250
Chartins, 30
Chemoaffinity hypothesis, 147
Chemotaxis, growth cone, regulation, 203
Chloroquine, acute CNS injury, 283–287
Choline acetyltransferase
  nerve growth factor in partial fimbrial transected rats, 106, 107, 109–112
  neuron rescue, CNS lesions, 69–72
Cholinergic neurons
  forebrain, basal, 69
  reinnervation, hippocampus, NGF in partial fimbrial transected rats, 105, 106, 109–112

septum, 70–71
  NGF in partial fimbrial transected rats, 105–109, 112
Chondroitinase ABC, 191
Chondroitin sulfate, 191, 192
Chromatolysis, 3, 36–37
Coaptation. *See* Spinal cord stump coaptation by spinal column shortening, rat
Colchicine, 49, 61
  mononuclear phagocytes in acute CNS injury, 283–287
Collagen(s), 139
  IV, 120, 122, 123
  nerve fiber growth, 147–149, 152, 155
Collagenase, 272
ConA, 297
Conditioned medium, trophic factor hypothesis, visual system
  concentration, 97–99
  hippocampus cf. diencephalon, 99–100
Conduction velocity, spinal motoneurons, 56, 57, 59
Coordinated bursting, spinal cord transection recovery, *Petromyzon marinus* (lamprey), 389, 393–395
Corticospinal tract, 344
Cranin (laminin-binding protein), 150, 152–153, 155
Creatine kinase, 24
Creutzfeldt-Jakob disease, reactive astrogliosis, 248, 250
CSAT, 212
  band 3, 120
Curare, spinal cord transection recovery, *Petromyzon marinus* (lamprey), 389
Cutaneous pectoral muscle, removal, axon terminals at synaptic sites, maintenance, frog NMJ, 168–169
Cyclic AMP, astrocyte responses to, early molecular events, 258, 260, 265
  dibutyryl, 258, 265
  forskolin and, 265
Cycloheximide, 260, 262
Cytochalasin B, 154
Cytochrome c, cf. nerve growth factor in partial transected rats, 106
Cytoskeleton, regenerating motoneuron axon, 3–5, 13–20, 23–30

actin, 13–20, 24–28, 30
  axotomy and transport changes, 24–25
  calmodulin, 24, 26, 28, 29
  facial nucleus, rat, axotomy, 14–20
  glial cells, surrounding, 16–17
  glial fibrillary acidic protein, 14, 16
  in situ hybridization for mRNAs, 16–20
  intermediate filaments, 23
  microfilaments, 13, 23
  microtubule-associated proteins, 24, 26, 28, 30
  microtubules, 13, 16, 23–24, 26, 30
  myosin, non-muscle, 24
  neurofilaments, 14–16, 20, 23–25, 27
    -68, 15, 17–19
    -150, 15, 17
  phosphorylation, 16, 19
  retrograde trophic factor, 15–16
  sciatic nerve, 25–27
  slow transport
    conditioned daughter axons, 26–30
    mature and daughter axons (sprouts), 24–26
  spectrin, 24
  tubulin, 14–20, 25–28
  vesicles, synaptic, 23
  see also specific components
Cytotactin receptor, 212

Decay accelerating factor, 193
Dedifferentiation, 58
Degeneration, Wallerian, 379
^{14}C-2-Deoxyglucose uptake, GM$_1$ effect on rat rubral neuron axotomy response, 33–34
Dexamethasone, in acute CNS injury, 283–287
DFP pretreatment, nerve growth factor in partial fimbrial transected rats, 106
1,2-Diacylglycerol, 194, 195, 201
  phospholipases C, 195
Diencephalon, 99–100
Dopaminergic pathway, nigrostriatal, 109
Dorsal root fiber regeneration into adult mammalian spinal cord, induced, 311–324
  abnormal terminal formation, 321, 323
  astrocytes, reactive, 311

dorsal root entry zone, 312–315, 317, 319, 323
  glial fibrillary acidic protein, 314, 315
  Millipore implants, embryonic astrocyte-coated, 311, 313, 315–319, 322
  phagocytes, 317, 318, 323
  scar tissue, 315, 319
  surgery and HRP histochemistry, 313–315, 317, 318, 321, 322, 324
D2 protein, 237
DRG neurons, 76, 184, 217
Drosophila, 133
DSP-2 antigen, 237

Edema, spinal cord stump coaptation by spinal column shortening, 362
Electrogenesis and action potential transmission, neurons, response to injury, 4–8
Electrophorus electricus, 190
Embryo, chick. *See* Fibronectin–neuronal growth interactions, chick embryo; Laminin–neuronal growth interactions, chick embryo
Embryonic astrocyte-coated Millipore implants, dorsal root fiber regeneration into spinal cord, 311, 313, 315–319, 322
Embryonic-cell-derived NTFs, trophic factor hypothesis, visual system, 93–100
Encephalomyelitis, experimental allergic. *See* Experimental allergic encephalomyelitis *entries*
Enolase, neuron-specific, 24
En passant synapse, spinal cord transection recovery, *Petromyzon marinus* (lamprey), 379, 381
Entactin, 149
Epidermal growth factor, astrocytes responses to, early molecular events, 258
Epidermal growth factor receptors, rat brain, astrocyte injury, 301–309
  EGF and, 302
  events after injury, 308–309
  glial fibrillary acidic protein, 303, 306, 307
  mitogen inhibitors, EGFR-related, 303–307, 309

Epithelial cells, basal surfaces, two-dimensional neural network, insect wing graft experiments, 133, 135
EPSPs, spinal motoneurons, target-dependence, 56–58, 60–61
Experimental allergic encephalomyelitis, 250, 251
Experimental allergic encephalomyelitis, gliotic plaque, 291–299
  astrocyte activation, 292
  extracellular matrix, astrocytes, 297, 298
  glial fibrillary acidic protein, 292–295, 297, 299
  radioautography, 293–296
    acute, 293, 295
    chronic, 296
Experimental allergic uveitis, 250
Extracellular matrix, 147–150, 153–155
  astrocytes, EAE gliotic plaque, 297, 298
  central cf. peripheral, 148, 153
  receptors, 150–153, 155
  see also specific components
Extracellular matrix–cell surface interactions in regeneration, 119–124
  central cf. peripheral, 119
  integrin family of heterodimers, 120–122
    listed, 120
  nerve growth factor, 119, 121
Extrinsic neurons, intrinsic vs., 33–34, 42

Facial nucleus, rat, axotomy, cytoskeleton of regenerating motoneuron axon, 14–20
F11 adhesion molecule, 212
Fetal spinal cord transplant, target-specific requirements, immature axotomized CNS neurons, rats, 77
  target cf. nontarget transplants, survival time, 80–84
Fibrin, 139
Fibroblast growth factor, astrocyte responses to, early molecular events
  acidic, 258, 301–302
  basic, 258, 259, 301
Fibroblasts, plasminogen activator and PA inhibitor production, 276
Fibronectin, 120
  nerve fiber growth, 147–149, 151, 155
  receptor, 212

Fibronectin–neuronal growth interactions, chick embryo, 137–144
  central cf. peripheral, 138–139, 143
  interactions with different FN domains, 139–140, 143
  domain-specific probes, 140–141
  neurite elongation, 142
  synthetic petpide studies, 142–143
Fictive locomotion/swimming, *Petromyzon marinus* (lamprey), 371, 388
Filamin, 215
Fimbrial transected rats. *See* Nerve growth factor in partial fimbrial transected rats
Fink-Heimer stain for degenerating axons, 354
Fish, spinal cord, regenerative capacity, 331–339
FNR β, 120
Fodrin (spectrin), 215
Forebrain, basal, cholinergic neurons, 69
Freeze-fracture, fine structure, axon terminals at synaptic sites, maintenance in absence of muscle fibers, frog NMJ, 171–173
Functional regeneration, 332–333
  spinal cord transection, *Petromyzon marinus* (lamprey), 390–395

GABAergic neurons, nerve growth factor in partial fimbrial transected rats, 109
GABA, spinal cord injury, rat, plasticity, 348, 349
GAD
  nerve growth factor in partial fimbrial transected rats, 109
  spinal cord injury, rat, plasticity, 348
Ganglia, leech segmental, 49
Ganglioside GM_1, astrocyte responses to, 265
Ganglioside GM_1 effect on rat rubral neuron axotomy response, 33–43
  ^{14}C-2-deoxyglucose uptake, 33–34
  morphometry, 34, 38
  neuronal programming, 41
  RNA, 34–36, 39–41
    microspectrofluorometry, 36
  tractotomy effect, 39–40
  neuron number and somatic size, 40

Gastrocnemius-soleus muscles, spinal motoneuron target-dependence, electrophysiology in cat, 55–56
Giant axon structural environment, spinal cord transection recovery, *Petromyzon marinus* (lamprey), 379–382
Glia, adhesion, 210, 211, 213, 216, 220; *see also* Nexins, glia-derived (GDNs), neurite outgrowth and
Glial cells, surrounding, cytoskeleton of regenerating motoneuron axon, 16–17
Glial fibrillary acidic protein, 248, 249
  astrocytes, responses to GFs and hormones, early molecular events, 258–260
  cytoskeleton, regenerating motoneuron axon, 14, 16
  dorsal root fiber regeneration into adult mammalian spinal cord, induced, 314, 315
  epidermal growth factor receptors, rat brain, astrocyte injury, 303, 306, 307
  experimental allergic encephalomyelitis, gliotic plaque, 292–295, 297, 299
Glial growth factor, astrocyte responses to, early molecular events, 258
Glial scar/gap, 301
  target-specific requirements, immature axotomized CNS neurons, rats, 76, 77
  see also Scar tissue
Glia maturation factor, 301, 302
Glioma, 159
  NG108 cell line, 151
Gliosis, 119, 122
Glucuronic acid 3-sulfate, 191, 219
D-Glutamate, spinal cord transection recovery, *Petromyzon marinus* (lamprey), 388, 389
Glutamine synthetase, 248
  astrocyte responses to, early molecular events, 258–260, 265
Glycogen, 248
Glycoprotein(s)
  myelin-associated, 209–212, 216–218, 221, 238
  neuronal surface, structure, 189–191

NILE, 191, 212, 217, 237
Thy-1, 193, 195
trypanosomal variant surface, 193
see also specific glycoproteins
Glycosaminoglycans, 192
Glycosylation, N-CAM and L1, development regulation, 239, 240
GM_1. *See* Ganglioside GM_1 *entries*
Goldfish, 40, 333–339
Grafts. *See* Neural network, two-dimensional, insect wing graft experiments
Granule cells, cerebellar, 213, 220
Growth-associated protein GAP43, 200
Growth cone, 13, 16, 24, 30, 121–123, 144, 149
  N-CAM, 230–231
  neural network, two-dimensional, insect wing graft experiments, 134, 135
  particles, 199–203
  spinal cord transection recovery, *Petromyzon marinus* (lamprey), 379, 382
Growth cone, regulation, 199–204
  chemotaxis, 203
  growth cone particles, 199–203
  protein kinase C activity regulation, 201–203
    calcium, 201–203
  protein kinase substrates
    calcium-calmodulin dependent, 200–201
    calcium-phospholipid-dependent, 200–201
    pp40, 201, 202
    pp46, 200–201, 203
    pp80ac, 201–203
Growth factors. *See* Astrocytes, responses to GFs and hormones, early molecular events; *specific growth factors*

Hemicholinium-3-binding site, 111
Heparan sulfate, 191–194
Heparin, 139–142, 149
Heparin-binding domain, N-CAM, 219
Hindlimb motor behavior, spinal cord injury, rat, plasticity, 349–352
Hippocampal cholinergic reinnervation, nerve growth factor in partial fimbrial transected rats, 105, 106, 109–112

Hippocampus, trophic factor hypothesis, 99–100
Hormones. *See* Astrocytes, responses to GFs and hormones, early molecular events; specific hormones
HRP
  retrograde and anterograde, sensory neuron responses to peripheral nerve injury, rat, 48
  sensory neurons, two-dimensional neural network, insect wing graft experiments, 132
  spinal cord injury, rat, plasticity, 350, 354
  spinal cord transection, recovery, *Petromyzon marinus* (lamprey), 370, 377, 378, 381
Human, alternate leg stepping spastic response, spinal cord, vertebrate, regenerative capacity, 339–340
Huntington's disease, reactive astrogliosis, 248
Hyaluronic acid, 139, 192
Hydrocortisone, astrocyte responses to, 259, 265
Hyperpolarization, spinal motoneurons, 57–59, 61

Imaginal disc, two-dimensional neural network, insect wing graft experiments, 131–133, 135
Immunoglobulin superfamily, 218
Immunosuppressive therapy and mononuclear phagocytes in acute CNS injury, 281, 283–285
Inositol 1,4,5-trisphosphate (IP$_3$), 201, 202
Input resistance, spinal motoneurons, 56, 57
Insect wing. *See* Neural network, two-dimensional, insect wing graft experiments
In situ hybridization for mRNAs, cytoskeleton, regenerating motoneuron axon, 16–20
Insulin, 202
  astrocyte response to, 258, 259, 265
Insulin-like growth factor-1 (IGF-1), astrocyte response to, 258
Integrins, 141, 144, 150–155, 212
  extracellular matrix–cell surface interactions in regeneration, 120–122
  listed, 120

Interleukin-1, 121, 247, 251, 297
  astrocyte responses to, early molecular events, 258, 302
  mononuclear phagocytes in acute CNS injury, 282–284
Intermediate filaments, 248, 249
  astrocyte responses to GFs and hormones, early molecular events, 258
  cytoskeleton, regenerating motoneuron axon, 23
Intestinal tract, L1 antigen, 214
Intrinsic vs. extrinsic neurons, 33–34, 42
Ion channels, neurons, response to injury, 4–5

J1 antigen, 210–212, 220, 238

Laminin, 120, 121, 123
  nerve fiber growth, 147–149, 151, 152, 155
  receptor, 150–152, 155
Laminin-binding protein (120 kDa, cranin), 150, 152–153, 155
Laminin–neuronal growth interactions, chick embryo, 137–144
  laminin fragments, 141–143
  synthetic peptide studies, 142–143
Lamprey. *See* Spinal cord transection, recovery, *Petromyzon marinus* (lamprey)
L1 antigen, 121, 123, 191, 209, 212–214, 218, 221
  N-CAM, interdependence with, 214–217, 237–242
  intestinal tract, 214
  nerve growth factor, 217–218
L2 antigen, 209–212, 219–221, 238
L3 antigen, 220–221
LDL receptor, 302–303, 306, 308
Leech segmental ganglia, 49
Leg-stepping, alternate, spastic response, human, 339–340
LGN
  neurons, target-specific requirements, immature axotomized CNS neurons, rats, 86
  trophic factor hypothesis, 91–92, 94–101
lin gene, 303

Lipoprotein, low-density (LDL), receptor, 302–303, 306, 308
α_2-Macroglobulin, 276
Manduca sexta, 127, 133, 135
Mauthner axons, 377
Melatonin, astrocyte response to, 258
Membrane assembly, neuron response to injury, 5
Microfilaments, 154
 cytoskeleton, regenerating motoneuron axon, 13, 23
Microglial response in acute CNS injury, 282
Microspectrofluorometry, GM_1 effect on rat rubral neuron axotomy response, 36
Microspikes, glia-derived nexins, neurite outgrowth and, 162
Microtubule-associated proteins, cytoskeleton of regenerating motoneuron axon, 24, 26, 28, 30
Microtubules, cytoskeleton of regenerating motoneuron axon, 13, 16, 23–24, 26, 30
Millipore implants, embryonic astrocyte-coated, dorsal root fiber regeneration into adult mammalian spinal cord, induced, 311, 313, 315–319, 322
Mitogen inhibitors, EGFR-related, rat brain, astrocyte injury, 303–307, 309
Molecular genetics
 N-CAM and L1, development regulation, 237–238
 nexins, glia-derived (GDNs), neurite outgrowth and, 160–161
Mononuclear phagocytes in acute CNS injury, 281–287
 arachidonic acid metabolites, 283
 immunosuppressive therapy, 281, 283–285
  AraC, 285
  chloroquine, 283–287
  colchicine, 283–287
  dexamethasone, 283–287
  penetrating injury, 285–286
  promethazine, 285
 interleukin-1, 282–284
 intrinsic cf. extrinsic, 281, 282
 cf. microglial response, 282
 superoxide anion, 283, 284

Morphometry, GM_1 effect on rat rubral neuron axotomy response, 34, 38
Motoneuron axon. *See* Cytoskeleton, regenerating motoneuron axon
Motoneurons, spinal, regenerative capacity, vertebrates, 336, 338
Motoneurons, spinal, target-dependence, electrophysiology in cat, 55–62
 afferent synaptic efficiency, 60–61
 conduction velocity, 56, 57, 59
 EPSP, 56–58, 60–61
 gastrocnemius-soleus muscles, 55–56
 hyperpolarization, 57–59, 61
 input resistance, 56, 57
 muscle functional connection, 59, 60
 neurofilament protein, 58
 neuromuscular synapse, 61
 rheobase, 56, 57, 62
Motor nerve phase delays, spinal cord transection recovery, *Petromyzon marinus* (lamprey), 392
Muller axons, 377, 379, 381
Müller cells, 259
Multiple sclerosis, 251
Muscle functional connection, spinal motoneurons, target-dependence, electrophysiology in cat, 59, 60; *see also* Axon terminals at synaptic sites, maintenance in absence of muscle fibers, frog NMJ
Myelin-associated glycoproteins, 209–212, 216–218, 221, 238
Myelin, P_0, 212, 217
Myosin, non-muscle, cytoskeleton, regenerating motoneuron axon, 24

N-CAM. *See* Cell adhesion molecule, neural (N-CAM)
Nerve growth factor, 148, 191, 202, 203
 extracellular matrix–cell surface interactions in regeneration, 119, 121
 L1 antigen, 217–218
 cf. nexins, glia-derived (GDNs), neurite outgrowth and, 159, 161
 rescue, neuron, CNS lesions, 67, 69–72
 sensory neuron responses to peripheral nerve injury, rat, 50–52

high-affinity receptors, 51, 52
target-specific requirements, immature axotomized CNS neurons, rats, 76
trophic factor hypothesis, visual system, 90, 99
Nerve growth factor-inducible large external (NILE) glycoprotein, 191, 212, 217, 237
Nerve growth factor in partial fimbrial transected rats, 105–113
  acetylcholinesterase, 106, 107, 111
  choline acetyltransferase, 106, 107, 109–112
  cf. cytochrome c, 106
  GABAergic neurons, 109
  GAD, 109
  hippocampal cholinergic reinnervation, 105, 106, 109–112
  rescue of septal cholinergic neurons, 105–109, 112
Nerve growth factor receptor expression on Schwann cells after axonal injury, 121, 123, 179–185
  induction in CNS, 184–185
  kinetic properties of induced receptors, 182–184
  reversibility of expression, 180–182
  Schwann cells not ensheathing NGF-responsive axons, 182
  ultrastructural localization, 180
Neural adhesion molecules, families, 209–221
  family traits, 218–220
  regeneration, 216–218
  see also specific molecules
Neural crest cells, 76
Neural network, two-dimensional, insect wing graft experiments, 127–135
  axonal growth, substratum organization, 127–129
    cell surface affinity hierarchies, 128–129
    proximodistal axis, 127–130, 133
  Drosophila, 133
  Manduca sexta, 127, 133, 135
  pioneering neurons, guidance, 130–135
    epithelial cells, basal surfaces, generality, 133, 135

growth cone, 134, 135
HRP, sensory neurons, 132
imaginal disc, 131–133, 135
substratum changes, regenerating axon response to, 130
Neurite(s)
  elongation, fibronectin–neuronal growth interactions, chick embryo, 142
  outgrowth. *See* Nexins, glia-derived (GDNs), neurite outgrowth and spinal cord transection, recovery, *Petromyzon marinus* (lamprey), 375, 376, 378, 380
Neuroblastoma cells, 143, 159, 189, 191
Neuroblastoma-glioma cell line, NG108, 151
Neurofilament(s)
  cytoskeleton, phosphorylation, regenerating motoneuron axon, 14–16, 20, 23–25, 27
  perikarya, 6
  protein, 215
    motoneurons, spinal, target-dependence, electrophysiology in cat, 58
  slow components
    a, 13, 20, 24–27
    b, 13, 19, 24–28
Neuromuscular junction, 211
  synapse formation, 123
  see also Axon terminals at synaptic sites, maintenance in absence of muscle fibers, frog NMJ
Neuromuscular synapse, spinal motoneuron target-dependence, electrophysiology in cat, 61
Neuron(s), 258, 260
  programming, ganglioside GM_1 effect on rat rubral neuron axotomy response, 41
  rescue. *See* Rescue, neuron *entries*
  surface
    glycoprotein structure, 189–191
    proteoglycans structure, 192–193
Neuron response to injury, 3–8
  axon regrowth, cytoskeleton, 3–5
  duration of response, 6
  electrogenesis and action potential transmission, 4–8

ion channels, 4–5
membrane assembly, 5
morphology, 6–7
sprouting, 7–8
Neuron-specific enolase, 24
Neurotrophic factors (NTFs), neuron rescue, CNS lesions, 67–70, 72
Neurotrophic hypothesis, 67; *see also* Trophic factor hypothesis, visual system
Nexins, glia-derived (GDNs), neurite outgrowth and, 159–164
microspikes, 162
molecular genetics, 160–161
cf. nerve growth factor, 159, 161
NG108 neuroblastoma-glioma cell line, 151
NHK-1, 218–220, 238
Nidogen (entactin), 149
Nigrostriatal dopaminergic pathway, 109
NILE glycoprotein, 191, 212, 217, 237
NMDA, spinal cord transection recovery, *Petromyzon marinus* (lamprey), 388
Nodes of Ranvier, 13, 211
notch gene, 303
Nucleus basalis, 105

Olfactory nerve, 122
Oligodendrocytes, 257, 258
adhesion, 210
Oligodendroglia, 184
Optic nerve, 211, 249

PC 12 cells, 120, 151, 152, 179, 189, 191–193, 195, 203, 217, 261, 267
3A3 antigen, 152
Penetrating injury, mononuclear phagocytes in acute CNS injury, 285–286
Perikarya, 3–7, 199
neurofilaments, 6
Peripheral nervous system, extracellular matrix–cell surface interactions in regeneration, 119; *see also* Central cf. peripheral nervous system; Sensory neuron responses to peripheral nerve injury, rat
Permissive hierarchies, N-CAM, 234
Petromyzon marinus. See Spinal cord transection, recovery, *Petromyzon marinus*

Phagocytes, dorsal root fiber regeneration into adult mammalian spinal cord, induced, 317, 318, 323; *see also* Mononuclear phagocytes in acute CNS injury
Pheochromocytoma, 143; *see also* PC 12 cells
Phosphatidylinositol, 201–203
anchor, N-CAM and L1, development regulation, 239
membrane protein anchors, 193–196
Phosphatidylinositol 4,5-bisphosphate (PIP$_2$), 201–203
Phospholipase C, 202
1,2-diacylglycerol, 195
Phosphorylation
cytoskeleton, regenerating motoneuron axon, 16, 19
N-CAM and L1, development regulation, 239–242
Physiological regeneration, 332
Pioneering neurons, guidance, insect wing graft experiments, 130–135
Piromen stimulation of regeneration, 324
Plasmin, 272, 277
inhibitors, 278
Plasminogen activator, 160, 161, 251
and PA inhibitor production, fibroblasts, 276
production, Schwann cells, 272, 274
cell migration, 277, 278
see also Astroglia and plasminogen activator, rat
Platelet IIa, 120
Platelet-derived growth factor, astrocyte responses to, 258
Poliomyelitis, 7
Polygonal-shaped astrocytes, responses to GFs and hormones, early molecular events, 258, 265
Poly(*N*-acetyllactosaminyl)glycan, 191
Polysialation, N-CAM and L1, development regulation, 239, 240
Polysialic acid (PSA) content, cell adhesion molecules, N-, 229–234
P$_0$ myelin, 212, 217
Post-polio syndrome, 7

Post-translational modifications, N-CAM, and L1, development regulation, 238–239
Potassium, 271
Potassium channels, 4
pp40, growth cone regulation, 201, 202
pp46, growth cone regulation, 200–201, 203
pp80ac, growth cone regulation, 201–203
Promethazine, in acute CNS injury, 285
Propriospinal circuit, spinal cord injury, rat, plasticity, 351, 352
Prostaglandin E, astrocyte responses to, 258
Protease, calcium-dependent, 162
α-1-Protease inhibitor, 160
Protease nexin, 122, 276
  type I, 160
Protein kinase C, 195
  growth cone, regulation, 201–203
Protein kinases. *See under* Growth cone, regulation
Proteoglycans, neuronal surface, 192–193
Proximodistal axis, two-dimensional neural network, insect wing graft experiments, 127–130, 133
Pyruvate kinase, 24

Radioautography, EAE, gliotic plaque, 293–296
  acute, 293, 295
  chronic, 296
Red nucleus
  ganglioside GM_1 effect on, axotomy response, 33–43
  rubrospinal tract neurons, 69–70
  target-specific requirements, immature axotomized CNS neurons, rats, 77–84
Regeneration
  anatomical, 332
  functional, 332–333, 390, 395
  physiological, 332
Rescue, neuron, CNS lesions, 42, 67–72
  acetylcholinesterase, 69, 72
  choline acetyltransfersae, 69–72
  endogenous and exogenous requirements for survival/sequestration, 68
  nerve growth factor, 67, 69–72
    septal cholinergic neurons, in partial fimbrial transected rats, 105–109, 112
  neuron death, 70
  neurotrophic factors (NTFs), 67–70, 72
    target territory, 68, 69
Reticular nuclei, spinal cord injury, rat, plasticity, 351
Reticulospinal axons, spinal cord transection, recovery, *Petromyzon marinus* (lamprey), 370, 375, 378
Retina, 40, 259
Retrograde trophic factor, cytoskeleton, regenerating motoneuron axon, 15–16
Reversibility of NGF expression on Schwann cells after axonal injury, 180–182
RGDS (Arg-Gly-Asp) sequence, 139–143, 151
RNA
  ganglioside GM_1 effect on rat rubral neuron axotomy response, 34–36, 39–41
  messenger (mRNA), in situ hybridization, cytoskeleton, regenerating motoneuron axon, 16–20

Scar tissue
  dorsal root fiber regeneration into adult mammalian spinal cord, induced, 315, 319
  spinal cord transection recovery, *Petromyzon marinus* (lamprey), 370, 371, 374, 375, 377–379, 380, 387–388, 393–394
Schwann cells, 13, 50, 149
  adhesion, 210, 216–218
  axon terminals at synaptic sites, maintenance in absence of muscle fibers, frog NMJ, 173–174
  nerve growth factor receptor, 121, 123
  plasminogen activator production, 272, 274
    cell migration, 277, 278
  see also Nerve growth factor receptor expression on Schwann cells after axonal injury
Sciatic nerve
  crush, sensory neuron responses to peripheral nerve injury, rat, 47–51
    vs. transection, 50, 51
  cytoskeleton, regenerating motoneuron axon, 25–27

Secretin, astrocyte responses to, 258
Sensory neuron responses to peripheral nerve injury, rat, 47–52
 HRP, retrograde and anterograde, 48
 nerve growth factor, 50–52
  high-affinity receptors, 51, 52
 sciatic nerve crush, 47–51
  vs. transection, 50, 51
Septal cholinergic neurons, 70–71
 rescue, NGF in partial fimbrial transected rats, 105–109, 112
Serotonergic projections
 descending reticulospinal, spinal cord injury, rat, plasticity, 347
 target-specific requirements, immature axotomized CNS neurons, rats, 83
Serotonin, 202
Slow transport, cytoskeleton, regenerating motoneuron axon
 components a and b, 13, 19, 20, 24–28
 conditioned daughter axons, 26–30
 mature and daughter axons (sprouts), 24–26
Sodium channels, voltage-sensitive, 4, 7, 58, 189–190
Somatostatin, astrocyte responses to, 258
Spastic response, alternate leg-stepping, human, 339–340
Specificity, spinal cord transection recovery, *Petromyzon marinus* (lamprey)
 axonal pathfinding, 372–376
 synaptic regeneration, 370–372
Spectrin (fodrin)
 brain, 215
 cytoskeleton, regenerating motoneuron axon, 24
Spinal cord injury, rat, plasticity, 333, 339, 343–356
 hemisections, bilateral, newborn cf. weanling, 349–355
  brainstem, 351
  hindlimb motor behavior, 349–352
  HRP, 350, 354
  propriospinal circuit, 351, 352
  reticular nuclei, 351
 transection during postnatal development, 344–349, 352, 355
  functional sparing, 344, 345, 347–348, 352

functional sparing, critical period, 347
GABA, 348, 349
GAD, 348
serotonergic descending reticulospinal projections, 347
supraspinal influences, 345, 348
see also Dorsal root fiber regeneration into adult mammalian spinal cord, induced
Spinal cord stump coaptation by spinal column shortening, rat, 361–366
 cord-cord apposition, 361
 cf. cord sutures or dura suturing, 365–366
 edema, 362
 spinal shock, 362
 surgery, 362–365
Spinal cord transection, recovery, *Petromyzon marinus* (lamprey), 369–382, 387–395
 central pattern generator for locomotion, 388, 391
 en passant synapse, 379, 381
 fictive locomotion/swimming, 371, 388
 functional recovery, adults, 390–395
 functional recovery, larvae, 369, 370, 388–390, 393, 394
  coordinated bursting, 389, 393–395
  fiber length, 393–395
  motor nerve phase delays, 392
  prey catching, 391
  restrained vs. unrestrained, 371–373
  synapse function, 391
 giant axon structural environment, 379–382
  growth cones, 379, 382
 D-glutamate, 388, 389
 HRP, 370, 377, 378, 381
 neurites, 375, 376, 378, 380
 NMDA, 388
 reticulospinal axons, 370, 375, 378
 scar/lesion, 370, 371, 374, 375, 377–379, 380, 387–388, 393–394
 specificity
  in axonal pathfinding, 372–376
  in synaptic regeneration, 370–372
 tangled regenerated fibers, pictured, 390

Spinal cord, vertebrate, regenerative capacity, 331–340
  age, decrease with, 333
  fish, 331–339
    axons, long, 338, 339
    motoneurons, 336, 338
    somata, 336–338
    terminals, 335, 336, 338
  human, alternate leg stepping spastic response, 339–340
Spinal shock, spinal cord stump coaptation by spinal column shortening, 362
S100 protein, astrocyte responses to, 258
Sprouting, neurons, response to injury, 7–8
Stellate-process bearing astrocytes, responses to GFs and hormones, early molecular events, 258, 259, 265
Sternarchus albifrons, 5
Stroke, 281
Stump coaptation. *See* Spinal cord stump coaptation by spinal column shortening, rat
Substance P, astrocyte responses to, 258
Substratum changes, regenerating axon response to, insect wing graft experiments, 130
Sulphation, N-CAM and L1, development regulation, 239–242
Superior cervical ganglion, 182–183
Supernumerary axons, 49
Superoxide anion in acute CNS injury, 283, 284
Synapse(s)
  formation, neuromuscular junction, 123
  function, spinal cord transection, recovery, *Petromyzon marinus* (lamprey), 391
  see also Axon terminals at synaptic sites, maintenance in absence of muscle fibers, frog NMJ
Synapsin I, 215
Synthetic peptide studies, chick embryo, laminin- and fibronectin-neuronal growth interactions, 142–143

T_3, astrocyte responses to, 258, 265
Talin, 154
Tangled regenerated fibers, pictured after spinal cord transection, *Petromyzon marinus* (lamprey), 390

Target dependence. *See* Motoneurons, spinal, target-dependence, electrophysiology in cat
Target-specific requirements, immature axotomized CNS neurons, rat, 75–84
  axonal elongation, raphe spinal projection, 82–83
  serotonergic projections, 83
  DRG neurons, 76
  fetal spinal cord transplant, 77
    target cf. nontarget transplants, survival time, 80–84
  glial scar or gap, 76, 77
  LGN neurons, 86
  nerve growth factor, 76
  red nucleus neurons, 77–84
  time course of cell loss, 79–80
Target territory, neuron rescue, CNS lesions, 68, 69
Tau factors, 30
T-cell receptor complex, 215
Tetrodotoxin, 56–58, 61, 211
Thalamus, trophic factor hypothesis, 96
Thrombin, 160, 161
Thrombospondin, 139
Thy-1 glycoproteins, 193, 195
Tibialis anterior muscle, 181
12-0-tetradecanoylphorbol 13-acetate (tPA) 201, 203
Tractotomy, rubral, and GM_1 effect on axotomy response, rat, 39–40
  neuron number and somatic size, 40
Transiently-induced sequences (TIS) genes, astrocyte responses to GFs and hormones, early molecular events, 260–267
  cf. c-fos, 261–263
  TPA-induction, 260, 262–264
Trauma, 281
Triiodothyronine (T3), astrocyte responses to, 258, 265
Trophic factor hypothesis, visual system, 89–101
  conditioned medium
    concentration, 97–99
    hippocampus cf. diencephalon, 99–100
  embryonic-cell-derived NTFs, 93–100
  dLGN, 91–92, 94–101

nerve growth factor, 90, 99
visual cortex lesions, 91–93
source of neurotrophic factors, 92–93
Trypanosomal variant surface glycoproteins, 193
D-Tubocurarine, spinal cord transection, recovery, *Petromyzon marinus* (lamprey), 389
Tubulin
α-, 17–20
β-, 215
cytoskeleton of regenerating motoneuron axon, 14–20, 25–28
Tumor growth factor, 302

Urokinase, 160, 161
Uveitis, experimental allergic, 250

Vesicles, synaptic, cytoskeleton of regenerating motoneuron axon, 23

Vimentin, 248
astrocyte responses to, 258, 259
Vinculin, 215
VIP, astrocyte responses to, 258
Visual cortex lesions, trophic factor hypothesis, visual system, 91–93
source of neurotrophic factors, 92–93
see also Trophic factor hypothesis, visual system
VLA, 120
Voltage-dependent calcium channels, 271
Voltage-sensitive sodium channels, 4, 7, 58, 189–190

Wallerian degeneration, 379
WGA, 231
Wing, insect. *See* Neural network, two-dimensional, insect wing graft experiments

3 9015 01380 0282
UNIVERSITY OF MICHIGAN

THE UNIVERSITY OF MICHIGAN

TO RENEW PHONE 764-1526

DATE DUE

JUL 2 8 1989

NEW BOOK SHELF

AUG 0 1 1989

JAN 1 2 1990